ACUTE CRITICAL EVENTS SIMULATION

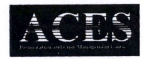

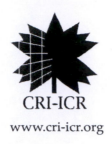

CRI-ICR

www.cri-icr.org

What is the Canadian Resuscitation Institute?

The Canadian Resuscitation Institute (CRI) is a non-profit corporation created to facilitate the development of peer-reviewed educational initiatives for healthcare professionals who practise acute care medicine in a wide variety of clinical settings. The CRI was federally incorporated on January 16th, 2004, but had its beginnings with the first Canadian national ACES (Acute Critical Events Simulation) course in 2001. In that year, in recognition of a need for improved multidisciplinary, hands-on training in acute medicine for healthcare professionals, a group of Canadian intensivists developed an innovative national educational training program known as ACES. By using high fidelity clinical simulation to create a real-life acute care environment, ACES courses offer challenging and stimulating, multidisciplinary training using novel skills modules that include Airway Management, Breathing, Circulation and other common clinical scenarios. This innovative training program for intensive resuscitation uses the latest technology, including simulator mannequins that resemble and function like real patients, to enhance the creation of an authentic clinical environment. Since December 2001, ACES courses have been offered nationally to community physicians, emergentologists, intensivists, anesthesiologists, surgeons, residents and other physicians and the ACES methodology has also recently been adapted for use in training registered nurses and respiratory therapists interested in the care of critically ill patients.

This book is the result of the collaborative efforts of the Canadian Resuscitation Institute and University Critical Care Training Program Directors across Canada and serves as a syllabus and reference source for the ACES course. Both the ACES courses and this book were developed by a group of intensivists who had identified common errors that were often made in the early treatment of the critically ill patient. CRI members believe that national collaboration and increased training opportunities like ACES will improve patient outcomes and safety by training healthcare professionals how to think and act critically and by significantly reducing medical errors. CRI is also committed to collaborative research and to lobbying for the adoption of best patient care practices in a wide variety of clinical settings despite varying personnel and resources.

ACUTE CRITICAL EVENTS SIMULATION

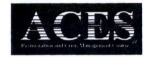

Course Syllabus

David T. Neilipovitz

University of Ottawa Press

This book has been published with financial contributions from Eli Lilly Canada Inc. *Lilly*, Bayer Inc., ORTHO BIOTECH, and Altana Pharma Inc. and in collaboration with the Canadian Resuscitation Institute.

The University of Ottawa Press gratefully acknowledges the support extended to its publishing programme by the Canada Council for the Arts and the University of Ottawa.

We also acknowledge with gratitude the support of the Government of Canada through its Book Publishing Industry Development Program for our publishing activities.

Library and Archives Canada Cataloguing in Publication

Acute resuscitation and crisis management : acute critical events simulation / David Neilipovitz ... [et al.].

Includes bibliographical references.
ISBN 0-7766-0597-6

1. Resuscitation--Simulation methods. 2. Critical care medicine--Simulation methods. I. Neilipovitz, David, 1969-

RC86.7.A27 2005   616.02′5   C2005-903451-3

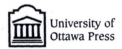 University of
Ottawa Press

Cover illustration: David T. Neilipovitz (photography) & Laura Brady (design)

Interior design and typesetting: Brad Horning

ISBN 0-7766-0597-6

Published by the University of Ottawa Press, 2005
542 King Edward Avenue, Ottawa, Ontario K1N 6N5
press@uottawa.ca / www.uopress.uottawa.ca

Printed and bound in Canada

Table of Contents

SECTION I
Crisis Resource Management

SECTION II
Airway Management

SECTION III
Respiratory Management

SECTION IV
Circulation

SECTION V
Sepsis

Detailed Table of Contents

SECTION I
CRISIS RESOURCE MANAGEMENT

Chapter 1

This chapter presents a general approach to the management of critically ill patients. It introduces the concept of crisis resource management and outlines the ACES strategies.

Chapter 2

Chapter 2 expands on the concepts of crisis resource management initially discussed in Chapter 1 and discusses important errors and strategies, including the ACES strategies.

Chapter 3

This chapter provides an introduction to medical simulation and discusses the role of medical simulation in the ACES Course.

Chapter 4

Chapter 4 provides an introduction to medical errors, including etiologies and the scope of the problem. Potential solutions are discussed, along with the role of the ACES Course.

SECTION II
AIRWAY MANAGEMENT

Chapter 5

Chapter 5 presents an approach to the assessment and management of an airway. It discusses basic airway skills and provides a description of how to confirm proper tube placement.

Chapter 6

This chapter discusses advanced airway devices and an approach to the failed intubation.

Chapter 7 presents the common medications used to facilitate airway management and the complications associated with them and discusses drug selection and dosing.

This chapter discusses the technique of rapid sequence intubation and its advantages and disadvantages. It also provides a discussion of cricoid pressure.

The dilemma of being unable to ventilate or intubate a patient is frightening. This chapter attempts to offer solutions.

SECTION III
RESPIRATORY MANAGEMENT

Chapter 10 introduces hypoxemia and hypercapnia with emphasis on their physiology and pathophysiology.

This chapter gives an overview of the approach to respiratory failure.

This chapter discusses non-invasive and invasive mechanical ventilation along with the different modes and strategies for using them. It also explores the role of PEEP and discusses the fundamentals of non-invasive positive pressure ventilation.

Chapter 13 covers the issues of compliance and resistance along with factors that contribute to changes in these parameters. It also explores the subject of the work of breathing.

This chapter discusses the concept of ventilator induced lung injury and techniques to prevent it. It also covers approaches to problems such as ARDS and obstructive lung disease and discusses the topic of patient ventilator dysynchrony.

SECTION IV
CIRCULATION

Chapter 15
Management of Shock

Chapter 15 is an introduction to shock with emphasis on early diagnosis and aggressive resuscitation. The chapter also provides an approach to management.

Chapter 16
Fluid Resuscitation: Theory and Practice

This chapter presents an approach to the complex and controversial topic of fluid resuscitation.

Chapter 17
Blood Products in Critically Ill Patients

Chapter 17 discusses the physiology of anemia along with the indications and dosing of presently available blood products and blood alternatives.

Chapter 18
Vasoactive Medications

This chapter presents a brief review of cardiaovascular physiology followed by a discussion of the various vasoactive medications and an approach to the rational use of these medications.

Chapter 19
Hemodynamic Monitoring

Chapter 19 provides an introduction to the common non-invasive and invasive hemodynamic monitors along with an approach to their use in managing patients.

SECTION V
SEPSIS

Chapter 20
Sepsis: New and Emerging Therapies

This chapter provides a review of sepsis, systemic inflammatory response syndrome and septic shock along with a discussion of management options and principles.

Chapter 21
Critical Points in Infectious Diseases

Chapter 21 provides a basic approach to patients with infections. It discusses the importance of underlying immunity defects and disease presentation and presents specific scenarios of some common types of infection.

Chapter 22
Fever in Critically Ill Patients

This chapter provides an approach to the investigation and management of patients presenting with fever and critical illness.

Chapter 23
Antimicrobial Therapy

Chapter 23 presents an approach to the rational use of antibiotics in the critically ill.

Preface

All of us can describe the sinking feeling we get when we are called upon to care for the patient who is quickly deteriorating in front of us. This can be especially troubling when you don't know where to start or what to do for the patient. Often there seem to be multiple problems to solve and several tasks to perform at once. Adding to one's anxiety is the chaos and confusion that occurs in this kind of situation. Although people shouting and monitors alarming makes for good television, it does not make managing the patient easier nor does it help the situation at all. Surprisingly, medical schools and residency programs do not usually provide training or instruction on how to handle these situations. Airline pilots and nuclear technicians receive extensive training, but for numerous reasons, physicians are usually expected to just cope.

The goal of the ACES Resuscitation Course is to help better prepare the physician for critical event situations. The course syllabus serves to complement the course sessions and provides the participants with important background information, allowing them to learn more during the course. The course takes a hands-on approach to teaching crisis resource management skills. It also provides participants with useful insights and strategies to improve their abilities to acutely resuscitate critically ill patients. ACES does not replace other life-saving courses but is there to complement them. The ACES Course strives to avoid numerous algorithms and magic solutions, focusing instead on simple principles and strategies that can be generalized to a majority of problems. Although ACES is still in evolution and development, we hope this course helps improve your ability to manage the critically ill patient and that you learn something useful.

Dave Neilipovitz
Pierre Cardinal

Contributing Faculty

Peter Brindley BSc MD FRCPC
Assistant Professor, Critical Care Medicine
Associate Residency Program Director
Co-director, General Systems Intensive Care Unit
University of Alberta Hospital
Edmonton, Alberta

Don Burke MD FRCPC FACP
Associate Professor
Department of Critical Care and Anesthesia
Sudbury Regional Hospital
Sudbury, Ontario

Pierre Cardinal MD FRCPC
Associate Professor
Program Director, Critical Care Medicine
Department of Medicine and Critical Care Medicine
University of Ottawa
The Ottawa Hospital
Ottawa, Ontario

Lois Champion MD FRCPC
Department of Critical Care Medicine
University of Western Ontario
London, Ontario

Michelle Chiu MD FRCPC
Assistant Professor
Department of Anesthesiology
University of Ottawa
The Ottawa Hospital
Ottawa, Ontario

Chris Christodoulou MBChB DA(UK) FRCPC
Assistant Professor
Department of Anesthesia
University of Manitoba
Winnipeg, Manitoba

William Gallacher MD FRCPC
Assistant Professor
Department of Anesthesia and Critical Care
Dalhousie University
Halifax, Nova Scotia

Richard Hodder MD FRCPC
Professor
Divisions of Pulmonary and Critical Care Medicine
University of Ottawa
The Ottawa Hospital
Ottawa, Ontario

Jon Hooper MD FRCPC
Assistant Professor
Departments of Anesthesiology and Critical Care Medicine
University of Ottawa
The Ottawa Hospital
Ottawa, Ontario

John Kim MD FRCPC
Assistant Professor
Department of Medicine and Critical Care Medicine
University of Ottawa
The Ottawa Hospital
Ottawa, Ontario

R. Bruce Light MD
Professor of Medicine and Medical Microbiology
Section Head, Critical Care Medicine
University of Manitoba
Winnipeg, Manitoba

Susan N. Nahirniak MD FRCPC
Medical Director, Transfusion Services
Division of Laboratory Medicine and Pathology
University of Alberta Hospital
Edmonton, Alberta

Dave Neilipovitz MD FRCPC
Assistant Professor
Departments of Anesthesiology and Critical Care Medicine
University of Ottawa
The Ottawa Hospital
Ottawa, Ontario

Editors	Dave Neilipovitz
	Pierre Cardinal
Assistants	Cynthia Habinski
	Karen Kinney

CRISIS RESOURCE MANAGEMENT

Objectives

1. Develop an approach to the critically ill patient.
2. Learn the components of and develop effective skills in crisis resource management.
3. Become familiar with the use of high-fidelity simulation in acute care medicine.
4. Gain an understanding of the scope of medical errors.

This chapter presents a general approach to the management of critically ill patients. It introduces the concept of crisis resource management and outlines the ACES strategies.

Chapter 2 expands on the concepts of crisis resource management initially discussed in Chapter 1 and discusses important errors and strategies, including the ACES strategies.

This chapter provides an introduction to medical simulation and discusses the role of medical simulation in the ACES Course.

Chapter 4 provides an introduction to medical errors, including etiologies and the scope of the problem. Potential solutions are discussed, along with the role of the ACES Course.

APPROACH TO THE CRITICALLY ILL PATIENT

**DAVE NEILIPOVITZ AND
PIERRE CARDINAL**

You are asked to assess a 64-year-old man on the medical ward who was admitted two days ago with mild pneumonia. The nurses were concerned about him because he was not looking well. You arrive to find him confused and somewhat combative. He is breathing very rapidly and is in considerable distress. He is pale and diaphoretic. The nurse tells you his heart rate is 140 bpm and his blood pressure is 75/45. The nurses would like to know what they should do.

The patient described above is obviously very sick and needs treatment quickly before he gets worse. The traditional approach[1] of taking a detailed history, performing a physical exam, ordering investigations and then deciding therapy is inappropriate. Time does not permit this approach since a patient's condition could irreparably worsen if treatment is delayed. This chapter describes an alternative approach to the acute resuscitation of critically ill patients. It describes the basic strategies for resuscitation: use concurrent management, follow the ABC's, and always reassess and re-evaluate. To employ these three strategies effectively, one first needs an understanding of crisis resource management.[2]

● Crisis Resource Management

Even though we all are not born as perfect leaders, with training we all can become effective leaders. The style of leadership depends upon many variables including your background, personality and training.[3] Regardless of your personal style, you need to take control of the situation and direct patient care.[4] While one can easily get caught up in the chaotic and stressful atmosphere, it is important to try to remain calm.[5] Your anxiety is contagious and could adversely influence the performance of your colleagues and assistants. It may be impossible to control your emotions. However, you do have total control over your attitude and demeanour. A calm and decisive demeanour will not only allow you to think more rationally, it will also help relax your assistants, thereby allowing them to better focus on the tasks you assign them. You will also become more confident and decisive as you perfect the basic management concepts discussed below and learn to trust your own skills.[3]

In crisis situations, effective communication between you and the rest of the health care team is essential.[6,7] Yelling orders and being confrontational is not effective in the situation. On the other hand, vague suggestions and ambiguous statements will often not be acted upon.[6,7] Thus, you must express yourself clearly and give specific orders. Each order must be directed at a single assistant. For example, "Dr. Smith, please intubate the patient's trachea" is the correct order as opposed to the vague suggestion "We should secure the patient's airway." One should listen carefully for input from the other health care professionals, but the person in charge should always make the final decisions. Conversely, if you are not the person directing the resuscitation, you should listen for instructions or offer your assistance to the person who is. When given an order, respond in a manner that leaves no doubt that you have understood the request (i.e., close the communication loop). For example, "I will place a central line in the patient" makes it clear that you have understood the assigned order.

A third component of crisis resource management is to effectively utilize all available resources.[2] Valuable resources include the other health care providers, monitors, documents, and investigations. Your attention is a valuable commodity but is a scarce resource and, thus, you must use it wisely. It is important that you remember always to *step back* and maintain a global perspective. Not only is the situation managed more efficiently when tasks and procedures are delegated to assistants, but it helps avoid a common mistake called a "fixation error."[2] Focusing your attention on performing a certain task will impair your ability to maintain a global perspective and may prevent you from identifying other important problems.[8] For example, focusing on inserting a central line may delay the diagnosis of a more acute life threatening problem such as ventricular tachycardia. You should only perform a procedure if you alone have the expertise for its correct or timely completion. Never be afraid to seek assistance from other specialists. If something is beyond your skill level or you simply need another set of hands, ask for assistance. For example, calling for the cardiac arrest team before the patient arrests is clearly better than waiting until the patient further deteriorates.

● Components to Resuscitation

The dilemma a physician encounters when presented with a critically ill patient is that there are often several conflicting issues and even multiple acute life threatening problems.[3,8] The approach to this complex situation can however be simplified by using three basic strategies: concurrent management, the ABC's approach, and reassess and re-evaluate (R&R). These strategies will allow you to quickly but effectively manage the situation (Table 1.1).

An important component of the resuscitation of a critically ill patient is the principle of simultaneous diagnosis and treatment (i.e., *concurrent management*).[3] Since time is of the essence, acute life threatening problems must be identified and treated immediately before they are allowed to deteriorate. Far too frequently, problems such as hypoxia and hypotension remain untreated while a patient is being transferred to a monitored unit. Delayed therapy causes end organ damage, which substantially increases a patient's risk of death. Remember that time is tissue.

Table 1.1 – Important Components of the Approach to a Critically Ill Patient

Crisis Resource Management
    a. Leadership
    b. Communication
    c. Resource Utilization

Concurrent Management

Manage the ABC's
    a. Airway
    b. Breathing
    c. Circulation

R&R Strategy
    a. Reassess
    b. Re-evaluate

The strategy of concurrent management enables therapy, even if only temporizing in nature, to be initiated while the etiology of the problem is still being investigated.

A simple but systematic approach is essential to avoid delays in identifying these life threatening problems. Where to begin and how to prioritize the problems can be overwhelming. The simplest approach is to use the *ABC's* strategy whereby airway, breathing and circulation are given top priority. As discussed below, the initial assessment of the ABC's should only take a couple of minutes at the most. Its purpose is to quickly identify and initiate treatment for all acute life threatening problems.

The final component is the strategy of reassess and re-evaluate (R&R). This is an ongoing process whereby the ABC's are repeatedly checked as other problems are evaluated and dealt with. Although the R&R strategy seems simple to do, it is often the component that is neglected in critical situations. The premise is that as the situation evolves or as new problems are encountered, one should always start over, i.e., check the ABC's. R&R helps prevent a second type of fixation error, which is the inability to question the diagnosis. For example, if a patient just recently intubated becomes hypoxemic, you should first verify that the endotracheal tube has not been displaced before moving on to assess whether another pulmonary complication has developed. It often takes repeated evaluations to identify more subtle signs that will point you to the correct diagnosis and allow you to institute a more definitive treatment. A lack of understanding of the underlying diagnosis should, however, not deter you from adequately resuscitating your patient.

● Initial Resuscitation Phase

The ABC's strategy is a simple yet effective approach to prioritize the acute resuscitation of a critically ill patient. The performance of the ABC's only requires a couple of minutes. The goal of this process is to identify acute life threatening problems and begin immediate therapy to rectify these problems.

A. Airway

A non-patent airway is incompatible with life and therefore must be quickly identified. The diagnosis is suggested by the presence of sternal indrawing, poor air movement and stridor. Simple manoeuvres such as a chin thrust or insertion of an oral airway usually can relieve the obstruction thereby temporizing the situation. Although rare, indications for immediate intubation involve situations where a patent airway will be lost if intubation is delayed (e.g., anaphylaxis, expanding neck mass or oral lesion, etc.). Though intubation in these situations can be difficult or even impossible, one must take immediate actions. Call for assistance, but proceed with intubation using the airway techniques you are most experienced with. Do not wait for someone else to come, but continue to do your best.

One must not confuse the need to open an airway with the need to protect an airway. Although patients who cannot protect their airway are at risk for aspiration, they do not need immediate intubation if their airway is patent. Once the airway is patent, proceed to life threatening breathing or circulatory problems. Although intubation may ultimately be required, it can be delayed until other more urgent problems are addressed.

B. Breathing

After establishing airway patency, breathing problems become the next priority. A quick assessment is performed to rule out acute life threatening problems such as a large pneumothorax. Ideally, the oxygen saturation should be measured continuously with a pulse oximeter.[9] Observe for the respiratory rate, chest movement and use of accessory respiratory muscles. Quickly auscultate to evaluate air entry or the presence of abnormal respiratory sounds. If there is any suggestion of an obstructed airway, one must go back and reassess the airway (i.e., go back to A).

The application of oxygen is indicated for all critically ill patients since it decreases the work of breathing, corrects hypoxia and can relieve myocardial ischemia.[10,11] Failing to administer oxygen in the hope of preserving a patient's hypoxic drive to breathe can lead to very serious complications. Even in patients with COPD, oxygen can be safely given by titrating its concentration to maintain an oxygen saturation of around 92%.[12]

Although the patient may ultimately require assistance from a ventilator, the situation can often be temporized by means of a bag and mask device connected to supplemental oxygen. The patient's respiration is then augmented by coordinating bag compression with the patient's inspiratory effort. An apneic patient can also be ventilated with gentle bag and mask ventilation. Once the breathing has been effectively temporized, quickly proceed to ensure adequate circulation (i.e., C).

C. Circulation

Assessment of the circulation begins once the airway and breathing have been addressed. Ideally, as you assess the circulation, your assistants are applying an ECG monitor and an automatic non-invasive blood pressure machine and obtaining intravenous access. The heart rate and blood pressure should be measured and the quality of the peripheral perfusion should be noted. Brief auscultation to simply note the quality of the heart sounds (e.g., distant suggestive of tamponade, displacement of the mediastinum by a tension pneumothorax) or the presence of loud murmurs is all that is initially required.

Any abnormal hemodynamic parameters should be considered an emergency and treated as such. Hypotension and tachycardia should be managed even in the relatively asymptomatic patient. A low blood pressure must be rapidly corrected to decrease the possibility of end organ injury.[13,14] Tachycardia indicates the presence of an underlying problem and may jeopardize viable myocardium. While the etiology of the abnormal hemodynamics is being investigated, corrective measures must be performed concurrently.

Virtually all hypotensive patients should receive a fluid bolus (e.g., 500 cc of saline). With the exception of a patient in florid pulmonary edema (a diagnosis that is usually easily made), most patients benefit from an augmentation of their volume state. Uncorrected hypovolemia is far more damaging than if a hypervolemic patient is given additional fluid. The fluid is given as a rapid bolus, which precludes the use of volumetric infusion pumps. Simply increasing the intravenous (IV) rate is inadequate. Select a fluid, which will increase the circulating blood volume. Hypotonic fluids such as D5W or 2/3^{rds} 1/3^{rds} are inappropriate. Colloids and isotonic fluids such as normal saline or Ringer's solution should be selected. Blood product administration should be considered if significant blood loss has occurred. Failure to even transiently respond to a fluid bolus implies the presence of serious underlying pathology.

Vasoactive medications are often required even while the etiology of the hypotensive state is being investigated. The blood pressure can be temporarily stabilized by intermittent boluses of various drugs such as phenylephrine (50–200 mcg bolus) or ephedrine (5–15 mg). These drugs can be administered via peripheral IVs to rapidly correct hypotension, albeit temporarily, thereby allowing the patient assessment to proceed (i.e., concurrent management). Once the circulation has been temporized, one can proceed to the ongoing resuscitation phase where more definitive care is given and a thorough assessment and investigations are conducted.

● Ongoing Resuscitation

The ongoing resuscitation process almost imperceptibly blends in with the initial resuscitation phase. This is the time to perform more definitive treatment of the ABC's and conduct a focused history and physical. Obtain information pertinent to the presenting problem along with medications, allergies and coexisting medical problems. Make arrangements for additional monitoring, IV access and investigations. Quickly decide if you should transfer the patient to a more appropriate setting. By the completion of this phase, you should formulate and act upon a management plan.

A. Definitive Airway Management

The decision to intubate a patient can be difficult, and often experienced physicians will hesitate to do so. Table 1.2 lists common indications for intubation. Several principles, however, can facilitate the decision whether or not to intubate the patient. If the patient is likely to deteriorate further, intubate early. A semi-elective intubation is safer than one that is performed in a crisis.[15] A hemodynamically unstable

Table 1.2 – Indications for Intubation

1. Airway Protection
2. Airway Patency
3. Respiratory Failure
4. Pulmonary Toilet

patient should be intubated and mechanically ventilated to reduce the oxygen cost of breathing. A physician's experience, the available personnel and the technical resources all influence this difficult but important decision.

B. Definitive Breathing Management

The oxygen saturation should improve with institution of positive pressure ventilation. If oxygen saturation does not improve, the patient must be thoroughly re-examined and a chest x-ray must be ordered. Correct endotracheal tube placement must be confirmed. Except in a cardiac arrest, the presence of carbon dioxide by a detection device is the *sine qua non* of correct tube placement within the trachea. If there is any doubt, remove the tube. Bag and mask ventilation is not ideal but is obviously preferable to an incorrectly placed tube (i.e., in the esophagus). Confirm bilateral air entry since the tube could be in too far (e.g., a right mainstem intubation). The possibility of a pneumothorax must always be considered especially when there is positive pressure ventilation (an undetected pneumothorax can become large once positive pressure is instituted). Other reasons desaturation may persist are failures to connect oxygen to the bag system or to administer 100% oxygen and occlusion of the endotracheal tube either from secretions or from a patient biting down. If ideal tube placement is confirmed and no problem is readily apparent, one must consider the possibility that there is worsening of the underlying pathologic process or that the patient aspirated during intubation.

Failure to find a readily correctable reason for the low oxygen saturations requires that changes to the mechanical ventilation be made. The addition of positive end expiratory pressure (PEEP) is useful to improve the oxygen saturation. Start with 7–10 cm H_2O of PEEP and increase by 2–3 cm H_2O every 20 minutes. A PEEP level above 15 cm H_2O is rarely required. Hypotension with higher PEEP levels usually suggests hypovolemia but always rule out the presence of a pneumothorax.[16,17] A struggling hypoxic patient may benefit from light sedation but be ready to manage the hypotension it may cause. Occasionally, a patient requires paralysis to improve ventilation and to reduce muscle oxygen consumption thereby improving their oxygenation. A patient with poor cardiac output often has poor oxygen saturation, which can be difficult to correct until the cardiac output improves. Thus, a hypoxic patient in shock should have the shock corrected concurrently with the institution of additional manoeuvres designed to improve oxygenation. Correction of the shock state invariably improves oxygenation even if the underlying pulmonary problem has remained unchanged.

C. Definitive Circulation Management

Although the definitive therapy for circulation abnormalities is to treat the underlying process, repeated fluid boluses and vasoactive medications may be required while the problem is being investigated. Useful information can be obtained from questioning the patient and examining their peripheral perfusion and central venous pressures and by chest auscultation. Obstructive forms of shock such as a tension pneumothorax or cardiac tamponade are rare but require specific treatments and thus should be ruled out. The possibility of ongoing blood loss should be determined and appropriate therapies instituted. The possibility of myocardial injury should be excluded. Septic shock is the most common form of distributive shock although less common forms such as anaphylaxis should be considered and excluded. It is often difficult to make a diagnosis of distributive shock initially since the classical manifestations of distributive shock (bounding pulses, warm extremities, wide pulse pressure) only become apparent once the patient's volume status has been fully restored.[18]

Although blood and fluid administration may ultimately rectify the patient's hemodynamics, temporary use of vasoactive medications may be needed. Impaired perfusion can quickly cause end organ damage and must therefore be minimized.[19,20] Unfortunately, delays in initiating vasoactive medications are common. Potential reasons for this are numerous but include physician inexperience in their use and poor IV access. Though it is preferable that these drugs be administered via a central line, they can be given peripherally if required until central access is obtained.

The selection of a vasoactive drug to use can be guided by several general principles. If the primary goal is to increase the blood pressure, then it is preferable to use a drug with vasoconstricting properties. Transient elevations can be obtained by intermittent boluses of phenylephrine (50–100 mcg) or ephedrine (5–10 mg). If a patient requires repeated boluses or has a process whereby a vasopressor is likely to be needed (e.g., septic shock), then a continuous infusion of a vasopressor such as dopamine, phenylephrine or norepinephrine is appropriate. Although vasopressors are not the treatment of hypovolemia, they can be used to transiently raise the pressure until adequate fluids are administered. Inotropes are selected if the goal of therapy is to increase the cardiac output. Although some inotropes are also vasopressors (e.g., dopamine, norepinephrine), most are not. Dobutamine and milrinone are inotropes that also vasodilate the peripheral vasculature, which can further reduce the blood pressure. These drugs should therefore only be used with extreme caution in hypotensive patients. In general, inotropes are rarely required in the acute resuscitation stage but have a very important role once euvolemia and blood pressure have been restored.[20,21]

D. Monitoring and Intravenous Access

Appropriate monitoring and IV access are crucial and should be initiated as soon as it is feasible. An ECG, pulse oximeter and automatic blood pressure device should be used for all patients if they are available. At least one IV line, preferably large bore in diameter, should be placed in all acutely ill patients. Although the insertion of invasive monitors carries some risks, these monitors can provide invaluable information.[21] An arterial line allows for continuous measurement of the blood pressure, which facilitates the titration of vasoactive drugs. Repeated blood tests including blood gases can be performed from the arterial line without the need for repeated venipunctures or arterial punctures. Large bore central lines such as an introducer sheath can allow for the rapid administration of fluids. In general however, fluid is more rapidly infused via a large peripheral catheter than via a central line, such as a triple lumen catheter. The longer the catheter, the greater the resistance to flow. Central venous lines provide information about the central venous pressure and are the preferred route for infusion of vasoactive medications and other products that can damage peripheral veins (e.g., some antibiotics, TPN, etc.). A pulmonary artery catheter can provide information about pressures in the pulmonary vasculature and is used to measure the cardiac output. The measured pressures in the central vasculature can be used to estimate the state of a patient's fluid volume status. However, a pulmonary artery catheter is rarely if ever needed in the acute resuscitative phase.

E. Transfer

The decision to transfer a patient can be difficult. Numerous variables must be considered when deciding to either transfer a patient or to continue with the resuscitation at its present location. The characteristics of the medical facility including the available support staff, specialists, equipment, access to investigative tools and even policies of the institution are some of the many factors that can influence the decision to transfer a patient. The most important factor however is the natural course of the patient's illness. A patient who is likely to deteriorate to a state that exceeds the facility's capacity should be transferred as soon as it can be done safely.

Case Summary

Let's now use this approach to resuscitate our 64-year-old man who is hypotensive and in respiratory distress.

The patient is able to talk, albeit incoherently, which suggests that his airway is patent. Since there are two nurses present, you specifically ask one of them by name to immediately call for a respiratory therapist and to bring the cardiac arrest cart. You tell the second nurse to place the patient on a 100% non-rebreathing oxygen mask. You auscultate the chest, which confirms bilateral air entry but reveals marked adventitial sounds on the right. You are confident that there is no significant pneumothorax. While listening to the chest, you also confirm the presence of heart sounds but do not hear any loud cardiac murmurs. A feel for a peripheral pulse reveals it to be thready and very rapid. The skin is warm. The blood pressure is still 75/45 and the rate is well over 120 bpm. You then ask the nurse who placed the oxygen, to start a large bore IV and give 500 cc of normal saline under pressure.

* * * * *

The cardiac arrest cart has arrived and you ask the nurse to hook the patient up to its monitors. From the cart, you obtain phenylephrine and dilute it appropriately. The patient is given 100 mcg of phenylephrine to temporarily improve his blood pressure while the fluid is infusing. You suspect that the patient is in septic shock and will require transport to an intensive care setting. You specifically ask a nurse to inform the ICU of the patient's need to be transferred and to immediately call for hospital porters. While these arrangements are confirmed, you reassess the patient's ABC's. Again the airway is patent and the breathing has improved a bit with the administration of oxygen since the respiratory rate has decreased and pulse oximeter has a reading of 88%.

When the respiratory therapist arrives, you ask them to prepare oxygen for transport including a bag and mask. The circulation is reassessed, which again reveals a low blood pressure of 80 systolic. A second 500 ml bolus of saline is given along with another dose of phenylephrine. A quick inquiry of the patient suggests he is also having chest pain and is short of breath. You ask the nurse to read off the patient's present medications and allergies while you quickly review the chart for the admission history and investigations.

The porters arrive and you quickly recheck the ABC's prior to transport. Although the patient will require intubation, you believe that the management instituted for the ABC's is adequate to stabilize the patient for transport. The patient will be intubated upon arrival to the intensive care unit. You bring the phenylephrine to correct hypotension should it reoccur during transport.

Key Points

- Remaining calm but decisive in crisis situations is an essential leadership quality.
- Communication must be clear, concise and specific (i.e., close the communication loop).
- It is important to make efficient use of all available resources.
- It is important to use a strategy of concurrent management whereby diagnosis and treatment are conducted simultaneously.

- Reassessment and re-evaluation is crucial for effective management in critical situations.
- ABC's is a simple yet effective approach to identify acute life threatening problems.
- ABC's is done to start temporizing therapy.

References

1. Bates B: Clinical thinking: From data to plan. p. 635–48. In Bates B (ed): *A guide to physical examination and history.* 6th ed. JB Lippincott, Philadelphia, 1995.
2. Gaba DM, Fish KJ, Howard SK: *Crisis management in anesthesia.* Churchill Livingstone, New York, 1994.
3. Schull MJ, Ferris LE, Tu JV, et al: Problems for clinical judgement: 3. Thinking clearly in an emergency. *Can Med Assoc J* 2001;164:1170–5.
4. Chambers R, Wall D, Campbell I: Stresses, coping mechanisms and job satisfaction in general practitioner registrars. *Br J Gen Pract* 1996;46:343–8.
5. Houston DM, Allt SK: Psychological distress and error making among junior house officers. *Br J Health Psychol* 1997;2:141–51.
6. Donchin Y, Gopher D, Olin M, et al: A look into the nature and causes of human errors in the intensive care unit. *Crit Care Med* 1995;23:294–300.

7. Howard SK, Gaba DM, Fish KJ, et al: Anesthesia crisis resource management training: Teaching anesthesiologists to handle critical incidents. *Aviat Space Environ Med* 1992;63:763–70.

8. Xiao Y, Hunter WA, Mackenzie CF, Jefferies NJ: Task complexity in emergency medical care and its implications for team coordination. *Hum Factors* 1996;38:636–45.

9. Mower WR, Myers G, Nicklin EL, et al: Pulse oximetry as a fifth vital sign in emergency geriatric assessment. *Acad Emerg Med* 1988;5:858–65.

10. Section 3: Adjuncts for oxygenation, ventilation, and airway control. *Circulation* 2000;102(suppl I): I95–I104.

11. Hussain SN, Roussos C: Distribution of respiratory muscle and organ blood flow during endotoxic shock in dogs. *J Appl Physiol* 1985;59:1802–8.

12. Gomersall CD, Joynt GM, Freebairn RC, Lai CK: Oxygen therapy for hypercapnic patients with chronic obstructive pulmonary disease and acute respiratory failure: A randomized, controlled pilot study. *Crit Care Med* 2002;30:113–6.

13. Walley KR, Wood LDH: Shock. p. 277–301. In Hall JB, Schmidt GA, Wood LDH (eds): *Principles of Critical Care*. 2nd ed. McGraw-Hill, New York, 1998.

14. Schuster DP, Lefrak SS: Shock. p. 891–908. In Civetta JM, Taylor RW, Kirby RR (eds): *Critical Care*. JB Lippincott, Philadelphia, 1988.

15. Schwartz DE, Matthay MA, Cohen NH: Death and other complications of emergency airway management in critically ill adults: A prospective investigation of 297 tracheal intubations. *Anesthesiology* 1995;82:367–76.

16. Ellman H, Dembin H: Lack of adverse hemodynamic effects of PEEP in patients with acute respiratory failure. *Crit Care Med* 1982:10:706–11.

17. Jardin F, Farcot JC, Boisante L, et al: Influence of positive end expiratory pressure on left ventricular performance. *N Engl J Med* 1981;304:387–92.

18. Carroll GC, Snyder JV: Hyperdynamic severe intravascular sepsis depends on fluid administration in cynomologous monkey. *Am J Physiol* 1982;243:R131–R141.

19. Claridge JA, Crabtree TD, Pelletier SJ, et al: Persistent occult hypoperfusion is associated with a significant increase in infection rate and mortality in major trauma patients. *J Trauma* 2000;48:8–14.

20. Rivers E, Nguyen B, Haustab MA, et al: Early goal-directed therapy in treatment of severe sepsis and septic shock. *N Engl J Med* 2001:343:1368–77.

21. Task Force of the American College of Critical Care Medicine, Society of Critical Care Medicine: Practice parameters hemodynamic support of sepsis in adult patients with sepsis. *Crit Care Med* 1998;26:1283–7.

CHAPTER 2

CRISIS RESOURCE MANAGEMENT

JOHN KIM AND
DAVE NEILIPOVITZ

> A 38-year-old woman has presented to you with a massive upper gastrointestinal bleed. She has vomited well over a litre of blood. Presently, she is agitated and combative. When she first presented, her heart rate was 140 bpm and her blood pressure was only 60/40. She has no intravenous access. There are a couple of nurses and other health care professionals around, but no one is presently doing anything. Everyone is looking at you to manage the patient. Where do you begin?

Education in the acute management of critically ill patients is an evolving field. Reviews of medical emergencies in the operating room (OR) during the 1980s reveal that physician error is a significant contributing factor in over half the cases.[1] Lack of medical knowledge was found to be an uncommon reason for such errors. Skills beyond medical knowledge were however identified as essential in effectively managing the actual crisis that occurs with the presentation of critically ill patients. These have become known as crisis resource management skills. Education in crisis resource management is often ignored in standard undergraduate and postgraduate training.[2-4] In addition, acquiring these skills as a team leader in an actual medical crisis exposes the patient to considerable risk. Thus, finding alternative methods for training in crisis resource management would be ideal.

● Crisis Resource Management

Examination of crisis resource management was first described after an extensive multi-centre review of crises in the operating room setting.[5] Gaba et al. identified risk factors for human error in medical crises.[5] Gaba and others have, however, reported that medical knowledge (or lack thereof) was an uncommon cause of human error in crisis situations.[5,6] The skills that are required can be collectively referred to as Crisis Resource Management (Table 2.1).

Table 2.1 – Important Components of Crisis Resource Management

1. Problem-Solving Approach
2. Situational Awareness
3. Resource Utilization
4. Leadership
5. Communication

Although the crisis resource management components will be discussed individually, it is clear that they are not mutually exclusive. One cannot be an effective leader without good communication skills, effective problem-solving skills and so on. We will present the important aspects of these issues and solutions to address them to help physicians improve their crisis resource management skills by expanding upon the skills presented in Chapter 1.

1. Problem-Solving Approach

The severity of illness with critically ill patients requires a problem solving approach that can be rapidly implemented. At the same time, since the underlying diagnosis is often unclear at the time of initial presentation, this approach must also be comprehensive. Thus, the approach used in these situations must take into account the need to act quickly and deal with the most life-threatening problems first while still remaining comprehensive.

Implementation of the *ABC's approach* is a well-recognized method for managing the most urgent life-threatening problems in a medical crisis. The goals should be focused and the timeline for their assessment and the implementation of life-saving treatment should be a couple of minutes at most.

Airway patency is clearly the first priority in all situations. Remember that patency is not synonymous with airway protection. The common misconception is that airway protection supersedes the remainder of the ABC assessment and primary evaluation. Intubation is appropriate once the remainder of the ABC and primary assessment are completed. The initial management of the breathing is primarily focused on initiating corrective therapy for hypoxemia and ruling out of a pneumothorax. The priority of circulatory management is to maintain central perfusion to the important organs but especially to the brain and heart. A high index of suspicion for shock must therefore be present when managing any patient who is critically ill. If there is even a slight suspicion of shock, intravenous fluid bolus is appropriate. If fluid therapy is insufficient at maintaining adequate central perfusion, then vasoactive therapy is indicated to ensure that there is an adequate organ perfusion.

The premise of *concurrent management* is another useful strategy for the approach to problem solving. The traditional problem-solving method of sequentially doing the history, physical examination and investigations before implementing therapy is not appropriate for a critically ill patient. An alternative is to use a parallel approach method whereby some history, physical exam and investigations (e.g., pulse oximeter) are performed simultaneously with the institution of therapy (e.g., insertion of an oral airway, application of oxygen). In essence, one is treating the patient immediately, even if the therapies are only temporizing in nature, prior to obtaining a definitive diagnosis.

The main advantage of a concurrent management approach is that it institutes life-saving treatment at the earliest possible time. Another advantage is the versatility of this strategy since it can be universally applied to problems, regardless of the etiology of the medical crisis. Furthermore, by implementing life-saving therapy, it can buy time for the remainder of the assessment to be completed. The disadvantages of this approach are that it can be disconcerting since therapy is often instituted before an underlying diagnosis is obtained and it mandates that frequent reassessments be done.

2. Situational Awareness

A physician must remain aware and alert during a crisis, because of the fluid nature of medical crises. One of the earliest errors Gaba described in managing crises is the failure to declare a crisis early.[5,7–9] There are several reasons for this delay, including the difficulty in diagnosing shock, especially in the context of so-called "normal" vital signs, and a physician's fear of being perceived as panicky, in declaring that "the sky is falling" when no readily apparent danger exists. However, the most recent literature demonstrates that aggressive early intervention in patients with shock dramatically improves mortality.[10] In other words, the adage "time is tissue" applies. For this reason, situational awareness in medical crises requires a physician to maintain a high index of suspicion and the willingness to declare an emergency early and institute therapy accordingly.

Critically ill patients are somewhat unique in that their condition can change dramatically within a very short period of time. This may be due to the progression of their underlying disease, response to life-saving treatment, or new problems that may arise. Therefore, situational awareness also requires one to monitor changes in the patient and their environment (i.e., monitoring equipment, laboratory data, etc.).

Another crucial element in situational awareness is the recognition of the potential to commit a fixation error.[5] This very common error occurs when a physician becomes fixated on a diagnosis, treatment, task, or another aspect of the crisis. The fixation occurs to the exclusion of other equally or even more important priorities for managing the crisis effectively — for example, focusing on the insertion of a central line rather than recognizing that the patient has removed their oxygen.

Fixation error occurs regardless of the level of expertise. There are many reasons that fixation error occurs.[5] The chaotic environment often seen in an acute resuscitation situation, the uncertainty of the underlying diagnosis, the need for multiple life-saving and temporizing treatments and the multiple sources of information that flood the physician's senses all can overwhelm a physician's ability to effectively manage a crisis in a logical and prioritized fashion.[11]

Situational awareness is improved by repeatedly using the *R&R strategy* (reassess and re-evaluate). For example, after completing the initial assessment of the ABC's and the institution of life-saving treatments, albeit temporizing in nature, one must repeat the ABC's to reassess the patient and re-evaluate the working diagnosis and treatment plan. While this may appear self-evident, this is often not the case. In fact, a common reason that fixation error occurs is that this process of reassessment and re-evaluation of the patient is often omitted.[5]

An additional benefit of the R&R strategy is the ability to detect new problems earlier during a medical crisis. Some problems are subtle in their initial presentation but become more apparent with repeated assessments. For example, breath sounds on one side of the chest could become more faint on repeated exams, heralding the presence of a pneumothorax and allowing its detection before it causes hemodynamic compromise. Furthermore, the majority of therapies used in resuscitation may have short durations of effect and, thus, repeated patient assessment allows for monitoring of response to treatment. In this manner, the use of the R&R strategy allows the initial treatments not only to be therapeutic but also to assist in the diagnostic process. For instance, transient response to a fluid bolus could signify the presence of substantial volume deficits. So the R&R strategy provides both protection against fixation error and improves patient care.

3. Resource Utilization

A medical crisis calls for urgent intervention, which can often translate into the performance of multiple tasks in order to resuscitate a critically ill patient. At the same time, one is often faced with the challenge of limited resources in attempting to implement temporizing measures and life-saving therapies. Managing the available resources in a crisis becomes another key element in effective crisis resource management.

Support staff is an essential resource in managing a crisis situation. Depending on the setting, however, not having enough help may be the most pressing concern. Conversely, in some situations having too many people present may hamper a team's effectiveness in resuscitating a critically ill patient. Furthermore, the quality of help can become just as important as the quantity. A skilled nurse trained in resuscitation may be worth more than multiple nurses and assistants. Similarly, other physicians may be able to reduce the physical workload that the team leader must assume when alone. Finally, expertise may be lacking for certain tasks. For these reasons, calling for extra help early is a crucial process in a medical crisis.

Other valuable resources include equipment for monitoring and ancillary investigations. Not only is obtaining such resources of paramount importance, but given that a limited number of tasks can be performed at any given time on a patient, prioritizing which resources are used first is also crucial.

Clearly, resource utilization is an extremely important component of crisis resource management. In this regard, one must use the available resources in the most effective manner possible. Delegation and direction of tasks to support staff whenever possible is the key aspect of resource utilization. Although occasionally the physician must perform a task when there is no other assistant who is capable of performing an essential task in a timely manner, usually delegation of a task is possible. Remember, the most valuable resource and the one that is in the shortest supply is the attention of the person directing the situation.

4. Leadership

Individual's personalities are directly tied into their leadership styles. Clearly there is no one mode of leadership that is appropriate for all physicians. Historical reviews of leadership, however, have identified some qualities that are essential in effective crisis resource management (Table 2.2).

Remaining calm in crisis situations is challenging. Anxiety is a normal reaction but it can be contagious. Remaining calm, even if only in appearance, will usually relax the people who are assisting and that will allow them to better concentrate and perform the tasks you assign them. Since there can only be one person ultimately directing the situation, it is crucial that that person maintain their leadership role throughout the crisis as much as possible. One should listen for input from the other assistants, but decisions should be clearly made by the person who is in control. Be decisive in your directions since ambiguity and hesitation can have detrimental consequences. Finally, it is essential that a leader always maintain a global perspective. One should know what is going on but should never lose track of the full picture. By maintaining a global perspective, one will be better able to anticipate future problems, thereby avoiding them or minimizing their detrimental impact.

Gaba described personal attitudes that may impair a person's leadership abilities.[1] Impulsiveness ("we have to do something—anything"), invulnerability ("I can intubate anyone"), anti-authority ("rules are for others") and resignation ("it's not my problem") have been identified as particularly common hazardous attitudes.

Although it is up to individuals to develop their own leadership style, physicians should strive to have the key qualities listed while attempting to avoid the detrimental attitudes. Awareness of one's own personality can be the most important aspect in improving leadership skills. Identification of personal strengths and weaknesses in such traits as demeanour, decisiveness and the ability to maintain a global perspective, as well as any tendency toward hazardous attitudes, may enable physicians to gain valuable insight into their own leadership style and improve and adjust it accordingly. In other words, physicians should work on developing a leadership style that utilizes their strengths during a crisis and, perhaps more importantly, guards against their particular weaknesses.

5. Communication

Lapses in communication were a significant cause of human error in Gaba's review of operating room critical incidents.[5] Interestingly, the communication errors demonstrated in Gaba's review were similar to those cited in other non-medical professions.[12] Giving vague instructions often have detrimental consequences. For example, "I think it would be good to intubate this patient" leaves it unclear as to whether the leader is asking someone to perform this task, is planning to perform it themselves, or is asking others if they think it should be done. The error of not directing commands is another important mistake to avoid. Simply saying, "Someone draw up some ephedrine" into thin air will result in either no one getting the drug or possibly several people getting it simultaneously, which is clearly an inefficient use of limited resources. A lack of confirmation of commands (thus producing uncertainty for both the leader and staff as to who is doing what) and lack of communication between the leader and support staff are other avoidable errors of communication.

Strategies that can assist in improving communication, thereby minimizing the occurrence of the above errors, are the three Cs: *clarity, cite names*, and *close the loop* (Table 2.3). *Clarity* refers to the fact that one should be clear with instructions and goals. For example, "Dr. Smith, intubate the patient now" is a clear and precise instruction that avoids the vagueness we previously described. *Cite names* helps

Table 2.2 – Ideal Leadership Qualities
1. Remaining Calm
2. Maintaining Control, Be Decisive
3. Maintaining Global Perspective

Table 2.3 – The Three C's of Communication

Clarity
Cite Names
Close the Loop

to avoid confusion of task assignment. If you do not know the name of an assistant, say that to them and then make it quite clear that they are the person to whom you are assigning a certain task. *Close the loop* refers to the interaction that occurs between support staff and the leader. Assistants should confirm the order, which informs the leader that the assistant has received and understood the assigned task. The assistant should also be instructed to report back to the leader when the task is complete (e.g., "Get the cardiac arrest cart and tell me when it is here"). *Close the loop* is a strategy that allows a leader to keep track of management and gives clear direction to assistants as to their responsibilities. Other important aspects of communication include listening; one can receive invaluable information and input from assistants. Again, as with leadership, personal styles of communication will differ, so self-awareness of personal strengths and weaknesses in the above areas will be extremely helpful.

● Improving Crisis Resource Management

Many readers will note that the concepts and strategies discussed in crisis resource management are not new.[5,7–9] Indeed, the principles behind the three basic ACES strategies—ABC's approach, concurrent management and the R&R strategy—are well known to most physicians. However, the fact that fixation error is common in medical crises and is committed by physicians at all levels of expertise suggests that these strategies are often overlooked or set aside during crisis situations.[5] Indeed, crisis resource management is a collection of skills that cannot simply be taught by reading or by lectures alone. In the end, the only way to improve such skills is through practice. Therefore, while this chapter is designed to introduce the physician to the concepts of crisis resource management and strategies to effectively deal with these situations, one must explore all available resources to improve one's skills. In this regard, the use of high-fidelity simulation will be a far more effective tool in improving crisis resource management skills than simply reading about the required skills.[13] Simulation offers physicians an opportunity to receive personalized feedback on their own style of leadership, problem solving skills, communication practice, situational awareness and resource utilization, which can assist them in improving their crisis resource management skills. Medical education has reliably demonstrated that there is no such thing as the perfect, all-knowing physician. Lifelong learning is a fact of life in present-day medicine. In the case of crisis resource management skills, it is even clearer that lifelong improvement is the goal for *all* physicians, and it is our belief that the ACES Program can assist in improving crisis resource management skills and, in the end, produce better physicians.

Key Points

- Crisis resource management includes situational awareness, problem solving, resource utilization, leadership and communication.
- The ABC's strategy is a concise and quick approach to acutely ill patients.
- Concurrent management (simultaneous diagnosis and therapy) allows for rapid institution of life-saving therapy.

- The R&R strategy is crucial to avoid fixation error and to identify problems early.
- Call for help sooner rather than later.
- Delegate and direct.
- Individual leadership and communication styles vary; learn your own strengths and weaknesses.

References

1. Khan FA, Hoda MQ: A prospective survey of intra-operative critical incidents in a teaching hospital in a developing country. *Anaesthesia* 2001;56:177–82.

2. Clarke GM: Training in critical care. *Curr Anaesth Crit Care* 1997;8:167–73.

3. Garcia-Barbero M, Such JC: Teaching critical care in Europe: Analysis of a survey. *Crit Care Med* 1996;24:696–704.

4. Harrison GA, Hillman KM, Fulde GO, Jacques TC: The need for undergraduate education in critical care. *Anaesth Intens Care* 1999;27:53–8.

5. Gaba DM, Fish KJ, Howard SK: *Crisis management in anesthesia*. Churchill Livingstone, New York, 1994.

6. Cooper JB, Newbowser RS, Kitz RJ: An analysis of major errors and equipment failures in anesthesia management: Considerations for prevention and detection. *Anesthesiology* 1984;60:34–42.

7. Gaba DM: Improving anesthesiologists' performance by simulating reality. *Anesthesiology* 1992;74:491–4.

8. Gaba DM: Dynamic decision-making in anesthesiology: Cognitive models and training approaches. In Evans DA, Patel VL (eds): *Advanced models of cognition for medical training and practice*. Sprinter-Verlag, Berlin, 1992.

9. Howard SK, Gaba DM, Fish KJ, et al: Anesthesia crisis resource management training: Teaching anesthesiologists to handle critical incidents. *Aviat Space Environ Med* 1992;63:763–70.

10. Rivers E, Nguyen B, Haustab MA, et al: Early goal-directed therapy in treatment of severe sepsis and septic shock. *N Engl J Med* 2001;343:1368–77.

11. Xiao Y, Hunter WA, Mackenzie CF, Jefferies NJ: Task complexity in emergency medical care and its implications for team coordination. *Hum Factors* 1996;38:636–45.

12. Billings CE, Reynard WD: Human factors in aircraft incidents: Results of a 7-year study. *Aviat Space Environ Med* 1984;55:960–5.

13. Issenberg BA, McGaghie WC, Hart IR, et al: Simulation technology for health care professional skills training and assessment. *JAMA* 1999;282:861–6.

CHAPTER 3

SIMULATION AND MEDICAL EDUCATION

JOHN KIM

The airplane you are in suddenly loses all the power due to a fire in two of the four engines. Outside, a major snowstorm rages on. The pilot needs to make an emergency landing. Nearby, the local nuclear plant suddenly has an emergency. A valve that allows water in to cool the rods in the reactor core is malfunctioning, and the backup cooling system is not working.

Fortunately, the pilot and the nuclear technician have practiced these scenarios through the use of simulation training. With prior experience, they quickly implement the proper solutions for each emergency, thereby averting catastrophic outcomes.

A 25-year-old lady arrives at the hospital after recently starting chemotherapy for acute myelogenous leukemia. She is having repeated convulsions. Her face is swollen and she is vomiting blood. She is hypotensive, tachycardic, tachypneic and has an oxygen saturation of barely 75%. She has no intravenous access. You are the physician who is called upon to manage this young lady. Would you not wish you had practiced this scenario before having one and only one chance to save her life?

The use of simulators in the instruction of crisis resource management dates back to the 1920s, with the use of rudimentary flight simulators.[1] Computer-assisted simulation was developed in the 1950s to make simulations more like real-life aviation. Simulation has now been widely incorporated by the airline, aerospace and nuclear power industries as a mandatory component of training and advancement. As it represents the only feasible alternative to actual real-life experience for these professions, the adoption of simulation is not surprising. Since real-life mistakes can also have disastrous outcomes in medicine, the appeal of computer simulation as a complementary method of skills training in medical education is obvious.

Due to the complexity of the human patient, computer simulation has only recently been used in medical education. Advances in computer technology over the past 20 years now make the use of simulation for skills training in medical emergencies possible. High-fidelity computer simulation forms an integral component of skills training in the ACES Program, with a focus on crisis resource management and resuscitation skills training.

In this chapter, we will briefly review the use of computer simulation in medicine, with an emphasis on its educational impact. We will discuss the various roles of high-fidelity simulation within medical education along with the benefits of participation in a high-fidelity simulation program. We will also explore barriers to successful implementation of simulation programs and discuss the emotional effects simulation has on participants. The ACES Program will be used to illustrate how high-fidelity computer simulation can be used to enhance the instruction of fundamental medical skills required in the resuscitation of critically ill patients.

● Simulation Fidelity

The extent to which the appearance and behaviour of the simulation correlates with that seen in real life is termed *fidelity*.[2] Fidelity is divided into *physical* fidelity and *psychological* fidelity.[3] Physical fidelity, also referred to as *engineering* fidelity, refers to the correlation of the physical characteristics of the training device and the environment it tries to reproduce. Psychological fidelity, or *functional* fidelity, describes the degree of similarity between the simulated tasks and skills performed and their real-life counterparts. The degree of fidelity necessary for a successful simulation depends not only on the recreation of the physical properties of a task, but also on the type of skills to be learned and the training level of the subject.[4] Thus, for training of the real-time skills necessary to manage crisis situations where interaction with a complex environment (e.g., monitors, personnel, equipment) is essential, *high-fidelity* simulations are required.

● High-Fidelity Simulation in Non-Medical Professions

The airline, aerospace and nuclear industries use high-fidelity computer simulation for two purposes: practice and evaluation. With the use of high-fidelity simulators, the participant has the opportunity to repeatedly practice managing life-threatening emergencies and acquire troubleshooting skills for rare yet catastrophic situations. Second, experts use high-fidelity simulation to assess a participant's performance during the simulator sessions. Successful simulation participation has become a mandatory component of airline pilot, astronaut or nuclear technician training. In addition, maintenance of certification in these professions requires periodic participation in high-fidelity simulations. Interestingly, the integration of high-fidelity simulation as a mandatory element in training and evaluation of competence has occurred despite the fact that simulation remains essentially unproven in these fields.[5-7] These industries have simply recognized simulation as a necessary component for skills training and evaluation.

● High-Fidelity Simulation in Medicine

In comparison to the aforementioned professions, medicine has only recently incorporated simulation into the training and assessment of health care professionals. The use of high-fidelity simulation has an even more recent genesis in medical education. Simulation programs in medicine began with the use of *part task trainers*,[8] or partial simulations of the environment. These were often used as anatomical models. Part task trainer simulators are still used today for the instruction of simple tasks or technical skills. Current examples include airway and venous access mannequins and laparoscopy and bronchoscopy simulators.

The next evolution in simulation design came in the form of *personal computer (PC) based* simulations. First started in the 1960s and 1970s, these instruction programs take the form of screen-based simulations of medical problems.[10] These simulations are well-suited for the instruction of the medical knowledge required to manage the crisis, but ill-suited for the development of crisis-specific skills.[10,11] Unfortunately, these programs do not recreate the real-life circumstances that accompany a medical emergency and thus are a form of *low-fidelity* simulation. PC-based simulations have been used for examination purposes in the past,[12,13] however, their greatest influence has been observed in medical education not evaluation. PC-based education programs form a vital component of present-day medical education; many cardiac arrest, trauma and various other resuscitation programs are available in this format.

The first *high-fidelity* simulation programs in medical education originated in the 1980s.[14–24] Originally, simulation programs were used almost exclusively in the specialty of Anesthesiology but their use has expanded to various other specialties including Critical Care Medicine, Surgery and Emergency Medicine.[25–29] The first high-fidelity simulators used a computer-controlled mannequin in a simulated operating room (OR) theatre. These simulated scenarios have all the monitoring equipment and personnel normally available in the OR. The first models, such as SIM 1 and CASE (Comprehensive Anesthesia Simulation Environment)[14,18] could recreate rare but recognizable OR emergencies (e.g., malignant hyperthermia, esophageal intubation, etc.). While these initial programs focused on the implementation of recognized solutions for specific OR emergencies, present day high-fidelity simulation programs now offer much more.

Simulation is a valid educational tool in several different medical settings. Training in surgical simulators clearly reduces the time required to achieve proficiency in certain skills. However, most literature concerning the use of high-fidelity simulation has been descriptive in nature, with only a few studies examining the utility of high-fidelity simulation as an educational tool. Moreover, almost all of the studies to date have been from the specialty of Anesthesiology. These studies use either measures of participant satisfaction or perception of utility (or both) as the main endpoints for evaluation of simulation as an educational tool.[24,30] Participants found simulation to be a more effective method of instruction and to be realistic.[14,18,23,31] Interestingly, most unplanned events in these simulations were due to human error;[16,19,20,22] however, additional training using the simulator decreased the number of these errors upon repeat performance.[21,23] Unfortunately, these studies had small numbers of participants, were specific to the OR environment and usually had clearly recognized "solutions" for each simulated emergency.

While little data exists for the use of high-fidelity simulation as an educational device, there are even fewer studies on its use as a formal evaluation tool. Prior to the year 2000, there were only four studies that examined the reliability and/or validity of high-fidelity simulation as an evaluation tool.[15,30–33] Since then, a few more studies have been published.[34–39] One

study did demonstrate differences between medical student and staff anesthesiologist performance but no differences were found between final-year residents and staff anesthesiologists.[38,39] In both earlier and more recent studies, significant limitations in study design exist. All the studies mentioned above are small, have only one simulator session per participant and use a limited number of evaluators (most unblinded) to perform the assessments. In all but two studies, the simulations deal with specific OR crises, which have a recognized "solution." These studies of specific OR emergencies can be reliably assessed by a checklist of "correct actions" for the emergency (i.e., best solution).[15,38,39] However, when evaluation is focused on more generic behaviours and actions performed in the crisis rather than the solution to the specific problem, poor inter-rater reliability was demonstrated.[15] Although there is some progress in developing a generic scoring system, it again is limited to evaluating actions in the OR environment.[36] Therefore, it is difficult to extrapolate the findings of these studies to more generic emergencies that occur outside of an OR environment. Investigations that examine the validity of high-fidelity simulation as an evaluation device indicate that simulator performance does not always correlate with standard written examination performance.[27] Given the evidence so far, there is presently little evidence to support the use of high-fidelity simulation as a formal evaluation device.

Limitations in the use of high-fidelity simulation as a mandatory component of training in medical education lie in the nature of the problems that can occur. Unlike non-medical professions, where a finite number of problems exist, in medicine a virtually infinite number of emergencies can occur under a countless number of circumstances. More importantly, for each "emergency" in the non-medical professions, a standard or ideal response exists. Thus, it is possible to set standards for curriculum development as well as formal evaluation of performance, given this finite number of emergencies and predefined responses for each emergency. Unfortunately, the vast majority of emergencies in medicine have multiple correct responses. Compounding this is that the solutions to a certain type of problem can change if the setting of the scenario changes. That is, an action deemed essential in one instance may be of secondary importance in another setting. Finally, the skill sets that are the focus of the simulation programs are not formally

Table 3.1 – Roles of High-Fidelity Simulation in Medical Education

1. Expose participants to rare events
2. Teach skills/knowledge in a more realistic context
3. Teach skills/knowledge not taught well through standard educational means
4. Provide opportunity for team training

examined by other means, thereby leaving no "gold standard" for comparison.

Despite the lack of evidence for the role of high-fidelity simulation as an educational or evaluation tool, it is nevertheless being integrated into multiple academic centres.[40] High-fidelity simulation programs can perform several unique and important functions in physician training for medical emergencies (Table 3.1). Simulation can provide participants with exposure to rare yet potentially disastrous events that they are unlikely to experience in their training. For example, an anesthesiologist can practice managing a patient experiencing a malignant hyperthermia crisis. Simulators can enable participants to learn certain skills and knowledge; more importantly, simulators can provide the context of when these skills would be required. Participants could, therefore, practice airway intubation in the presence of other conflicting medical emergencies, thus providing a more realistic learning experience. Simulation can educate participants on skills necessary to manage medical emergencies that are not taught through standard forms of medical education. A prime example of this is the crisis resource management skill set that is required to effectively manage critical events. Although one can discuss crisis resource management in didactic lectures, it is considerably more effective to have participants refine these skills in a lifelike scenario on a simulator. Finally, simulators have the ability to provide team training for health care professionals. Thus, multidisciplinary resuscitation teams have the opportunity to practice together for clinical situations they will experience as a group.

The key to the success of a high-fidelity simulation program lies in the determination of the role that it provides for participants, programs and institutions.[6] Given the variety of roles simulation can fulfill, it is of paramount importance that a centre identifies specific objectives and goals before starting a high-fidelity simulation program. Ultimately, at this time, as is the case in the non-medical professions, simulation may represent the only alternative to real-life resuscitation skills training, making it a very attractive tool in medical education.

● Available High-Fidelity Simulators

Presently, three companies produce high-fidelity simulator mannequins. Each offers similar features but has some unique qualities. Some aspects, however, are important for all types of simulators. All of the simulators are controlled by means of a PC linked remotely to the simulator mannequin. In most settings, a simulator instructor and PC operator are present, ideally located in an adjacent room that is shielded from view of the participants.

A. MedSim-Eagle Patient Simulator®

The MedSim-Eagle Patient Simulator® (PatientSim®) has loudspeakers in the head that provide communication through a link to an operator-controlled microphone.[41] PatientSim® includes an anatomically correct head and neck assembly; its eyes blink and change in pupillary size. Loudspeakers located in the chest provide heart and breath sounds that can be detected in the usual chest locations with a stethoscope. The lungs produce carbon dioxide using a computer-controlled gas metering system. The airway anatomy is such that endobronchial or esophageal intubation is possible. Palpable pulses at the carotid artery and radial artery are present using real-time hydraulics. There are also sites in the mannequin's arm into which intravenous lines can be inserted. A simulated twitch response in one of the mannequin's thumbs can be used for the assessment of neuromuscular blockade.

PatientSim® directly interfaces with the ventilator, respiratory gas analysis devices (e.g., capnograph, agent analyzer), pulse oximeters and other patient monitoring equipment. PatientSim® can thus provide information to all commercially available monitors. The information includes an ECG, arterial blood pressure, central venous pressure, pulmonary artery pressure, temperature, pulse oximetry and numerous other possible parameters.

PatientSim® scenarios progress by preprogrammed physiologic responses to the actions taken by the participant. PatientSim® operators enter these responses, which then trigger complex mathematic formulas simulating a human reaction to these changes (e.g., blood pressure decrease with the use of a vasodilator agent). The PC operator can alter the degree of response or can enter a second action to counteract the first response but cannot abort the initial sequence once it starts. Thus, the programming done prior to the simulation and the mathematical formulas used in the software program play a primary role in the course of events during the simulation. Since PatientSim® is able to simulate the effect of events or drugs by means of various complex mathematical formulas and relies less on operator input, it is often referred to as a "model-driven" simulator.

B. Laerdal SimMan™

SimMan™ has the advantage of being portable.[42] SimMan™ possesses multiple physical properties that can be directly observed by the participants. Direct communication between the participants and SimMan™ is available by means of internal and external speakers. Auscultation of the chest can reveal a wide range of lung and heart sounds. SimMan™ comes equipped with a full upper airway that allows for basic and advanced airway management including intubation, bronchoscopy, cricothyrotomy and even pneumothorax needle decompression. SimMan™ has several sites where peripheral pulses can be palpated. Unlike PatientSim®, SimMan™ is not able to move its thumb nor is it able to open its eyes. SimMan™ can however be treated with full chest compressions and direct DC cardioversion. Since fully functional defibrillators can be used, the risk of accidental defibrillation of staff is 100% real!

SimMan™ does not communicate directly with other monitoring equipment; all monitoring data can only be displayed on the monitor that comes with SimMan™. In addition, there are fewer preprogrammed responses to physiologic actions or drug effects and, thus, the reactions only occur by the direct input of the simulator operator. Due to these differences in monitor interaction and greater dependency on operator input to provide fidelity, SimMan™ has been termed by some to be an "intermediate-fidelity" or "instructor-driven" simulator mannequin. Although considered by some to be a disadvantage, the need for an instructor to directly control the physiologic parameters allows for

tighter operator control over the simulator scenario. The mannequins that have automated responses can have unpredictable changes that can interfere with the goals of the scenario (i.e., unexpected or undesired responses occur in the program). Furthermore, more recent versions of SimMan™ allow for preprogrammed physiologic responses to certain events or drugs thus decreasing the need for operator input. At the same time, the option for an operator to take complete control over a scenario without having to alter programmed responses exists. Thus, while on the surface SimMan™ may possess intermediate-fidelity hardware, with its preprogrammed response and use of a SimMan™ specific monitor, it is considered by most simulator instructors as a high-fidelity simulator.

C. METI Simulators

Medical Educational Technologies Incorporated (METI) offers two different types of high-fidelity simulators.[43] The Human Patient Simulator™ (HPS®) represents a model-driven, non-portable simulation mannequin comparable to PatientSim®. The second mannequin is the Emergency Care Simulator™ (ECS™), a portable model-driven simulation mannequin that is comparable to SimMan™.

The HPS® and ECS™ include loudspeakers located in the chest that provide heart and breath sounds that can be auscultated in the usual chest locations with a stethoscope. The lungs produce carbon dioxide using a computer-controlled gas metering system. Both HPS® and ECS™ provide a full upper airway that allows for basic and advanced airway management including intubation, bronchoscopy, cricothyrotomy and even pneumothorax needle decompression. The airway anatomy is such that endobronchial or esophageal intubation is possible. The HPS® and ECS™ have palpable pulses at the carotid artery and femoral artery. Peripheral intravenous insertion sites are present in both models. A simulated twitch response in the thumbs of both the HPS® and ECS™ can be used for the assessment of neuromuscular blockade.

HPS® directly interfaces with the ventilator, respiratory gas analysis devices (e.g., capnograph, agent analyzer), pulse oximeters, and other patient monitoring equipment. Thus, like PatientSim®, HPS® can provide information to all commercially available monitors. ECS™ uses a direct interface with a monitor that comes with ECS™ to provide this information. Thus, ECS™ sacrifices some of the physical fidelity in monitor interaction to provide a portable simulator mannequin.

● Simulator Environment

While providing a lifelike patient is important, recreating the actual environment of a medical crisis is essential to the success of high-fidelity simulation sessions.[4,18,44,45] For this reason, it is necessary to provide all of the equipment necessary for the acute management of a critically ill patient. Readily available equipment should include a crash cart, defibrillator, ventilator, intubation trays, medication carts, procedure trays, x-ray box and numerous other devices and equipment. A fully capable monitor that is directly linked to the simulator computer should be present to display simulated patient data.

Aside from the physical environment, another key element of high-fidelity simulation is the participation of support staff.[18] Normally there is at least one registered nurse and respiratory therapist present during each scenario. A scenario can, however, be tailored to mimic the environment a participant is likely to experience in real life. Thus, if a respiratory therapist would not present in real life, then only nurses would be present for the simulation scenario. The support staff can communicate with the instructor via a headset. These assistants are essential in that they can provide realistic responses to any actions or requests by the participants as well as facilitate development of the scenario. Although they are briefed for each case scenario, ideally they will simply provide the same reactions that support staff would have in real life.

● Benefits of High-Fidelity Computer Simulation

High-fidelity computer simulation offers many benefits to participants. Unlike in real life, simulator scenarios focus solely on the educational experience of the participants, not on patient outcome. The people in the simulation can thus act as team leaders throughout the entire medical emergency without having other senior physicians intervene or take over their roles (which often occurs in real life).

Thus, participants have the opportunity for *deliberate practice*.[46] Participants can also safely commit errors and can witness their consequences without concern of hurting real patients (i.e., they can learn from their mistakes). The acquisition of real-life experience can be a hit or miss phenomenon, often dependent on the on-call experience of physicians. Participation at regular intervals in a high-fidelity computer simulation program ensures a minimal level of exposure to common medical emergencies. A third benefit of simulation is that participants react in an *uncued manner*. Unlike didactic teaching sessions or small group discussions where participants can only answer questions, simulation creates a lifelike atmosphere where they are actively participating and responding to multiple stimuli. Another benefit this provides is that the reaction of participants occurs in *real time*. Unlike lectures, small group discussions or even examinations, the crucial temporal elements that occur in a crisis will be present in the simulator sessions. Physiologic responses to drugs, time required to institute life-saving therapy, the wait before any test results return are all recreated in a temporal sequence that mimics real life.

Simulation scenarios are normally videotaped. Videotaping allows debriefing and feedback during playback of the scenario. Although watching oneself can be intimidating and daunting, the use of videotape review is invaluable in that participants receive instruction in a *focused feedback* format. Previous participants of the ACES Program have cited the video review sessions as the most valuable aspect of participation. Simulation provides participants with the ability to perform self-assessment or *reflective learning*[47] by viewing their own performances, an opportunity not usually present in real-life events. The videotape review also provides an objective form for review and feedback by the instructor, thereby helping to *reduce bias* inherent in feedback. Finally, the review sessions ensure that there is *positive skills transfer* and that *negative skills transfer* is avoided.[4] During the video review, instructors can provide corrective feedback when errors occur and reinforce desirable behaviours (i.e., positive skills transfer). If wrong behaviours and approaches are not addressed (especially if the wrong action did not cause adverse consequence), these actions could be inadvertently reinforced (i.e., negative skills transfer).

Aside from the benefits participants receive from high-fidelity simulation programs, institutions also benefit considerably from these programs: Patient safety is improved by providing a complementary method for skill acquisition in the management of medical emergencies. The use of high-fidelity computer simulation programs may also create a public perception of increased patient safety at the institution. Furthermore, the use of regular practice, especially when combined with clearly defined objectives and appropriate feedback, can improve long-term skill acquisition.[11,48-50] Thus, high-fidelity simulation is a means of providing trainees with regularly scheduled practice and feedback, thus enhancing the quality of the institution's trainees. Finally, the reproducibility of computer simulation may offer institutions the ability to track the progress of a trainee. While simulators are not used as a formal evaluation tool, they nevertheless offer the opportunity to follow trainees as they progress and offer formative feedback to help assist them in skill acquisition during their training process.

● Barriers to Success for High-Fidelity Computer Simulation

Despite the many potential benefits to both participants and institutions, high-fidelity simulation has not been globally incorporated by medical education institutions. Barriers to successful implementation and maintenance of a simulation program exist from both participant and institutional perspectives.

Participants have three major barriers regarding high-fidelity computer program. The experience can be stressful for participants, especially for those unfamiliar with the simulator environment. In addition, because it is a simulation of a medical emergency, participants know some catastrophe is about to occur which compounds their stress levels. Anticipation of events may cause participants to perform in a manner they would not do outside of the simulator. The Hawthorne effect describes the changes in behaviour that participants display when they know they are being observed. The realization of participants that they are being videotaped for debriefing afterwards along with their self-expectation of their performance will add to their stress levels. Finally, simulations, by their very nature, are only imitations of real-life experience. No matter how sophisticated the technology, no present-day simulation program can fully recreate every aspect of a medical emergency. Thus, participants always recognize that they are in a simulation, not a real-life emergency. Despite this fact, most participants comment that scenarios tend to be realistic and are far superior to other educational formats. More importantly, reviews of high-fidelity simulation programs show error patterns in crisis resource management similar to those seen in real life.[16,22]

For medical institutions, a major barrier to high-fidelity simulation programs is the costs associated with such programs. The purchase costs of medical equipment and audiovisual equipment and even the space necessary to run these programs are quite high. Until recently, simulator mannequins cost hundreds of thousands of dollars. Although the cost of simulation equipment has become more affordable, cost is still a major barrier to simulation programs. Additional barriers to simulation programs are that they are labour intensive and time consuming. The required personnel includes an operator, instructor and several ancillary staff. The required time for debriefing and feedback for each 15-minute scenario participants experience in the simulator will translate into a 45-minute session. Finally, for a simulation program to succeed, its participants must be receptive to the program. Participants will be receptive if they perceive simulation as the best manner to learn important skills that are not available by other means. For this reason, the teaching of medical knowledge and technical skills is de-emphasized in the ACES Program. Instead, emphasis is placed on the acquisition of crisis resource management skills, which are harder to teach by traditional education techniques.

● Keys to Participating in Simulation Programs

Although there are barriers to the success of simulation programs, there are some keys things that participants should remember that can improve their experience in simulation programs.

1. Feeling Stress is Natural

It is commonplace for participants to feel stress throughout their high-fidelity simulation sessions.

Unfamiliar environments, being videotaped and reviewed, and the stress of knowing a crisis is about to occur are among the many sources of stress participants experience in simulation programs. Remember, stress is a natural reaction to these circumstances. Further, since a real emergency will produce a similar, if not more intense reaction, it is important to learn to deal with this feeling. So, while you may feel stressed, please remember that this is natural and that you are not alone in feeling this.

2. Simulation is not Perfect but still Useful

Although the simulation is designed to be as realistic as possible, some aspects will not be life-like. The mannequins are not perfect. Interestingly, though participants often cite this fact, they are almost unanimous in disclosing that this lack of perfection does not impede their ability to respond. Further supporting the utility of simulation, many participants in the ACES Program have noted that the feedback they receive during their review sessions often parallels feedback given to them in real life. How is this possible? The answer is simple, the feedback focuses on areas that the simulator environment can reproduce well and not on areas in which it is weak (i.e., crisis resource management instead of physical examination skills). In addition, feedback noting the difference between simulated responses and real-life responses may serve to overcome the lack of fidelity in some areas of the simulator sessions.

3. This is not an Exam

The main purpose of most simulation programs, such as the ACES Program, is to provide feedback and instruction, and not to evaluate participants. In order to provide feedback, programs are designed to encourage participants to behave as naturally as possible. Unlike examinations, nothing is meant to "trip you up" or complicate the scenario. For example, the ancillary staff tries to act as if it were a real life event and thus are there to help you, not to examine you. Participants will get more out of their scenarios if they focus on learning new and important skills rather than on thinking that they are being scored.

4. Confidentiality of Case Content is Essential

The key in providing effective and useful feedback after the simulation scenario lies in enabling participants to react as they would in real life. Clearly, the experience would be unrealistic if one knew the problem before it happened. Thus, confidentiality of scenario content benefits all present and future participants. Therefore, maintenance of strict confidentiality by everyone who participates in the ACES Program is expected, both before and after participation.

● Conclusion

Changes within the culture of medicine have led to a search for alternative methods of skills training for medical emergencies. While it may have been a time-honoured tradition to learn such skills on the job, a greater emphasis on patient safety has been the driving force behind the increasing appeal for simulation in medical education. Although someday simulation may be used as an evaluation tool, presently the main role of high-fidelity simulation is in teaching participants unique skills. However, it is important to remember that while simulation is a powerful educational tool, alone it will not succeed. Rather, it is the entire educational program that the simulator is designed for that will ultimately determine the success of any high-fidelity simulation program, and not the other way around. Presently, high-fidelity simulation remains a novel and largely untested tool in medical education. Despite this fact and despite the high costs and limitations associated with its use, high-fidelity simulation will likely play a pivotal role in the future education and evaluation of physicians. Ultimately, high-fidelity simulation's potential as a low-risk alternative to real-life medical emergency training will likely mandate further use and refinement over time.

Key Points

- Simulation is a risk-free alternative to real-life skills training.
- Realistic environments and support staff help ensure simulators are high-fidelity devices.
- Simulation in medicine is presently used for medical education.

- Review and feedback is an essential component of simulation training.
- Barriers to successful implementation include high financial and human resource costs.
- Simulation programs must have specific educational objectives to succeed.

References

1. Valverde HH: Flight simulators: a review of the research and development. Wright Patterson Air Force Base, OH, Aerospace Medical Research Laboratory, 1968.
2. Farmer E, van Rooij J, Riemersma J, et al: *Handbook of simulator-based training*. Ashgate Publishing, Aldershot, Hants, UK, 1999.
3. Miller RB: Psychological considerations in the design of training equipment. WADC-TR-54-453, AD71202. Wright Air Development Center, Wright-Patterson Air Force Base, OH, 1953.
4. Druckman D, Bjork RE: *Learning, remembering, believing, enhancing human performance*. National Academies Press, Washington, DC, 1994.
5. Hays RT, Jacobs JW, Prince C, Salas E: Flight simulator training effectiveness: a meta-analysis. *Mil Psychol* 1992;4:63–74.
6. Bell HH, Waag WL: Evaluating the effectiveness of flight simulators for training combat skills: a review. *Int J Aviat Psychol* 1993;8:223–42.
7. Koonce JM, Bramble WJ: Personal computer–based flight training devices. *Int J Aviat Psychol* 1998;8:277–92.
8. Maran NJ, Glavin R: Low to high fidelity simulation—a continuum of medical education? *Med Educ* 2003;37(Supp 1):22–8.
9. Piemme TE: Computer-assisted learning and evaluation in medicine. *JAMA* 1998;260:367–372.
10. Hmelo CE: Computer-assisted instruction in health professionals' education: a review of the published literature. *J Educat Tech* 1989;18:83–101.
11. Issenberg SB, McGaghie WC, Hart IR, et al: Simulation technology for health care professional skills training and assessment. *JAMA* 1999;282:861–6.
12. Woolridge N: The C-ASE Project: computer-assisted simulated examination. *J Audiov Media Med* 1995;18:149–55.
13. Norcini JJ, Meskauskas JA, Langdon LO, Webster GD: An evaluation of a computer simulation in the assessment of physician competence. *Eval Health Prof* 1986;9:286–304.
14. Schwid HA, O'Donnell D: The anesthesia simulator-recorder: a device to train and evaluate anesthesiologists's responses to critical incidents. *Anesthesiology* 1990;72:191–7.
15. Gaba DM, Howard SK, Flanagan B, et al: Assessment of clinical performance during simulated crises using both technical and behavioural ratings. *Anesthesiology* 1998;89:8–18.
16. Gaba DM, Fish KJ, Howard SK: *Crisis management in anesthesia*. Churchill Livingstone, New York, 1994.
17. Gaba DM: Improving anesthesiologists' performance by simulating reality. *Anesthesiology* 1992;74:491–4.
18. Gaba DM, DeAnda A: A comprehensive anesthesia simulation environment: re-creating the operating room for research and training. *Anesthesiology* 1988;69:387–94.
19. Gaba DM: Human error in anesthetic mishaps. *Int Anesthesiol Clin* 1989;27:137–47.
20. DeAnda A, Gaba DM: Unplanned incidents during comprehensive anesthesia simulation. *Anesth Analg* 1990;71:77–82.
21. DeAnda A, Gaba DM: Role of experience in the response to simulated clinical incidents. *Anesth Analg* 1991;72:308–15.
22. Cooper JB, Newbowser RS: An analysis of major errors and equipment failures in anesthesia management: considerations for prevention and detection. *Anesthesiology* 1984;60:34–42.

23. Chopra V, Engbers FH, Geerts MJ, et al: The Leiden anesthesia simulator. *Br J Anaesth* 1994;73:287–92.

24. Swank KM, Jarhr JS: The uses of simulation in anesthesiology training. *J La State Med Soc* 1992;144:523–7.

25. Saliterman SS: A computerized simulation for critical care training: new technology for medical education. *Mayo Clin Proc* 1990;65:968–78.

26. McLellan BA: Early experience with simulated trauma resuscitation. *Can J Surg* 1999;42:205–10.

27. Gilbart MD, Hutchison CR, Cusimano MD, Regehr G: A computer-based trauma simulator for teaching and testing. *Am J Surg* 2000;179:223–8.

28. Small SD, Wuerz RC, Simon R, et al: Demonstration of high-fidelity simulation team training for emergency medicine. *Acad Emerg Med* 1994;6:312–23.

29. Cavanaugh S: Computerized simulation training technology for clinical teaching and testing. *Acad Emerg Med* 1997;4:939–43.

30. Byrne AJ, Greaves JD: Assessment instruments used during anaesthetic simulation: review of published studies. *Br J Anaesth* 2001;86:445–50.

31. Morgan PJ, Cleave-Hogg D: Evaluation of medical students' performance using the anaesthesia simulator. *Med Educ* 2000;34:42–5.

32. Devitt JH, Kurrek MM, Cohen MM, et al: Testing the raters: inter-rater reliability of standardized anaesthesia simulator performance. *Can J Anaesth* 1997;44:924–8.

33. Devitt JH, Kurrek MM, Cohen MM, et al: Testing internal consistency and construct validity during evaluation of performance in a patient simulator. *Anesth Analg* 1998;86:1160–4.

34. Morgan PJ, Cleave-Hogg D, Guest C: A comparison of global ratings and checklist scores from an undergraduate assessment using an anesthesia simulator. *Acad Med* 2001;76:1053–5.

35. Weller JM, Bloch M, Young S, et al: Evaluation of high fidelity patient simulator in assessment of performance of anesthetists. *Br J Anaesth* 2003;90:43–7.

36. Fletcher G, Flin R, McGeorge P, et al: Anaesthetists' non-technical skills (ANTS): evaluation of a behavioural marker system. *Br J Anaesth* 2003;90:580–88.

37. Schwid HA, Rooke GA, Carline J, et al: Evaluation of anesthesia residents using a mannequin-based simulation. *Anesthesiology* 2002;97:1434–44.

38. Devitt JH, Kurrek MM, Cohen MM, Cleave-Hogg D: The validity of performance assessments using simulation. *Anesthesiology* 2001;95:36–42.

39. Morgan PJ, Cleave-Hogg D, Guest C, Herold J: Validity and reliability of undergraduate performance assessments in an anesthesia simulator. *Can J Anaesth* 2001;48:225–33.

40. Morgan PJ, Cleave-Hogg D: A worldwide survey of the use of simulation in anesthesia. *Can J Anaesth* 2002;49:659–62.

41. MedSim Corporate website. 2004.

42. Laerdal Corporate website. 2004.

43. METI Corporate website. 2004.

44. Holzman GB: Clinical simulation. p. 240–3. *The medical teacher*. Churchill Livingstone, London, 1998.

45. Ker J, Mole L, Bradely P: Early introduction to interprofessional learning: a simulated environment. *Med Educ* 2003;37:248–55.

46. Ericsson KA, Krampe RT, Tesh-Romer C: The role of deliberate practice in the acquisition of expert performance. *Psychol Rev* 1993;100:363–406.

47. Knowles M: *The adult learner: a neglected species.* Gulf, Houston, TX, 1984.

48. Maguire P, Fairbairn S, Fletcher C: Consultation skills of young doctors—1. Benefits of feedback training in interviewing as students persist. *BMJ* 1986;292:1573–8.

49. Liddell M, Davidson S, Taub H, Witecross L: Evaluation of procedural skills training in an undergraduate curriculum. *Med Educ* 2002;36:1035–41.

50. Regehr G, Norman GR: Issues in cognitive psychology: implications for professional education. *Acad Med* 2004;71:988–1001.

MEDICAL ERRORS

Dave Neilipovitz

Headlines were made around the world when the Institute of Medicine estimated that up to 98 000 people die each year in the United States as direct result of medical errors.[1] Dramatic analogies to a 747 jetliner full of patients dying daily[2] or a major motor company losing an employee every day[3] were used to describe a problem of astonishing proportions. Not surprisingly, the topic of medical errors has now become one of the leading public concerns. Although this issue is not a new one, it is clear that society is demanding dramatic changes and improvements in this area. The "head in the sand" attitude that has hitherto been taken to this taboo subject will no longer be tolerated.[4] An exhaustive review on medical errors in this chapter is clearly not feasible. Rather, the goal of this chapter is to introduce some of the important aspects of the problem and illustrate how some of the strategies advocated by the ACES Program may help reduce the impact of medical errors.

● Definition of Medical Errors

Historically, the circumstances that have resulted in adverse events in patients have been called "medical errors." A leading researcher in this topic suggests that the use of the term has been unfortunate. Dr. Troyen Brennan suggests that this term has negative connotations: some synonyms would include blooper, blunder, goof—and numerous other derogatory names.[5] Although few would question calling horrific mistakes such as amputating the wrong limb or transplanting an incompatible organ as nefarious errors, these are not representative of the vast majority of circumstances that result in adverse events.[6,7] Regardless of the appropriateness of the term, medical error will be used in this review. Thus, it becomes crucial to understand what constitutes an actual medical error before embarking on a discussion of the topic.

The definition of what constitutes a medical error unfortunately differs substantially depending upon who is defining it. The Institute of Medicine defines medical error both as the failure of a planned action to be completed as intended or as the use of a wrong plan to achieve an aim, whether or not the error results in harm.[1] Wu et al.[8] modified this definition by describing a medical mistake as a "commission or an omission with potentially negative consequences for the patient that would have been judged wrong by skilled and knowledgeable peers at the time it occurred, independent of whether there were any negative consequences." They thus included inaction as an important source of error and, most importantly, suggested that actions must be judged in the context of when they were made rather than through retrospection. Thus, medical errors are the result of an action or an inaction and their being judged to be errors should not be dependent on whether a patient is harmed— in spite of the fact that it is often the severity of the injury that will bias individuals in determining whether or not an error has occurred.[9] Some authors argue that only mistakes that have adverse consequences should be the focus of error reduction programs. On the contrary, we will argue that although an error that has no adverse consequences is certainly not as devastating as one that results in someone dying, the end result should not diminish the fact that an error occurred. Small and seemingly unimportant mistakes left unaddressed could potentially proceed to what ultimately becomes a catastrophe. As discussed below, solving the cause of the problem often involves changing the environment in which it occurred. Thus, all errors should be addressed in some manner.

One last issue in the discussion of medical errors is the subject of negligence. Negligence is often defined as the failure of a health care professional to meet the standard of care that would be expected within their community resulting in injury or harm.[10] Negligence is certainly related to the topic of medical errors but the two should not be regarded as synonymous. Although negligence will often result in an event that would be termed a medical error, not all medical errors are the result of negligence. Furthermore, the term *negligence* again arouses numerous negative responses in most health care professionals, which could inhibit open and fruitful discussion about medical errors. Therefore, the following discussion of medical errors will attempt to address this topic in general rather than focusing on the potentially divisive and litigious topic of negligence.

● Scope of the Problem

Since we do not have a uniform definition of medical error, it is not surprising that the exact incidence of medical errors is difficult to quantify. The vast majority of medical errors have no adverse consequences and are therefore not easily detected. Most studies that have attempted to determine the incidence are retrospective and are subject to the inherent limitations of this kind of study design.[7] The two largest studies, the Harvard Medical Practice Study (HMPS)[10] and the Utah-Colorado Medical Practice Study (UCMPS),[11] had trained physicians use a standardized review of selected charts. The process determining which charts to review has been challenged as having the potential to create selection bias. More important, however, is the potential for problems associated with the review process itself. These studies relied on the implicit judgment of the reviewers that a medical error had, indeed, caused the adverse event—rather than explicit judgment.[12] Indeed, the judgment of reviewers can often be a source of overestimation, which can bias the results.[6] The unavoidable bias inherent in the hindsight nature of a retrospective approach compounds the review process further. The studies also did little to account for the baseline risk of death that these patients already had.[13] However, despite these potential sources of overestimating the actual number of medical errors, most evidence would support the opposite premise: that medical errors are actually more frequent than retrospective reviews suggest.

Most prospective studies support the premise that medical errors occur at a higher rate than reported in retrospective reviews.[14,15] The reasons are numerous but often relate to the fact that events are not documented in the medical record in a way that would allow adverse events to be identified retrospectively.[7] A potential solution for better identifying the actual incidence is to have physicians self-report medical errors with a similar system to that employed by the airline industry: Pilots are expected to report episodes where mistakes have possibly been made. This process is protected by anonymity and has numerous guarantees of protection from retribution. Despite demands for this process in the landmark report from the Institute of Medicine, experts are skeptical that this process will succeed in medicine unless changes to the litigious context in which medicine is practised are made concurrently.[5] Physicians and health care professionals will obviously be reluctant to admit making any form of mistake if they are then to be held liable and accountable for these errors, which are often beyond their control to prevent. Therefore, any estimates of the scope of the problem are indirect, imprecise and likely an underestimation of the real number. However, let us assume for the sake of our exploration of the issue that the numbers from the report from the Institute of Medicine can be used to estimate the potential impact of the problem on society.

The number of deaths in the United States attributable to medical errors is said in the report to range from 44 000 to 98 000 annually, with an estimated resulting financial burden of 17 billion dollars.[5] It was based on these figures that newspapers presented their terrifying analogies to jet liners of patients crashing daily and wrote that medical error is the fourth leading cause of death. It should come as no surprise that these and other analogies have frightened the public into demanding immediate changes. However, it is important to determine the origin of these figures. These staggering values were primarily derived from extrapolation of the numbers from the HMPS and the UCMPS studies. The data from these reports suggested that the rate of injury from medical error was between 2.9 and 3.7% of hospitalized patients.[10,11] The process of extrapolating population-based figures from these numbers, however, has dubious statistical merit and

was performed despite the cautions against doing so put forth by the actual authors of these same studies.[5,10,11]

More important than the accuracy of the numbers cited by the Institute of Medicine, is the implied corollary to these statements: that if these errors had been prevented all these deaths would have been avoided.[16] While it is a reasonably safe assumption that preventing an airplane crash would save the lives concerned, the assumption that all deaths that are attributable to medical error would be prevented if all errors are prevented is not correct. A study by Hayward and Hofer[16] reported similar numbers of preventable deaths as the HMPS and several other alarming studies. However, this study differed in that it went on to question what the likelihood of death was in the absence of the error. Their results supported the premise that the majority of deaths attributed to medical errors occur at the end of life or in critically ill patients in whom death was the most likely outcome in any case. The adjustment reduced the estimate of preventable death from 6.0% to 1.3%.

Even if we assume that the staggering numbers put forth in the Institute of Medicine report may be inflated and have created an overestimation of the actual impact of the problem, the more conservative figures are still significant. Although the belief that patients would likely have died regardless of whether or not an error occurred may reduce the guilt burden experienced by physicians, it should not diminish the concern of health care professionals regarding this subject.[7] Medical errors undoubtedly will have a significant negative impact on patient outcome and have substantial costs associated with them. Prevention and strategies to minimize their impact must, therefore, proceed with considerable effort and support from all health care professionals.

● Etiology of Medical Errors

The etiology of medical errors, as with most aspects of this subject, is not straightforward. The vast majority of errors are complex and lack readily apparent etiologies; even the circumstances that generate them can be extremely hard to identify. Indeed, most complications are not due to one mistake but rather are the cumulative effect of smaller errors from multiple sources.[17] Our understanding is further limited by the narrow parameters for investigation of the majority of adverse events: Investigations most often focus on the last minutes of a situation rather than the days preceding it.[17] Unfortunately, the circumstances that created the milieu in which an adverse event was likely to occur are not usually described and thus are not addressed to prevent future complications. Compounding the difficulty in determining the etiology of medical errors is the punitive approach that can surround these events, which limits the co-operation of those involved. In spite of these challenges, numerous lists and classifications of medical errors have been created. While an exhaustive description of these lists is not possible here, we will conduct a brief examination of the categories of errors.

Broadly speaking, the causes of medical errors can be divided into two main categories: failures of the personnel involved and failures of the system. The errors attributable to personnel failure are usually due to physiological and psychological limitations.[18] These human factors include habits, fatigue, workload, cognition, attitudes, imperfect processing of information, flawed decision making, communication problems and countless other aspects of human behaviour.[12] However, despite the fact that historically most blame has been attributed to the individuals involved in the adverse event, emerging evidence indicates that system failures are the largest source of error.[7,17]

Why is the blame usually directed towards health care professionals even when they are not the prime cause of the adverse event? The reasons for this are numerous and somewhat complex. The medical legal approach, with its emphasis on malpractice and negligence, has instilled the belief that adverse events only occur because someone was careless or negligent. Quite often, patients and their families have a limited perspective when they gauge an adverse event, as they can only assess the situation in a context with which they are familiar or that they have experienced[17] (for instance, they only know the specific circumstances of how their loved one presented but may be unfamiliar with the overall medical and organizational context; nor might they be familiar with the relative rarity or commonness of the patient's condition). Further, physicians are often limited by the information and resources that are available to them in a given situation. For

example, an elderly man presents with confusion to an emergency room in a small rural hospital. The physician, working in an understaffed area, is a bit slow in assessing him and, when the patient is finally seen, decides the situation does not require immediate therapy and elects instead to observe the patient. Unfortunately, the patient suddenly collapses and dies. The cause of death is a large subdural hematoma that occurred when he fell several days ago. In this kind of case, fault is most often attributed to the physician's inaction. However, there could have been numerous other contributors to the situation: Limited information may have been presented to the doctor, with no information at all regarding the fall or other risk factors for subdural hematoma. The lack of resources (including radiographic imagery), an exceptionally busy emergency room due to a local physician shortage, and countless other contributing factors are not assigned blame by the family for the unfortunate adverse event. The family believes that the doctor made a mistake. Even the doctor will often believe this. This kind of belief is an illustration of what Westrum called the *fallacy of centrality*:[17] the idea that one is the centre of an information network rather than just another participant in a complex and interdependent system. The unfortunate reality is that it is rarely the individual who is the prime reason mistakes occur; rather it is the design and the conditions of the system they are working in that are the root of the problem. Leape aptly said that medical errors are primarily due to faulty systems, not faulty people.[7]

The contribution of systems to errors in general was first appreciated in the 1950s by the manufacturing industry. When errors that occurred in their industry were investigated, roughly 85% of errors turned out to be due to problems in the system itself as opposed to mistakes by individuals.[3] Research demonstrated that problems formerly attributed to human fallibility, incompetence or negligence could often be traced back to pre-existing organizational (e.g., work environment, financial resources) or institutional factors (e.g., national standards, regulatory bodies); these are often referred to as *latent conditions*.[17] Latent conditions are events and circumstances, including the various organizational aspects of the medical system, that are in place long before accidents develop.[17] The physician is expected to operate in the presence of these latent conditions but is essentially powerless to directly change or influence these conditions. The vast majority of adverse events are thus the consequence of flaws within the medical system itself and not of the actions of the individuals who participate in it. The actual number of problems in the system is virtually countless but includes problems with the design of the hospital, training shortfalls, inadequate staffing, untenable governmental and hospital policies, failure to integrate preventive strategies, poorly structured organizations and numerous other possibilities.[17] Thus, any attempt to solve the problem of medical errors will need to focus on improving medical systems rather than on trying to make health care professionals better.

Potential Solutions to a Complex Problem

The issue of medical errors is huge and highly complex and offers no simple solutions. The inability to easily solve this issue is an extension of the initial challenge to even try to accurately define what constitutes a medical error, let alone try to identify all circumstances predisposing and causing medical errors to occur. Despite the magnitude of the task, it is necessary to try to formulate an approach to the problem. To assist in this endeavour, the solutions created by other industries may serve as sources of guidance and assistance. The airline industry has so far been the area where most comparisons are made.

Although direct comparisons between the discipline of medicine and the aeronautic field may be somewhat simplistic and unrealistic, there appears to be some value in the undertaking. The airline industry had a reported fatality rate of 1.18 per million passengers in 1950, which was reduced to 0.57 by 1990.[3] To effect this improvement, analyses of events were studied in detail to discover the possible faults of the system rather than focusing on personnel performance.[19] This approach to adverse events is virtually the opposite of medicine, where mistakes are dealt with in a primarily punitive fashion with minimal attention given to investigating why an event occurred.[19] It would seem logical that medical errors should all be investigated to determine if they were solely due to individual human failure or if factors within the system contributed to the event (thus indicating a risk of reoccurrence). Unfortunately, the majority of medical errors are never addressed in such a thorough and potentially insightful fashion.

The airline industry assumes that human errors are inevitable and attempts to redesign systems to have the capability to absorb their impact.[19] One measure this industry has used to make the system proof against individual error is the creation and institution of standard practices, which have been demonstrated to be an important mechanism for mitigating error.[3] Critics will counter this proposition by saying that standardizing practice in medicine is unfeasible. The argument is that patients are infinitely more complex than even the most sophisticated jet plane. Indeed, the classic belief is that medicine is both a science and an art. However, if it is indeed the deviation from certain standards that kills patients, it is imperative that we ensure that the scientific side of this partnership is the stronger component.[3] The airline industry also provides personnel with highly developed and structured training, which includes an ongoing re-certification process.[19] Finally, the American airline industry has not one, but rather two agencies to oversee the safety of the industry. These agencies allow pilots to report adverse events or concerns in a confidential and non-punitive fashion.[12] The agencies then have the opportunity to address their concerns and make changes to the system before a catastrophe occurs.

If we use the solutions put forth by the airline industry, some changes to the health care system should be considered. Although the unique characteristics of patients will dictate the customization of therapy they receive, there appears to be some merit in attempting to simplify and even standardize professional health care practices.[20] Physicians unfortunately can become isolated in their practices with little opportunity for interaction with colleagues and thus minimal refinement of their skills.[3] Providing them with readily accessible sources of practice standards for common afflictions or situations may serve to reduce the number of medical errors. Redesigning the medical system to be more robust and resistant to mistakes by reducing the need for significant operator vigilance and reliance on memory would be invaluable.[20] Better and more readily available patient monitoring devices could lessen the burden placed on physicians. Internet websites that are simple to access but contain valid and regularly updated information for physicians could lessen their need for memorization of numerous facts. Even the placing of vital patient information such as allergies and past medical problems on the magnetic strip of their health cards, could reduce medical errors by decreasing reliance on a patient's recall. Redesigning the health care system is obviously a complex undertaking, but it is likely to have the greatest impact on reducing medical error. That said, attention to the training of physicians may have a positive impact as well.

Aside from the investment of time and effort to improve both the engineering of airplanes and the system in which they operate, the airline industry has also attempted to improve how airline crews work together through the development of Crew Resource Management (CRM) strategies. Although it can be argued that we are not likely to be able to improve individuals much more than we already have,[20] we could profitably examine the issue of how health care professionals interact. In particular, surprisingly few physicians are trained to have the necessary knowledge and skills to effectively manage crisis situations. So in addition to redesigning aspects of the medical system itself, there is still a vital role for providing individuals with additional knowledge and skills to improve their role in managing patients, especially those that are critically ill.

The Acute Critical Events Simulation (ACES) Program will obviously not prevent the occurrence of all medical errors, but it may help contribute some solutions to this complex problem. The management of critically ill patients can be a challenging and confusing process. Overt errors will hopefully be reduced by the specific knowledge and techniques discussed in the various chapters of this book. More important, however, are the discussions surrounding the topic of *crisis resource management* (the medical CRM). Remember, not all medical errors are solely acts of commission but also include acts of omission. An inability to make decisions can delay life-saving therapy and thereby seriously compromise the welfare of patients. The ACES Program advocates certain strategies that should improve physicians' skills in managing critically ill patients. These strategies are simple, easy to remember and effective.

The first and most important strategy in emergency situations is the ABC's approach. Although the ABC's approach is old and often taken for granted, it can be highly useful. But simply saying one should do the ABC's is not enough. Unfortunately, many physicians do not have the necessary knowledge or skills to effectively perform the ABC's. The following chapters are therefore designed to help one develop the necessary skills to effectively perform the ABC's. The Concurrent Management strategy, which stresses simultaneous treatment and diagnosis of problems, results in therapy being instituted earlier. Finally, the Reassess and Re-evaluate strategy (R&R) is often neglected but is invaluable in the prevention and minimization of the impact of medical errors. Mistakes in initial management strategy will invariably occur. However, when physicians use the R&R strategy, smaller problems are identified earlier and at a more readily reversible stage than if the R&R strategy is omitted. Thus, aspects of crisis resource management and the other strategies advocated in the ACES Program will hopefully enable physicians to make the most of their small yet integral role in minimizing the problem of medical errors.

● Conclusions

It has been said that medical errors are excusable, but ignoring them is not.[7] Medical errors have long been a problem and will likely continue to be an issue until profound changes in the medical system occur. The medical system needs to be redesigned so as to be robust enough to absorb and minimize the impact of the mistakes that will inevitably occur. Until such major revisions in the medical system are made, initiatives like the ACES Program may have a role in reducing the impact, and possibly the occurrence, of medical errors.

Key Points

- Medical errors are a common occurrence.
- The consequences of medical errors are costly in terms of lives lost.

- Most errors are due to failings of the medical system as opposed to individual failings.
- Initiatives to improve the medical system are sorely needed.

- Although the main problem is with the design of the system, there is some merit in improving individual physician training, particularly in the area of crisis resource management.

- The ACES Program may help reduce medical errors and their impact by offering crisis resource management education and strategies.

References

1. Kohn LT, Corrigan JM, Donaldson MS (eds): Committee on quality of health care in America, Institute of Health. To err is human: Building a safer health system. National Academy Press, Washington, DC, 2000.
2. Preventing medical errors. *New York Times.* December 1, 1999:A22.
3. van Amerongen D: Error management and patient safety: A managed care competency. p.117–36. In Rosenthal MM, Sutcliffe KM (eds): *Medical error: What do we know? What do we do?* Josey-Bass, San Francisco, 2002.
4. Blumenthal D: Making medical errors into medical treasures. *JAMA* 1994;272:1867–8.
5. Brennan TA: The Institute of Medicine report on medical errors—could it do harm? *N Engl J Med* 2000;342:1123–5.
6. Hayward RA, Hofer TP: Estimating hospital deaths due to medical errors: Preventability is in the eye of the reviewer. *JAMA* 2001;286:415–20.
7. Leape LL: Institute of Medicine medical error figures are not exaggerated. *JAMA* 2000;284:95–7.
8. Wu AW, Cavanaugh TA, McPhee SJ, et al: To tell the truth: Ethical and practical issues in disclosing medical mistakes to patients. *J Gen Intern Med* 1997;12:770–5.
9. Studdert DM, Brennan TA, Thomas EJ: What have we learned since the Harvard Medical Practice Study? p. 3–33. In Rosenthal MM, Sutcliffe KM (eds): *Medical error: What do we know? What do we do?* Josey-Bass, San Francisco, 2002.
10. Brennan TA, Leape LL, Laird NM, et al: Incidence of adverse events and negligence in hospitalized patients. Results of the Harvard Medical Practice Study I. *N Engl J Med* 1991;324:370–6.
11. Thomas EJ, Studdert DM, Burstin HR, et al: Incidence and types of adverse events and negligent care in Utah and Colorado. *Med Care* 2000;38:261–71.
12. Heimreich RL: On error management: Lessons from aviation. *BMJ* 2000;320:781–5.
13. McDonald CJ, Weiner M, Hui SL: Deaths due to medical errors are exaggerated in Institute of Medicine Report. *JAMA* 2001;284:93–5.
14. Classen DC, Pestonik SL, Evans RS, Burke JP: Computerized surveillance of adverse drug events in hospital patients. *JAMA* 1991;266:2847–51.
15. Bates DW, Cullen DJ, Laird N, et al: Incidence of adverse drug events and potential adverse drug events. *JAMA* 1995;274:29–34.
16. Hayward RA, Hofer TP: Estimating hospital deaths due to medical errors: Preventability is in the eye of the reviewer. *JAMA* 2001;286:415–20.
17. Weick KE: The reduction of medical errors through mindful interdependence. p. 175–99. In Rosenthal MM, Sutcliffe KM (eds): *Medical error: What do we know? What do we do?* Josey-Bass, San Francisco, 2002.
18. Amalberti R: *La conduite de systèmes à risques.* Presses Universitaires de France, Paris, 1996.
19. Leape LL: Errors in medicine. *JAMA* 1994;272:1851–7.
20. Bates DW, Gawande AA: Errors in medicine: What have we learned? *Ann Intern Med* 2000;132:763–7.

AIRWAY MANAGEMENT

Objectives

1. Learn how to assess the airway and identify difficult intubations.
2. Develop an approach to airway problems including planning and preparation.
3. Learn the fundamentals of basic airway management.
4. Develop a knowledge of the drugs commonly used in airway management.
5. Create an approach to difficult and failed airways.

Chapter 5 presents an approach to the assessment and management of an airway. It discusses basic airway skills and provides a description of how to confirm proper tube placement.

This chapter discusses advanced airway devices and an approach to the failed intubation.

Chapter 7 presents the common medications used to facilitate airway management and the complications associated with them and discusses drug selection and dosing.

This chapter discusses the technique of rapid sequence intubation and its advantages and disadvantages. It also provides a discussion of cricoid pressure.

The dilemma of being unable to ventilate or intubate a patient is frightening. This chapter attempts to offer solutions.

CHAPTER 5

BASIC AIRWAY MANAGEMENT

DAVE NEILIPOVITZ

A man in his late 50s has arrived at the hospital and you are the physician who is responsible for his care. He has a history of respiratory problems due to smoking. He was on 2 l/min home oxygen but has had to increase it to over 4 l/min for the last week. He had a non-productive cough. He is now in respiratory extremis with a respiratory rate over 40 and oxygen saturation levels of around 78%. Supplemental oxygen was attempted but did not work. He will not co-operate for non-invasive ventilation. Clearly, he will need intubation. What should you do?

One of the most important but unnerving situations is having to secure a patient's airway. Many questions come to mind. Will I be able to secure the airway? What drugs should I use? What will happen if I am unable to do it? The goal of this and the following chapters is to prepare you for this scenario, by helping you develop a strategy to deal with the problems associated with airway management. The primary theme for the chapter will be preparation. A physician should have a primary plan and several backup plans for each of the different problems that may arise as the airway is secured. Table 5.1 outlines this review. The reader is encouraged to read each section in succession but the sections are designed so that they can be individually referenced when a specific question or issue arises.

Table 5.1 – Overview of Chapter
I   Indications for Airway Intubation
II   Airway Anatomy and Assessment
III   Preparation
IV   Bag and Mask Ventilation
V   Intubation
VI   Confirmation of Correct Endotracheal Tube Placement

I. Indications for Airway Intubation

The decision to intubate a patient's airway is not always an easy decision to make (Table 5.2). Although a patient often requires intubation for several different reasons, some patients present a dilemma to even the most experienced physician. The most common reason for inserting an endotracheal tube (ETT) is respiratory failure. Airway intubation is usually required if positive pressure ventilation is going to be instituted. Although the use of non-invasive ventilatory support with a BiPAP® machine is gaining in popularity, airway intubation with an ETT is still a required skill for the resuscitation of critically ill patients.

Placement of a cuffed ETT is recommended if a patient is unable to protect their airway from aspiration of gastric contents. Airway protection is often required in patients with a decreased level of consciousness and an absent gag reflex. A rule of thumb is that patients with a Glasgow Coma Score below 8 usually require airway protection.[1] Early airway intubation to protect the airway is also recommended for patients who have the potential to obstruct their airway. Patients presenting with anaphylaxis, an enlarging neck mass or who have experienced an upper airway burn require early placement of an ETT to ensure airway patency, since complete airway obstruction can rapidly develop.

Patients unable to expel pulmonary secretions may require intubation to facilitate access to the bronchial tree to allow for their removal. Secretions that are not removed become a fertile environment for bacterial growth and put the patient at a greater risk of developing pneumonia. A hemodynamically unstable patient usually requires intubation and mechanical ventilation to reduce oxygen consumption from the work of breathing and to improve the oxygen delivery to other vital organs. Furthermore, shock will often be complicated by respiratory failure due to inadequate oxygen delivery to the respiratory muscles. The excessive work of breathing could overwhelm a patient in shock. Other indications for intubation include the need to induce hypocapnia to treat increased intracranial pressure. Finally, the ETT can be used as a conduit to administer cardiac arrest medications if there is no intravenous access.

II. Airway Anatomy and Assessment

A rudimentary knowledge of airway anatomy and airway evaluation is essential to avoid problems during intubation. The ideal view that should be seen during laryngoscopy is illustrated in Figure 5.1. Unfortunately, the vocal cords and other structures are not always easily visualized, making intubation difficult and sometimes impossible. The goal is therefore to learn to recognize patients in whom intubation may be difficult, thus alerting the physician to call earlier for more experienced assistance and to avoid the administration of drugs that could make the situation much worse (e.g., muscle paralyzing drugs). Although there is often an urgent need for ETT placement, it is recommended that airway assessment and preparation be performed prior to all intubations.[2] The time used to assess and prepare for intubation will easily be recovered by avoiding unexpected difficulties and complications that can occur with intubation. Airway assessment is not as simple as it sounds. Numerous studies have attempted

---

Table 5.2 – Indications for Airway Intubation

1. Airway Protection
2. Ensure Airway Patency (e.g., neck hematoma)
3. Respiratory Failure:
   a. hypoxic respiratory failure
   b. hypercapnic respiratory failure
   c. combined respiratory failure
4. Pulmonary Toilet
5. Hemodynamic Instability
6. Induce Hypocapnia for Increased ICP

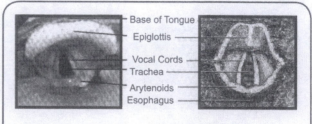

Figure 5.1 – Larynx and Vocal Chords

Photograph and drawing of the glottic opening. The tracheal rings can often be visualized through the vocal cords.

to identify features that predict increased difficulty during intubation.[2-7] Unfortunately, no single test or feature in and of itself is sufficient to identify a difficult airway.[2,7] Several different characteristics have, however, been found to help predict which patients may be difficult to intubate. As the number of abnormal airway characteristics on examination increases, so does the probability that the intubation will be difficult. A simple acronym to remember is TUMS (something you often need after being asked to intubate a patient). *TUMS* refers to teeth, uvula, mandible and spine (Table 5.3).

The first characteristic one should look for is the presence or absence of teeth. Large protruding teeth make intubation difficult whereas the absence of teeth makes it easier. A patient's dentures should always be removed prior to intubation. The next important predictor is how much of the uvula and posterior pharynx can be visualized when the patient's mouth is open. Although a classification system exists (the modified Mallampati class),[3,4] it is simpler to remember that the more the uvula can be seen, the easier the intubation (Figure 5.2). The third characteristic that should be assessed is the size of the mandible.[6,7] A larger jaw is favourable since there is more space to displace the tongue with the laryngoscope thereby facilitating larynx visualization. The thyromental distance assesses the jaw size, which is simply the space between the chin and the thyroid cartilage. Normally this space is at least three finger breadths (approximately 6–7 cm). Difficulty during intubation is more likely to occur in patients whose thyromental space is less than three finger breadths.[6,7] Cervical spine movement should be assessed since a reduction in flexion and especially in extension will make intubation more difficult[7] (do not assess

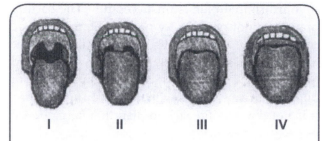

Figure 5.2 – Modified Mallampati-Samsoon Class

The classification of the pharyngeal structures. The class is determined with the patient sitting erect with the mouth as wide as possible and tongue protruded. The patient does not say anything. In Class I, the entire soft palate, tonsillar pillars and entire uvula are visible. In Class II only the tonsillar fauces are visible but the entire uvula and soft palate are still visible. In Class III only part of the uvula is seen, while in Class IV none of the soft palate is visible. The level of intubation difficulty increases from Class I to Class IV.

movement of the cervical spine in patients suspected of having a cervical spine injury). Inability to extend a patient's neck will make placement of a patient's head into the optimal intubating position more difficult (see sniff position in Section III). Additional characteristics that can impair your ability to intubate a patient include unusual masses in the mouth or neck (e.g., abscesses, hematomas), previous neck surgery or radiation and various other facial anomalies. A previous tracheotomy is usually not a problem but may require a slightly smaller ETT, since there may be an element of tracheal stenosis at the previous tracheostomy site that could impair the passage of the ETT.

● III. Preparation

Time spent planning for airway intubation can prevent life-threatening problems by avoiding complications associated with failed intubation. One should quickly formulate a plan on how the patient will be intubated. The plan can simply be to use the laryngoscope blade and a styletted tube. However, you should always have a backup plan

Table 5.3 – Assessment of Airway (TUMS)

T	Teeth – do they protrude or are they absent?
U	Uvula – how much of it is seen (so-called Mallampati class)?
M	Mandible – the size of it as assessed by the thyromental distance.
S	Spine – the flexion and extension movement of the cervical spine.

if your original plan is unsuccessful.[8] The backup plan does not necessarily need to be much more complicated than your initial plan. It could simply be to bag and mask the patient until more experienced help arrives. Conversely, it could involve the use of different airway devices with which you are familiar. It is not the specific backup plan that is important per se, but rather that a backup plan does exist. A common mistake made by physicians who have no backup plan is to perform repeated attempts to intubate with direct laryngoscopy.[9] Each intubation attempt leads to progressively more soft tissue injury. Eventually, a patient who would have been easy to bag and mask will no longer be so and can thus develop a life-threatening airway obstruction. A good rule of thumb is that the first attempt will be the best attempt. No more than three intubation attempts should be made.

Before embarking on intubation, one should always do a quick check that all the equipment is readily available. An oxygen source and the means to administer it must be available. A good selection of oral airways is important since they can facilitate bag and mask ventilation. The laryngoscope should be checked to ensure that the light works. While the laryngoscope blade is a matter of personal choice, most prefer the curved blade called the Macintosh blade (Figure 5.3). A Macintosh blade is generally recommended when there is less upper airway space to pass the ETT (e.g., a small mouth). A straight blade

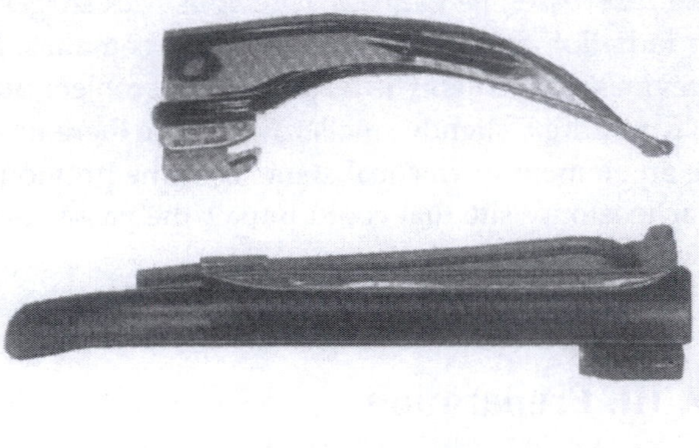

Figure 5.3 – Laryngoscope Blades

The Macintosh laryngoscope blade (the curved blade, above) is generally the blade of choice for most intubations. The Miller laryngoscope blade is the most commonly available straight blade.

like the Miller is generally regarded as the preferred blade in patients with a small mandibular space, large incisors or a long floppy epiglottis.

Proper blade size depends on patient size but usually a four is required for males and a three for females. The Macintosh blade must be long enough to place tension on the glossoepiglottic ligament while the Miller blade must be of sufficient length to trap the epiglottis against the tongue. An ETT whose balloon has been checked should be available. Again the size depends on patient size but a 7.0 to 8.0 is appropriate for most patients. A stylet in the ETT is recommended since it facilitates tube placement and can be easily removed if it's not required. The ability to suction secretions and vomitus is very important. Finally, means to inflate the ETT and secure the tube in place should be available.

Ideally a patient who is about to be intubated will have several monitors already applied or readily available. A pulse oximeter to measure oxygen saturation is invaluable. A device that measures for the presence of expired carbon dioxide is very useful to confirm the position of the ETT following intubation. ECG and blood pressure monitors can also be invaluable.

After selecting the required equipment, the patient should be optimally positioned. A major misconception is that the patient's pillow should be removed. Pillow removal will make intubation considerably more difficult. As illustrated in Figure 5.4, a pillow will help position the patient into the *sniff position*. The neck extension from a pillow will improve the alignment of a patient's pharyngeal axis and their laryngeal axis. The oral axis is then aligned with the laryngeal and pharyngeal axis by use of the laryngoscope. Airway intubation requires that the three axes be brought into alignment.

In an obese patient, proper positioning is even more important. Intubating an obese patient can be very challenging. The patient's chest can interfere with intubation by impinging upon the handle of the laryngoscope (Figure 5.5). Furthermore, the scenario is often complicated by difficulties with mask ventilation and rapid desaturation. Pillows and blankets should be used to create a ramp under the patient's shoulders and upper back to help displace the adipose tissue, which greatly facilitates airway intubation. Complete preparation also implies readiness to deal effectively with any possible complications that can result from the intubation

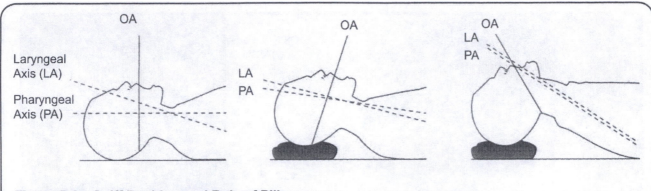

Figure 5.4 – Sniff Position and Role of Pillow

The diagrams illustrate the sniff position and the reason the use of a pillow is preferred in most intubations. The use of a pillow improves the alignment of the laryngeal and pharyngeal axes. The final diagram illustrates how pressure on the head is applied to improve the alignment of the oral axis to facilitate airway intubation.

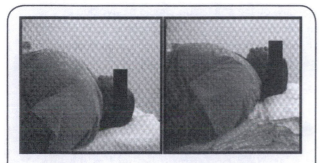

Figure 5.5 – Positioning in Obese Patients

The photographs illustrate the importance of, and technique for, obtaining an ideal sniff position even in obese patients. Without altering the patient's position, there is no space for the laryngoscope handle, and the adipose tissue and breasts may severely interfere with intubation. The placing of several blankets or pillows under the patient to create a ramp-like structure will markedly improve the ease of intubation.

process, whether related to failure to secure the airway or to other hemodynamic complications.

● IV. Bag and Mask Ventilation

The skill of bag and mask-ventilation saves lives, yet is rarely mastered by physicians. The ability to effectively bag and mask ventilate a patient can keep a patient alive even if they cannot be intubated.[10] The use of paralytic drugs requires that the physician be able to ventilate the patient even if the intubation attempts fail. Thus, the physician should routinely bag a patient prior to intubation to ensure they maintain and develop this essential skill.

The first component of bag and mask ventilation is correct placement of the mask. Two types of masks are commonly used. The black solid mask is often referred to as the *anesthesia mask* and while it is thought by some to be more difficult to use, it is more versatile. The anesthesia mask is first placed over the bridge of the nose and then down onto the chin. Pressure is then exerted on the nasal bridge with the thumb and below the tip of the nose with the index finger (Figure 5.6). The baby finger of the same hand is then placed behind the angle of the mandible. Avoid pushing underneath the patient's chin since this can obstruct the airway. Occasionally, obtaining a good seal with the mask is difficult and two hands are required. Although a second person must then squeeze the bag to ventilate the patient, the two-handed mask seal can be a valuable technique. The second type of mask is the clear mask. The clear mask is simply placed on top of the face thereby covering the nose and mouth. The mask is held in a similar manner as with the anesthesia mask.

Ideally, one should coordinate the bag ventilation with the patient's breathing if it is present. If the chest is not moving there are several manoeuvres that can be done to improve ventilation. The most common reason for poor chest movement is upper airway obstruction. The head can be repositioned into a better sniff position and a chin thrust can be performed with the finger behind the angle of the jaw. If these

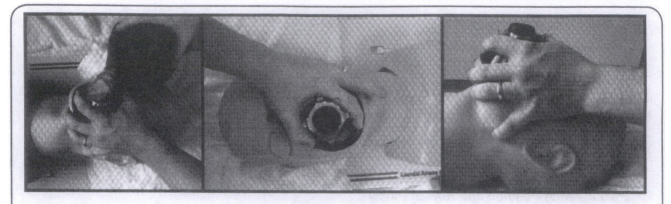

Figure 5.6 – Bag and Mask Ventilation

Figure 5.6 illustrates the correct hand placement for mask ventilation with the black anesthesia mask. Ideally, the little finger is behind the angle of the mandible to pull the jaw forward to open the airway. The thumb and index finger then place pressure on the mask to create a mask seal. The palm of the left hand is pressed against the face to also help create a seal. The common tendency to place pressure under the chin on the soft tissue should be avoided as this can obstruct the airway. Occasionally, a slight tilt to the right can improve the mask seal while a head tilt to the right may help open the airway. Other modifications include the use of two hands to hold the mask (the fingers of second hand are similar to the one-hand technique) with a second person required to squeeze the bag,

manoeuvres are unsuccessful, the insertion of an oral or nasal airway often relieves airway obstruction. The appropriate size of both oral and nasal airways should approximate the distance between the jaw angle and the chin. Both forms of airways should be well lubricated prior to insertion. The nasal airway is inserted by pushing it straight back through the nares. An oral airway is usually inserted upside down and run along the hard palate. Once it is past the back of the tongue it is rotated to its proper orientation. A potential problem with nasal airways is epistaxis, which can cause airway obstruction and may also render future attempts at intubation more difficult by impairing visualization of the airway. Oral airways can stimulate the gag reflex and cause vomiting. Conversely, a patient who tolerates an oral airway should probably be intubated since they are unlikely to be able to protect their airway.

Occasionally, even after oral airway placement, patients can be difficult to bag ventilate. This situation is potentially life-threatening. If the patient appears to be easy to intubate, proceed to intubation immediately (e.g., edentulous patients are easy to intubate but difficult to mask ventilate).[10] If intubation is not expected to be easy, one should call for help sooner rather than later. There are still other options available to you (see Chapters 6 and 9).

● V. Intubation

The laryngoscope should be held in the left hand since its phalange is designed to displace the tongue to the left. The act of intubation begins by opening the patient's mouth with the right hand. The right hand is then placed on the back of the patient's head to rotate the occiput backward thereby causing atlanto-occipital extension (omit this step if patient has an unstable cervical spine). Insert the blade into the right corner of the mouth rather than in the middle of the mouth (a common mistake). Insert the blade deeper by following the natural curvature of the tongue. Be careful as the blade is inserted to keep the tongue on the left side of the blade. Once the tip of the laryngoscope is at the base of the tongue, the blade is swept towards the middle thereby displacing the tongue out of the line of vision. The laryngoscope is then lifted upward and forward at an angle of approximately 45° from the patient. Avoid the urge to rotate the laryngoscope since this can damage the upper teeth and can actually worsen visualization. When the vocal cords and the laryngeal inlet (space between cords) have been clearly identified, pass the tip of the ETT through the inlet into the trachea.

If the view is suboptimal, there are several manoeuvres one may need to use. First and foremost ensure the patient is in an optimal sniff position and that the proper size laryngoscope blade is being used. If the tongue is in view then reinsert the laryngoscope blade such that the tongue is displaced to the left. An assistant can provide some BURP to assist visualization. BURP refers to back-up-right pressure, which is applied to the thyroid cartilage (i.e., it brings the larynx into view).[11] BURP should not be confused with cricoid pressure (Sellick's manoeuvre). Sellick's manoeuvre refers to downward pressure, which is applied upon the cricoid cartilage (a ring) towards the cervical spine in an effort to compress the esophagus and prevent passive regurgitation. Occasionally, the larynx inlet cannot be seen and the ETT must be inserted blindly using the epiglottis as a landmark. If visualization was limited during laryngoscopy, a *Ford manoeuvre* is recommended to help confirm correct tube placement. Prior to removal of the laryngoscope, a Ford manoeuvre is performed by downward pressure on the ETT, which displaces the glottis posteriorly thereby bringing the vocal cords into view if the tube has been inserted correctly. The balloon of the tube should only be advanced 2–3 cm past the cords. As the blade is carefully withdrawn, take note of the ETT marking at the lips. The usual distance is about 21–24 cm in adult males and 18–22 cm in adult females. The cuff should be inflated with just enough air to prevent air leakage around the tube during positive pressure ventilation.

The utilization of a stylet can assist the directing of the ETT into the glottic opening when the view of the glottic opening is suboptimal. Generally, it is recommended that a stylet be utilized for all intubations. If the stylet is always used then delays and repeated laryngoscopies are avoided should it turn out to be required on the first attempt. The stylet can easily be removed if it is deemed to be unnecessary. If a stylet is used, it should be removed once the tip of the tube has just passed the vocal cords to avoid causing damage to the tracheal mucosa. Special stylets are available and are discussed in Chapter 6.

VI. Confirmation of Correct Endotracheal Tube Placement

Patients have suffered severe brain damage and died from incorrectly placed ETTs in the esophagus. Confirmation of correct tube placement is therefore essential after all ETT placements. Absolute proof of correct placement is if the tracheal lumen is visualized through the ETT using a fiberoptic scope or if carbon dioxide is measured with each respiration.[2,12] If a patient is in cardiac arrest with zero cardiac output, however, CO_2 may not be measured even with correct tube placement. The presence of CO_2 should be ensured after at least five breaths since the presence of carbonated drinks in the stomach could falsely raise the CO_2 for the first breaths and mimic proper tube placement. All other signs and techniques are not perfect but rather are supportive signs and thus should not be relied upon.

Auscultation is an indirect technique to confirm correct tube placement. First listen over the epigastric area to rule out esophageal placement and to minimize stomach insufflation. After listening over the epigastrium, place the stethoscope near the axilla to auscultate the chest. The chest should be observed to rise and fall with each positive pressure breath. There have been numerous reports of "breath sounds" heard when the ETT was in fact in the esophagus. Hence auscultation is considered supportive evidence but not absolute proof. A correctly placed ETT will mist with exhalation, and air movement can be felt in a spontaneously breathing patient. A patient should not be able to talk with correct ETT placement since the vocal cords are unable to adduct to produce sound. A chest x-ray can help confirm correct positioning but it is not absolute proof and requires time to perform. A chest x-ray is, however, useful to confirm proper insertion depth of the ETT. The tip of the tube should be approximately 4–5 cm above the carina. If there is any doubt about whether the ETT is correctly placed the tube should be removed and the patient should receive mask ventilation with 100% oxygen. An incorrectly placed tube will subject the patient to a high risk of hypoxic injury and can potentially induce aspiration.

Key Points

- Take time to assess a patient's airway (TUMS) prior to all intubations.
- Prepare all equipment and medications prior to intubation .
- Know your approach to intubation but also plan strategies to manage failed intubation and other problems (e.g., hypotension).

- Always take time to optimally position the patient.
- Bag and mask ventilation is an essential skill.
- End tidal CO_2 and fiberoptic visualization are definitive means to confirm correct ETT placement.
- Call for help sooner rather than later.

References

1. King BS, Gupta R, Narayan RK: The early assessment and intensive care unit management of patients with severe traumatic brain and spinal cord injuries. *Surg Clin North Am* 2000;80:855–70.
2. Crosby ET, Cooper RM, Douglas MJ, et al: The unanticipated difficult airway with recommendations for management. *Can J Anaesth* 1996;43:30–4.
3. Mallampati SR, Gatt SP, Gugino LD, et al: A clinical sign to predict difficult tracheal intubation: A prospective study. *Can Anaesth Soc J* 1985;32:429–34.
4. Samsoon GLT, Young JRB: Difficult tracheal intubation: A retrospective study. *Anaesthesia* 1987;42:487–90.
5. Wilson ME, Spiegelhalter D, Robertson JA, Lesser RP: Predicting difficult intubation. *Br J Anaesth* 1988;61:211–6.
6. Butler PJ, Dhara SS: Prediction of difficult laryngoscopy: An assessment of the thyromental distance and Mallampati predictive tests. *Anaesth Intens Care* 1992;20:139–42.
7. El-Ganzouri AR, McCarthy RJ, Tuman KJ, et al: Preoperative airway assessment: Predictive value of a multivariate risk index. *Anesth Analg* 1996;82:1197–1204.
8. American Society of Anesthesiologists: Practice guidelines for management of the difficult airway. *Anesthesiology* 1993;78:597–602.
9. Caplan RA, Posner KL, Ward RJ, Cheney FW: Adverse respiratory events in anesthesia: A closed claims analysis. *Anesthesiology* 1990;72:828–33.
10. Adnet F: Difficult mask ventilation: An underestimated aspect of the problem of the difficult airway? *Anesthesiology* 2000;92:1217–8.
11. Takahata O, Kubota M, Mamiya K, et al: The efficacy of the "BURP" maneuver during a difficult laryngoscopy. *Anesth Analg* 1997;84:419–21.
12. Birmingham PK, Cheney FW: Incorrect tube placement: Prevention of a fatal complication. *Problems in Anesthesia* 1988;2:278–92.

CHAPTER 6

ADVANCED AIRWAY MANAGEMENT

**DAVE NEILIPOVITZ AND
WILLIAM GALLACHER**

You have attempted to intubate a patient who was in severe respiratory distress but were unsuccessful. Help has been called but is over 20 minutes away. You try to ventilate the patient with the bag and mask but this is not effective and the saturation levels are falling. What should you do?

Basic airway management skills are some of the most important skills one can develop. Unfortunately, there are occasions when these skills will be insufficient to manage a patient's airway. Many different devices are available to facilitate intubation and airway management when the basic skills are not sufficient. A complete review of these devices is not feasible here nor is it practical for the physician who performs only the occasional intubation. The goal in this chapter is to introduce some useful devices. A physician should chose only a couple of the devices and become proficient with their use. Do not try to learn how to use a new device during a crisis. However, familiarity with a special airway device can save the day (and the patient) in a situation when the usual devices and techniques fail. The chapter will also present the reader with various suggestions for specific problem situations.

● Laryngeal Mask Airway

A. LMA Classic™ (LMA™)

The LMA™ is a specialized airway device that when properly placed will rest above the vocal cords (Figure 6.1).[1] The LMA™ does *not* protect the patient from gastric aspiration and is therefore not a substitute for an endotracheal tube (ETT).[2] The utility of the LMA™ is that it can be used to ventilate and oxygenate a patient in whom intubation or mask ventilation is not successful. Insertion of an LMA™ is relatively easy with a very steep learning curve.

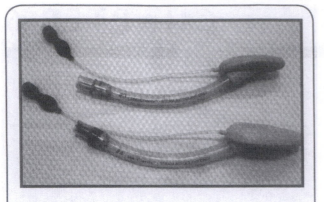

Figure 6.1 – Laryngeal Mask Airway

The Laryngeal Mask Airway (LMA™) is designed to encompass the glottic opening. The photograph is of the LMA Classic™, which is a reusable device. The blue pilot balloon is typically inflated with approximately 20–30 ml of air.

Although numerous insertion techniques have been described, only two will be discussed in this review. The LMA™ should be lubricated and deflated. The first technique involves pushing the solid side of the LMA™ up towards the top of the head along the hard palate. The LMA™ will slide against the palate and then down along the posterior pharynx. Advance the LMA™ until there is considerable resistance. The LMA™ is then inflated until the pilot balloon is firm or with 20–35 ml of air (amount varies depending upon the size of the LMA™). A second technique is very similar to the placement of an oral airway. The LMA™ is initially inserted upside down and then flipped as it is passed down along the posterior pharynx. The LMA™ is then inflated. Regardless of the insertion technique, the black line on the tube of the LMA™ should always be facing the upper incisors once it is in position. The laryngoscope may be used to help place an LMA™.

The value of the LMA™ lies in the fact that it is usually very easy to insert. In addition, it can provide a considerably better airway than a mask alone and can rescue the doctor and patient from a critical situation.[3,4] However, the LMA™ does not provide airway protection against gastric aspiration.[3] The need for high airway pressures to effectively ventilate a patient will limit the usefulness of an LMA™ because the pressures will risk gastric insufflation.

B. Intubating Laryngeal Mask Airway

The intubating laryngeal mask airway or ILMA (LMA Fastrach™) is a modified LMA™ that allows blind intubation of the trachea (Figure 6.2).[5,6] The ILMA differs from the traditional LMA™ in that it comes with an insertion handle. The ILMA is mounted on the handle and lubricated. The ILMA is inserted into the mouth and passed against the palate, around the tongue, in a motion similar to the insertion of a laryngoscope. Once inserted, the handle is then removed. The ILMA can now be used in a similar fashion to a traditional LMA™. However, the additional advantage of the ILMA is that an ETT can be inserted through the lumen. An ETT is not easily inserted through the traditional LMA™ because it has a web-like inner opening.

The insertion of an ETT through the ILMA can be done blindly by simply passing it through the lumen. Although Agro[5] et al. and Baskett[6] et al.

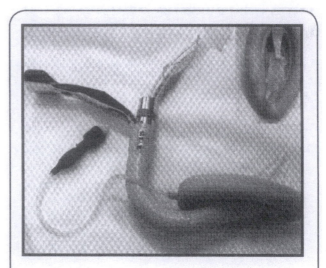

Figure 62 – Intubating Laryngeal Mask Airway

Figure 6.2 is a photograph of an intubating laryngeal mask airway or LMA Fastrach™ with an endotracheal tube inserted through the device. The insert demonstrates how the tube passes out the distal orifice of the Fastrach. The device is first inserted into the mouth in a similar fashion to the classical laryngeal mask airway device. The endotracheal tube is then passed down, either "blind" or with the assistance of a fiberoptic bronchoscope (see text for details).

reported success rates with blind insertion of over 95%, anecdotally the success rate may not be this high and there is a learning curve to this technique. Improved success with ETT intubation via the ILMA has been reported by concomitant use with a lighted stylet. Fan et al. reported a blind intubation success rate through the ILMA of 76%, which improved to a 95% rate when the ILMA was used in conjunction with a lighted stylet.[7] The advantage of the lighted stylet is that it can help one direct the ETT into the trachea.

The intubating laryngeal mask can also be used in combination with a fiberoptic bronchoscope. Pandit et al. reported a 95% first try success rate for bronchoscope-guided intubation via an ILMA versus a 75% first try success rate using the ILMA blindly.[8] In general, however, the use of a bronchoscope in emergency cases is limited because of the poor availability of bronchoscopes, a general lack of operator experience with their use, the possible presence of blood in the airway, which decreases visualization, and the set-up time required for a bronchoscope.

C. LMA ProSeal™

The LMA ProSeal™ is very similar to the LMA Classic™ but has some differences: The ProSeal has a small lumen that connects to the tip of the LMA™ and ideally sits near the esophagus. The purpose of the additional lumen is to minimize inadvertent passage of air and oxygen into the stomach by preventing the buildup of positive pressure in the esophagus. The additional lumen has also been reported to act as a conduit for gastric contents thereby potentially decreasing the risk of pulmonary aspiration.[9] The ProSeal also has an insertion handle, as described above with the ILMA. Although theoretically the LMA ProSeal™ would appear to be preferable to the LMA Classic™, the insertion of the ProSeal is not as simple as the traditional LMA™ and there is limited evidence that it prevents aspiration.

D. Combitube®

The multilumen esophageal airway device (Combitube®) is similar to the esophageal obturator airway device but with several improvements (Figure

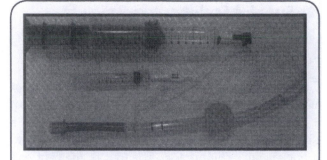

Figure 6.3 – Combitube® Airway Device

Figure 6.3 is a photograph of the Combitube® with the two syringes attached. Note the blue and clear lumens with standard connectors on the proximal end and the two black lines (see text for insertion details).

6.3). The advantage of the Combitube® is its ease of insertion.[10] The mouth is opened and the tube is inserted blindly until the upper incisors are between the two black lines. The large syringe is used to inflate the white balloon and the small syringe inflates the blue balloon (insertion volumes are written on the pilot balloons). The large balloon is in the oral pharynx. The ventilator bag is then connected to the ETT connector on the tube whose balloon was just inflated. The bag is squeezed while listening over the epigastrium. The vast majority of the time, air will be heard to enter the stomach and no CO_2 will be detected, thus confirming esophageal placement. Rarely, the tip will enter the trachea; auscultation then reveals bilateral air entry and CO_2 is detected. The Combitube® in this case is essentially a large ETT. When the Combitube® is positioned in the esophagus, the ventilating bag is reconnected to the other tube (blue tube) and the original tube (clear tube) is left opened to the atmosphere. Positive pressure ventilation will enter the lungs and any air that enters the stomach will escape through the esophageal tube, thus reducing the risk of gastric dilation. Aside from its ease of insertion, other advantages of the Combitube® include that it provides some protection against aspiration and can rescue the doctor and patient from a critical situation. The disadvantages are its cost and the fact that it cannot be left in place for a prolonged period of time.

● Special Stylets

A. Gum Elastic Bougie

The gum elastic bougie is a rigid stylet made of hard rubber that can facilitate the placement of an ETT during direct laryngoscopy. The bougie has a slight bend at its distal end making it look similar to a hockey stick (Figure 6.4). The idea of the bent end is that it can be blindly passed under the epiglottis when direct visualization of the vocal cords is not possible. As the bougie passes through the cords, tactile stimulation of the tip of the bougie passing over the tracheal rings confirms that the bougie has entered the trachea. The bougie is then lubricated and an ETT is passed over it into the trachea. Although some pass the ETT without keeping the laryngoscope in the mouth, it is generally recommended that the scope be left in the mouth. The presence of a scope facilitates passage of the tube around the tongue and allows a Ford manoeuvre to be performed, which can help confirm proper placement. The original bougie could be sterilized for repeated use but there are now single use disposable versions available. A variant exists that has a central lumen that can be used for jet ventilation if passage of an ETT is not possible.

B. Lighted Stylet

The lighted stylet or lightwand is a device that consists of a fiberoptic light source, a malleable stylet, a removable metal stylet and usually a handle onto which the ETT is placed (Figure 6.5). It relies on transillumination of the soft tissues to determine

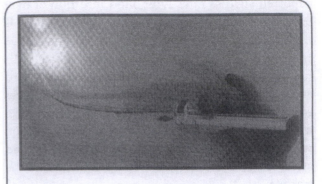

Figure 6.5 – Lighted Stylet

Figure 6.5 is a photograph of the lighted stylet. Suggested hand placement is demonstrated with the thumb on the handle and a finger on the metal stylet. During insertion, once light is visualized in the correct position in the neck, pressure is applied by the thumb. The finger should not pull back on the stylet but rather stay in place, thus preventing advancement of the metal stylet when the tip of the flexible stylet is advanced.

when the tip has entered the larynx. It is usually used for oral intubation but can be modified for nasal intubation. Although there is a learning curve to its use, with practice it has a high success rate. Hung et al. successfully intubated patients 99% of the time in a large trial involving 479 patients.[11] Similar intubation results were reported for patients with known difficult airways or failed direct laryngoscopy cases.[12]

The lightwand is most useful in situations where direct laryngoscopy is difficult, including for patients with limited mouth opening or facial trauma and in unstable cervical injuries. Caution is advised for use in morbidly obese individuals because it may not be possible to transilluminate the tissues. Likewise, upper airway pathology is a relative contraindication to its use.

The lightwand is designed to be used as an indirect method of intubating the patient. With the head placed in a relatively neutral position and the ETT placed onto the lightwand, the tube-stylet is placed into the midline position of the mouth. The lightwand should be held in the dominant hand with its light turned on, and dimming of the overhead lights is recommended (although the transillumination can often be visualized with the overhead lights on). Although handling depends on

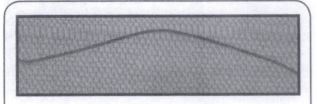

Figure 6.4 – Gum Elastic Bougie

Figure 6.4 is a photograph of the rigid gum elastic bougie. The distal end, seen above on the left, has a slight bend in it, like a hockey stick, to facilitate placement. The rigidity helps allow the intubator to palpate the tracheal rings to help confirm correct placement.

the specific type of lighted stylet used, when using the Laerdal Trachlight® the index finger should be placed on the metal stylet and the thumb at the top of the handle (Figure 6.5). The non-dominant hand can then be used to pull the jaw forward by placing the thumb in the mouth. The tube-stylet combination is then passed around the tongue. Passage through the opening of the vocal cords is detected by a change in the pattern of transillumination. The light pattern in the neck changes to a conical pattern (the apex is cephalic) when it passes through the cords. Once the cone of light is seen, the tube-stylet is advanced by pushing down with the thumb which is on the handle. The finger on the stylet is held at the same level. The action of the thumb forces the tube–malleable stylet combination caudally but the finger keeps the metal stylet from entering the trachea. Thus, the tube and the soft malleable stylet enter the trachea, but the potentially damaging rigid metal stylet does not enter the trachea where it could injure the trachea mucosa. Once advanced, the ETT is held and the lightwand is pulled out of the mouth and tube confirmation is performed. Although the above sequence may sound complicated, with practice one can quickly become proficient with its use. Although the lightwand is designed to be used as an indirect method of intubation, it can be used in conjunction with direct laryngoscopy. The lightwand in this scenario serves as a second light source to facilitate intubation.

● Trans-tracheal Procedures

A. General Principles

All of the trans-tracheal techniques have a similar initial procedure whereby a catheter is inserted through the cricothyroid membrane (Figure 6.6). The cricothyroid membrane can be found immediately below the thyroid cartilage. Using aseptic technique, a 14G intravenous catheter is inserted through this space using a saline filled syringe. When bubbles are seen in the syringe, the trachea has been entered and the catheter is advanced into the lumen of the trachea. The needle and the syringe are then removed. The catheter can then be used for the various trans-tracheal procedures.

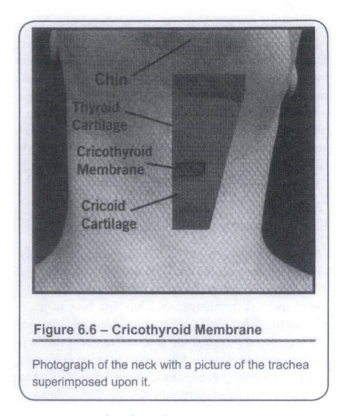

Figure 6.6 – Cricothyroid Membrane

Photograph of the neck with a picture of the trachea superimposed upon it.

B. Trans-tracheal Catheter

The trans-tracheal catheter–based strategies simply use the 14G catheter that was placed into the tracheal lumen. The classic recommendation is to use this catheter with a 3 cc syringe and the connector from a 7.0 ETT. The plunger from the syringe is removed and discarded. The connector from the ETT is inserted into the syringe where the plunger was. The syringe is then connected to the catheter in the neck. A bag apparatus with an oxygen source is connected via the ETT connector and attempts to oxygenate the patient should commence. Although anecdotal success with this technique has been described, the ability to oxygenate patients with significant lung pathology can be questioned. In preference to the bag and syringe setup, the catheter can be directly connected to a hand-operated valve system that can supply an intermittent source of oxygen delivered at 50 psi pressure. Oral and/or nasal airways should be inserted to insure a patent upper airway, which will allow air to expire from the lungs and reduce the danger of barotrauma, which can occur if the upper airway becomes obstructed. During delivery of the high pressure oxygen, the chest is observed for appropriate inspiratory movements. After each second of inspiration, two seconds for expiration is allowed and the chest should again be observed. The position of the catheter is maintained by hand. Despite calling this jet ventilation, the ability to ventilate the patient (i.e., remove CO_2) using this technique is limited. However, jet ventilation is an effective method for oxygenating the patient. The above techniques should be considered to be only temporizing solutions to airway problems. Once they have been performed, a more definitive airway management solution should be found.

C. Cricothyrotomy and Surgical Airway

Despite being recommended as the final emergency airway in many publications, a needle cricothyrotomy and other surgical airways are not routinely performed. A tracheostomy is not the best surgical airway to perform in an emergency situation. Instead, the preferred surgical airway is a cricothyrotomy. Various cricothyrotomy kits, which utilize a Seldinger insertion technique, are available and can be used to quickly insert this emergency airway. The catheter is placed into the tracheal lumen. A wire from a central line kit is then passed caudally down the trachea. The catheter is removed and a small incision in the skin by the wire is performed. A small forcep or the back end of the scalpel is used to dilate the skin. A lubricated small ETT (e.g., 4.0–5.0) or tracheotomy tube is then inserted over the wire into the trachea. Tests to confirm proper tube placement are then performed. The prepared cricothyrotomy kits have a dilator, which aids insertion.

D. Retrograde Intubation

Retrograde intubation has the advantage of securing the airway without performing cricothyrotomy and, therefore, may reduce the risk of long-term sequelae that occur secondary to the surgical airway. It has been successfully used in the management of maxillo-facial trauma, cervical spine injuries and temporo-mandibular ankylosis and in the presence of upper airway pathology.[13]

Retrograde intubation again begins with placing the catheter in the trachea. The catheter is directed in a cephalic direction. A wire from a central line kit is passed through the catheter into the larynx and the oropharynx in a retrograde fashion. It is retrieved from the oropharynx either by hand or with the aid of McGill forceps (one can use direct laryngoscopy to aid retrieval). A forcep is used to secure the wire at the skin insertion site. Since the wire in the oropharynx is no longer sterile, ideally it should not be allowed to contaminate the tissues by moving back. While maintaining tension on the wire, an ETT is threaded over the catheter with the wire being passed through Murphy's eye (a small hole at the tip of an ETT). The Murphy's eye is used because most wires are not long enough to pass through the entire tube length. If an extra long wire is obtained, well over 60 cm, then the wire can be passed through the entire tube. The ETT is then inserted using the wire to help direct it into the trachea. Direct laryngoscopy during this stage is recommended. Advance the ETT over the wire until resistance is met. In order to determine that the ETT has indeed entered the larynx and is not snagged on the epiglottis, the wire should show tension as the tube is advanced. The wire is then withdrawn through the ETT. Tests to confirm proper tube placement are then performed.

Alternative to using the above, the use of an epidural anesthetic kit has been described. The Tuohy needle replaces the intravenous catheter and the epidural catheter is used in lieu of the central line wire. Commercially available kits are now procurable that include all the necessary equipment. Most kits include a long guide wire, small scalpel, forceps and an introducer sheath. The wire passes through the middle of the introducer sheath. An ETT is then threaded over the sheath with the sheath being used to direct the tube into the trachea (similar to using it as a bougie).

A further refinement of this technique involves the use of an extra long guide wire (e.g., 125 cm, 0.025 cm Teflon-coated J-wire). A fiberoptic bronchoscope that has an ETT loaded onto it is then passed over the wire (the wire goes through the suction port of the scope). The advantage of this approach is that it gives visual confirmation of tube placement. The retrograde approach to intubation has also been modified by Hung et al. to incorporate the use of the lightwand to confirm positioning of the ETT in the larynx. Transillumination of the cricothyroid membrane confirms that the ETT has entered the larynx.[14]

● Fiberoptic Intubation

Fiberoptic intubation is not usually useful for emergency situations because of the time required to set up the bronchoscope and because blood in the airway makes this technique difficult. Further, patients with a decreased level of consciousness are also more difficult to perform fiberoptic intubation upon. This is because the soft tissue in the mouth is more relaxed, which impairs visualization, and because of the absence of patient co-operation. Fiberoptic intubation, however, is considered to be the gold standard for management of difficult airways on an elective or semi-elective basis.

The secret to successful fiberoptic intubation is good anesthesia of the oropharynx and larynx, along with good sedation. The anesthesia can be further augmented by superior laryngeal nerve blocks. Under sterile precautions, these nerves are blocked by injection of 2 cc of 2% lidocaine just inferior to the hyoid bone using a 23 gauge needle. The process is repeated on the opposite side. Alternatively, the superior laryngeal nerves can be anesthetized by the insertion of pledgets, first soaked in a local anesthetic solution, placed in the valleculae of the oropharynx. Topicalization with local anesthetic can be achieved with nebulization of 4% lidocaine or by having the patient swish around 10 ml of EMLA® anesthetic cream. The anesthesia can be further augmented by superior laryngeal nerve blocks. These nerves can be blocked by insertion of local anesthetic—soaked pledgets in the oropharynx. Alternatively, under sterile precautions, the superior laryngeal nerves are blocked by injection of 2 cc of 2% lidocaine just inferior to the hyoid bone using a 23 gauge needle. The process is repeated on the opposite side. An injection of 4 cc 2% lidocaine through the cricothyroid membrane will block the recurrent laryngeal innervation of the trachea below the glottic opening. Glycopyrrolate 0.4 mg given intravenously is useful to dry secretions, which aids topicalization and helps reduce visually impairing secretions. A bite block is used to prevent damage to the bronchoscope. Once the bronchoscope has been successfully introduced into the trachea, the ETT is slid over the scope into the trachea. Occasionally, the tube needs to be advanced in a corkscrew fashion to help it pass around the epiglottis.

● Special Situations

Many different situations can occur and a complete review is beyond the scope of this book. The assistance of a physician skilled in airway management is recommended. The goal of this section is to introduce some suggestions and considerations for the following situations.

A. Failed Intubation

Although the topic is explored in more detail in Chapter 9, several important principles will be discussed here. The inability to intubate is a life-threatening situation. Even in the operating room with optimal conditions, there is still a failed intubation rate of between 5 and 35 per 10 000. Unanticipated difficult intubations reportedly occur in 1 to 3% of cases with an even higher rate in emergency situations.[15–17] Although many complex algorithms have been developed for this situation, most require skills that exceed all but the most experienced physicians'.[3,4] A simple and practical approach is outlined in Figure 6.7. The principle of the approach is to keep the patient oxygenated until more

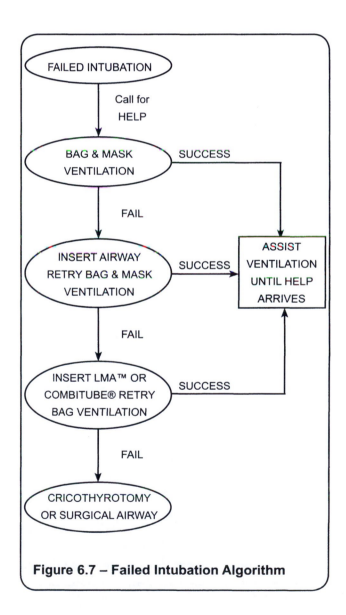

Figure 6.7 – Failed Intubation Algorithm

experienced help arrives. Do not persist with attempts to intubate a patient since each attempt causes tissue trauma, which can greatly worsen the situation.[18] A patient with a patent albeit unprotected airway is better than a patient with no airway at all.

B. Vomiting and Gastrointestinal Bleeds

Regurgitation may make it very difficult to secure an airway in a patient who is vomiting. The risk for aspiration is considerable in this situation. The ideal position is debatable for such a patient. While the head up position may decrease regurgitation, the extreme head down position may decrease aspiration. Turning a patient onto their left side may reduce the risk of aspiration, but renders intubation more difficult due to the lack of familiarity with this position. At least one or two suction devices should be employed to maximize visualization. The use of cricoid pressure in an actively vomiting patient is not recommended but may be useful to reduce passive regurgitation.

C. Heart Failure

A patient in congestive heart failure is often in considerable respiratory distress. After intubation the patient can become quite hypotensive for reasons that have been discussed previously. Acute reductions in preload and decreased sympathetic tone are the primary reasons for the onset of hypotension with the institution of positive pressure ventilation. Thus, you should anticipate that the patient will become hypotensive and be ready to treat it. Discontinuing nitroglycerine prior to intubation is advisable in non-ischemic patients. A syringe containing phenylephrine or ephedrine should be readily available to treat hypotension.

D. Trauma

A multitude of different intubation scenarios arise in trauma situations. Although patients tend to be younger, the dose requirements of the commonly used medications should be reduced. Pre-existing shock and decreased circulating blood volumes are some of the reasons for lower dose requirements. Avoidance of cervical spine movement is mandatory due to potential cervical spine injury. In line stabilization, not traction is recommended during oral intubation in patients with potential cervical spine injury. The presence of head injury and increased intracranial pressure is discussed below. A burn patient who potentially has burns to the upper airway should be intubated early before edema develops and intubation becomes virtually impossible.

E. Difficult Airway

A patient with a difficult airway is best managed by an experienced airway physician. Avoidance of respiratory depressants and paralytic drugs is mandatory in this patient population. If the airway must be secured, the safest approach is to topicalize the upper airway with lidocaine and proceed with direct laryngoscopy. Fiberoptic intubation and other airway devices can be used but should be reserved for physicians who are experienced in their use.

F. Rapid Sequence Intubation (RSI)

As further discussed in Chapter 8, a lot has been written about rapid sequence intubation. In brief, this is typically used in patients in whom there is considerable risk of aspiration. The drug doses are determined prior to administration rather than titrated in. The technique involves the bolus dosing of an induction drug and a rapidly acting muscle relaxant so as to give the best possible intubating conditions. Cricoid pressure is performed to prevent passive regurgitation of stomach contents and aspiration. This technique has the advantage of quickly protecting the airway.

RSI has some major drawbacks, however. Firstly, drugs are not titrated to effect. The doses to be administered are prejudged and delivered as boluses. This can result in over- or under-dosing. Secondly, the adverse hemodynamic effects of this manoeuvre may be significant in terms of hypotension. Thus, the physician must have considerable knowledge of the medications used during intubation. Most importantly, however, the physician must have proficient airway intubation skills. Failure to intubate may result in a rapidly deteriorating situation with the potential for severe hypoxemia, aspiration and even death. Different levels of skill will therefore define the options open to an individual. The individual making the plan must recognize his or her limitations and either work within those limitations or get appropriate help. Since paralytic agents are used, the physician must be sure they can intubate the patient. The use of RSI is therefore best reserved for physicians with considerable experience with airway management. As with all airway management strategies, it is especially important when RSI is used that the physician has an effective alternative plan to use in the event of failure to intubate. The basic premise of the ACES approach to airway management is very simple. It is based on a step-wise progression of simple airway techniques with emphasis on careful assessment of each case and always being prepared for the unexpected difficult airway. Careful titration of drugs and avoiding "burning bridges" may cost a little more time but can usually be done in most cases. The place of RSI in this approach to airway management is thus limited. Although this technique has become more popular for the management of emergency intubations, the widespread use of RSI remains controversial and it should be used with caution in most critically ill patients.

G. Increased Intracranial Pressure

Ideally, in these situations one would obtain assistance from a physician with the most experience in airway management. The goals of the intubation are to avoid hypertension, hypotension and coughing, all of which can exacerbate cerebral ischemia. The use of the RSI is recommended with cervical spine precautions if there is potential cervical spine injury. The use of lidocaine, beta blockers and higher doses of narcotics can be helpful. If an airway physician is not immediately available, progress as you normally

would but take the extra time to topicalize. This is not an ideal alternative but it is safer than administering drugs you are not familiar or comfortable with.

H. Changing Endotracheal Tubes

Typical indications for exchanging one ETT for another include the need for a larger ETT, replacing an ETT with a damaged balloon or the fact that an existing ETT is occluded by secretions. Since the procedure can be life-threatening, it is best left to experienced physicians. Thus, unless it is an emergency situation, the exchanging of an ETT should be conducted in a semi-elective fashion.

Several different types of tube exchange catheters exist that can help for this procedure. A patient is pre-oxygenated on 100% oxygen for at least five minutes and all preparations for intubation including positioning, are conducted before embarking on the tube exchange. The tube exchange catheter is passed through the existing ETT. The existing ETT is then withdrawn, with care taken to maintain the position of the exchange catheter. The exchange catheter is lubricated and the new ETT is passed over it into the trachea. Although the use of a laryngoscope during this procedure is considered optional, it is recommended, since it greatly facilitates passage of the tubes around the tongue, making the procedure safer. Once the new ETT has passed into the trachea, the exchange catheter is removed and tube placement confirmation is performed. Most tube exchange catheters have a central lumen that allows for jet ventilation should tube replacement be difficult and time consuming.

Key Points

- Numerous airway adjuncts for intubation are available.

- Select a few devices to become proficient with rather than trying to master all of the devices.
- Call for help sooner rather than later.

References

1. Brain AIJ: The laryngeal mask: a new concept in airway management. *Br J Anaesth* 1983;55:801–4.

2. Rabey PG, Murphy PJ, Langton JA, et al: Effect of the laryngeal mask airway on lower oesophageal sphincter pressure in patients during general anaesthesia. *Br J Anaesth* 1992;69:346–8.

3. Crosby ET, Cooper RM, Douglas MJ, et al: The unanticipated difficult airway with recommendations for management. *Can J Anaesth* 1996;43:30–4.

4. American Society of Anesthesiologists: Practice guidelines for management of the difficult airway. *Anesthesiology* 1993;78:597–602.

5. Agro F, Brimacombe J, Carassiti M, et al: The intubating laryngeal mask: Clinical appraisal of ventilation and blind tracheal intubation in 110 patients. *Anaesthesia* 1998;53:1084–90.

6. Baskett PJ, Parr MJ, Nolan JP: The intubating laryngeal mask: Results of a multicentre trial with experience of 500 cases. *Anaesthesia* 1998;53:1174–79.

7. Fan KH, Hung OR, Agro F: A comparative study of tracheal intubation using an intubating laryngeal mask (Fastrach) alone or together with a lightwand (Trachlight). *J Clin Anesth* 2000;12:581–5.

8. Pandit JJ, MacLachlan K, Dravid RM, Popat MT: Comparison of times to achieve tracheal intubation with three techniques using the laryngeal or intubating laryngeal mask airway. *Anaesthesia* 2002;57:128–32.

9. Evans NR, Llewellyn RL, Gardner SV, James MF: Aspiration prevented by the ProSeal laryngeal mask airway: A case report. *Can J Anaesth* 2002;49:413–6.

10. Frass M, Frenzer R, Rauscha F, et al: Evaluation of esophageal tracheal combitube in cardiopulmonary resuscitation. *Crit Care Med* 1986;15:609–11.

11. Hung OR, Pytka S, Morris I, et al: Clinical trial of a new lightwand device (Trachlight) to intubate the trachea. *Anesthesiology* 1995;83:509–14.

12. Hung OR, Pytka S, Morris I, et al: Lightwand intubation II: clinical trial of a new lightwand for tracheal intubation in patients with difficult airways. *Can J Anaesth* 1995;42:826–30.

13. Barriot P, Riou B: Retrograde technique for tracheal intubation in trauma patients. *Crit Care Med* 1988;16:712–13.

14. Hung OR, al-Qatari M: Light-guided retrograde intubation. *Can J Anaesth* 1997;44:877–82.

15. Foley LJ, Ochroch EA: Bridges to establish an emergency airway and alternate intubating techniques. *Crit Care Clin* 2000;16:429–44.

16. Samsoon GL, Young JR: Difficult tracheal intubation: a retrospective study. *Anaesthesia* 1987;42:487–90.

17. Tse JC, Rimm EB, Hussain A: Predicting difficult endotracheal intubation in surgical patients scheduled for general anesthesia: A prospective blind study. *Anesth Analg* 1995;81:254–8.

18. Caplan RA, Posner KL, Ward RJ, Cheney FW: Adverse respiratory events in anesthesia: A closed claims analysis. *Anesthesiology* 1990;72:828–33.

CHAPTER 7

MEDICATIONS FOR AIRWAY MANAGEMENT

DAVE NEILIPOVITZ

You have been managing a 38-year-old man who was admitted two days ago with mild pneumonia. His condition, however, has deteriorated substantially and he is in severe respiratory distress. His oxygen saturations are only 83% despite receiving 100% oxygen. He is combative and will not keep his oxygen mask on. His heart rate is 140 bpm and his blood pressure is 75/45 despite repeated fluid boluses. Clearly, he requires intubation but he is unlikely to allow you to intubate him. What should you do?

The above patient obviously requires respiratory assistance. He is unlikely to be a candidate for non-invasive ventilation since he is uncooperative and hemodynamically unstable. Thus, he needs the institution of positive pressure ventilation via an endotracheal tube. The problem will be to get him to allow you to place the tube. Invariably, there is a need for medications to facilitate this. The big challenge is to select the best drug or drugs to allow you to safely place the endotracheal tube. Unfortunately, there is no perfect drug for this purpose nor is there a perfect cocktail that is appropriate for all patients. The physiologic variability of patients along with the different kinds of situations that require drugs for the facilitation of airway management prohibit one from recommending specific drug recipes. Instead, the goal of this chapter is, firstly, to introduce different airway management drugs but, secondly and more importantly, to present principles that should not only guide drug selection but assist with dosing.

● Introduction

The difficulty in discussing medications to facilitate intubation is that physicians have varying backgrounds and training. Two important principles for this section should, however, always be adhered to (Table 7.1): The first is to "use what *you* know and know what

> **Table 7.1 – Guiding Principles for Drug Administration**
>
> A. Know what you use ... use what you know.
> B. You can always give more .... but you can't take it back.

> **Table 7.2 – Rationale for Drug Administration during Intubation**
>
> I. Physiologic Indications
>   1. Coronary Artery Disease
>   2. Increased Intracranial Pressure
>   3. Reactive Airway Disease
>   4. Risks for Aspiration
>
> II. Technical Indications
>   1. Patient Compliance
>   2. Improve Visualization
>
> III. Psychological Indication

you use." Although there will always be the first time you use a drug, you should understand how the drug works and know the dosing and what the complications with its use are. You should never use a drug that is recommended for a certain situation if you do not have knowledge of that drug. Inexperience with a drug is considered an absolute contraindication to the use of that drug, since life-threatening problems could result if the drug is administered incorrectly. Ideally, a drug should be used in less critical situations first to obtain experience with its use. The second very important principle is that you can always administer more drug but you cannot take back drug that has already been given. A relative overdose is often inadvertently administered to a critically ill patient, which can cause life-threatening cardiovascular collapse. Drug reversal with naloxone or flumazenil is not a reliable option and these drugs have their own unique problems associated with their use.[1,2] Thus, the best therapy for drug overdose is prevention.

● Rationale for Airway Drugs

The indications for using drugs to facilitate airway intubation usually fall into one of three categories: physiologic, technical or psychological (Table 7.2). The physiologic indications are primarily a reflection of the adverse responses a patient can experience during and immediately following intubation. Although direct laryngoscopy with the insertion of an endotracheal tube can sometimes initially cause a vagal response, it is virtually always followed by a marked sympathetic response if no drugs are administered to blunt the response. This adrenergic response may cause tachycardia and hypertension, which has life-threatening consequences in a patient with coronary artery disease or increased intracranial pressure.[3–5] Manipulation of the airway in a patient not pre-treated with medications can

be a potent stimulus for bronchospasm, which can have adverse consequences in the asthmatic patient.[6] Laryngoscopy stimulates the gag reflex, which can cause regurgitation of gastric contents and possible aspiration if this reflex is not blunted by drugs. Thus, avoidance of medications to facilitate intubation can have adverse consequences.

The use of drugs during intubation can make the act of intubation technically easier.[7,8] Although spontaneous airway patency and protection can be lost secondary to the effects of various drugs, the patient can become an easy intubation. A patient who is biting down or has a strong gag reflex can be extremely difficult to intubate. The judicious use of various drugs can ease the insertion of the laryngoscope. Paralysis, although very controversial,[8,9] usually can improve visualization of the larynx during intubation thus increasing the probability of success[7,8] (but, of course, failure to intubate or be able to bag ventilate in a paralyzed patient is an acute life-threatening problem).

A final reason to use drugs is to minimize the psychologic impact intubation can have on a patient. When already struggling for breath, to be forced to lie flat on one's back and have a mask thrust upon one's face would raise the anxiety of most people. Typically, the situation is chaotic with the patient's well-being often in danger. Compounding this, intubation can be very painful. Thus, to minimize these effects, drug administration is often a compassionate and considerate act.

Complications of Drug Administration

Although any drug can have unpredictable complications such as allergic reactions, most of the drugs used to facilitate intubation have predictable problems associated with their use. The beneficial effects of these drugs can also be their drawbacks. Apnea and the loss of airway protective reflexes can facilitate intubation but would jeopardize the patient's well-being if one were unable to secure the airway. Reduction of a patient's anxiety and blunting the adrenergic response to intubation is often a desirable effect of the medications. However, a reduction in the patient's sympathetic outflow, along with the myocardial depressant effects of certain drugs, could also cause catastrophic hypotension and cardiovascular collapse. Along with the reduction in a patient's level of consciousness, the tone of the lower esophageal sphincter decreases, which predisposes the patient to regurgitation and possible aspiration. Although paralysis may improve visualization of the larynx, it should never be used without drugs to alter a patient's level of consciousness; to be awake but paralyzed can have grave psychologic effects on the patient. Finally, certain drugs have rare but predictable complications associated with their use. For example, administration of succinylcholine to a patient with a previous spinal cord injury or recent burn could cause life-threatening hyperkalemia and thus should be avoided in these circumstances.[10–12] Thus, one must know *all* the complications and contraindications to a drug *before* deciding to use it.

Factors Influencing Dose Selection

Once a drug or a combination of drugs is selected, the actual dose to administer must then be determined. The principle that "you can always give more but you can't take it back" is always useful to keep in mind but a starting dose must be chosen. Although textbooks often include recommended doses, one must be aware of which patient population was used to determine these values. For the most part, these drugs were tested in patients presenting for elective surgery. Typically these study patients are young, healthy individuals who are usually in a state of euvolemia. Clearly, this population is not the same as that of patients requiring emergent airway management. Many factors must therefore be accounted for when

Table 7.3 – Variables That Influence Drug Dosing

1. Coexisting Pathology (e.g., cardiac disease, liver disease, etc.)
2. Patient Age
3. Body Weight
4. Volume Status
5. Potential Drug Interactions
6. Desired Goals of Drugs

selecting the dose of a drug to administer. Table 7.3 lists some of the important factors; most focus on the patient and their underlying physiology.

Although most of the factors make intuitive sense, volume status is not often considered. A patient who is in a volume contracted state, be it actual or relative, will require a reduced dosage of drug. The reason is that their cardiac output will be primarily directed to the brain and the heart. Respectively, this is where the desired effects (e.g., anxiolysis, sedation) and the most common complications (e.g., cardiac depression, hypotension) occur. Thus, a trauma patient with hypovolemia or the patient in cardiogenic shock both require reduced doses of drugs.

An obvious determinant is the patient's weight. A very small patient typically requires much less than a patient who is considerably larger. Although drugs should be administered on a per kilogram basis, the proper weight to use can be debatable: Although obese patients require higher drug doses than non-obese patients, one should not use their actual weight. Various formulas have been proposed but a simple one is to use their ideal body weight plus 50% of their weight above the ideal value. For example, for the 120 kg patient who has an ideal weight of 80 kg, the dosing weight would be approximately 100 kg (i.e., 80 + 0.50 [120–80]).

An older patient will usually require lower doses than a younger patient: The reasons for this are multiple but are not solely related to coexisting physiologic problems.[13–15] The patient who has underlying cardiac problems will also require lower doses and be more susceptible to the complications associated with the drugs used for airway management. Likewise, a patient with renal or liver disease is less likely to clear drugs and thus can experience a prolonged duration of drug effects.[15,16]

Drug interactions are another very important determinant for drug dosing. Many drugs have synergistic reactions. For example, benzodiazepines and narcotics individually have minimal cardiovascular depressant effects. Together, however, they can cause profound hypotension.[17] Although the synergistic responses may be problematic, when used correctly together, they can reduce the requirements of both drugs thereby potentially minimizing complications associated with each.

A final factor, which does not directly affect dose selection but should be remembered when administering drugs, is that of circulation time. This is the time it takes for the drug to pass from the entry vein and travel through the heart up to the brain (i.e., arm to brain time). A rapid circulation time may be seen in young trauma patients. A more important problem however is a reduced circulation time, which commonly occurs in elderly patients or those with cardiac disease. A very slow circulation time (often over a minute) in these patients mandates that one must wait for the initial dose to circulate before deciding that more drug is required. A common mistake is that an appropriate dose is given initially but insufficient time is allotted and additional drug is given. Once the initial dose takes effect, it would provide the desired effect (e.g., sedation). However, when the second dose exerts its actions, it typically causes complications (e.g., hypotension). Thus, one should always account for a potential reduced circulation time before determining that the administered dose is insufficient.

● Factors Influencing Drug Selection

Many different drugs are available that can be used to facilitate intubation of the airway. Unless the patient is in special circumstances where the stress of intubation could have serious repercussions (such as if there is increased intracranial pressure), the safest and easiest approach to intubation is to simply use topical lidocaine spray and administer minimal amounts of a sedative such as midazolam. Unfortunately, this simple strategy does not always work and additional medications can be required. A simple approach to drug selection, however, is to choose drugs that address the specific needs of the patient. These needs or goals can be divided into the A's and

Table 7.4 – Goals of Airway Drugs (A's and R's)
1. Amnesia
2. Anesthesia
3. Analgesia
4. Blunting of Autonomic Reflexes
5. Muscle Relaxation
6. Rescue Drugs
n.b. Some drugs address more than one goal.

R's (Table 7.4). The amnestic drugs interfere with the formation of long-term memories. Airway intubation can be an unpleasant experience and drugs that have amnestic effects can be useful to help patients avoid experiencing disturbing recollections. Anesthesia is the lack of sensation, which, when generalized, is a state of unconsciousness. Amnesia and general anesthesia are usually achieved using either the anesthesia induction drugs (e.g., propofol) or a benzodiazepine, either alone or in some combination. Benzodiazepines are particularly useful since they cause minimal depression of the cardiovascular system if used alone.[17–19] Midazolam is a rapid acting benzodiazepine, which is usually administered in 0.5–1.0 mg aliquots. Diazepam and other benzodiazepines can be used but they have much slower onset times, which limit their usefulness. The problem with the anesthetic induction drugs is that they tend to cause more adverse cardiovascular effects and have a higher propensity to cause respiratory arrest. Occasionally, the anticholinergic drug scopolamine, given intravenously in a dose of 0.2–0.4 mg, can provide amnestic effects with minimal adverse cardiovascular side effects.

Airway intubation can be quite painful and thus the use of analgesia to reduce perception of the painful stimuli is important. Narcotics are the mainstays for this purpose. Fentanyl is an opioid that is often administered in 25–100 mcg aliquots. And lidocaine spray can also be used to decrease the discomfort of intubation. Each puff of the spray will result in the administration of approximately 10 mg of lidocaine and thus one should be aware of potential lidocaine toxicity from overzealous spraying (toxic topical dose 5–7 mg/kg). Ketamine is the only anesthetic induction drug, however, that has analgesic properties.

Table 7.5 – Drugs to Facilitate Intubation

Drug	Incremental	Induction	Indications	Complications	Comments
Midazolam	0.5–1.0 mg	0.1–0.3 mg/kg	amnestic, sedation	hypotension, apnea	synergy with opioids
Propofol	10–20 mg	0.5–3.0 mg/kg	sedation, anesthesia	hypotension (++), apnea	decreases ICP
Thiopental	N/R	3–5 mg/kg	anesthesia	hypotension, apnea	decreases ICP
Ketamine	10–25 mg	1–2 mg/kg	anesthesia, analgesia	delirium, hallucinations	minimal BP decrease
Fentanyl	25–50 mcg	2–20 mcg/kg	analgesia	apnea, chest rigidity	blunts sympathetics

Aside from reducing pain, analgesic drugs are very important in blunting the autonomic reflexes to intubation (e.g., hypertension, tachycardia, bronchospasm). The blunting of these responses is particularly important in patients with increased intracranial pressure and coronary artery disease. Aside from analgesic drugs, several other medications can be used for this purpose. Intravenous lidocaine (1–1.5 mg/kg), given approximately three minutes before intubation, is classically used for patients with high intracranial pressure (ICP). Although there is controversy surrounding its use for elevated ICP and a number of other indications,[20] many physicians believe it is beneficial if used properly (i.e., enough circulation time is allocated). Lidocaine can however be used in other patients where the response to intubation should be blunted (e.g., asthma). Esmolol (0.25–0.5 mg/kg) is a short-acting beta blocker that is very useful for blunting the hemodynamic response to intubation. Finally, a small bolus of intravenous nitroglycerine (25–100 mcg bolus) can be used in patients with coronary artery disease. Nitroglycerine is however contraindicated in patients with elevated ICP, since it can raise the ICP and detrimentally decrease cerebral perfusion.

The use of muscle relaxants to facilitate intubation is a controversial subject.[8,9] Paralysis will improve visualization during laryngoscopy thus increasing the probability of intubation being successful.[7,8] Unfortunately, paralysis can make a bad airway situation into a no airway situation, which is obviously incompatible with life. An absolute contraindication to the use of muscle relaxants is if there is high probability that you will be unsuccessful in trying to intubate the patient. Although succinylcholine is a relatively short acting muscle relaxant, it can cause paralysis of sufficient duration to cause permanent hypoxic brain damage. Further, the list of contraindications (Table 7.6) and problems associated

Table 7.6 – Some Conditions Associated with Hyperkalemia from Succinylcholine

A. Denervation Injuries (over 24 hours old) – this includes:
   a. Spinal Cord Transection
   b. Cerebral Vascular Accident/Stroke
   c. Peripheral Denervation Injuries
B. Trauma – especially crush trauma
C. Burns – extensive burns greater than 1st degree burns (vulnerable period after 3–4 days)
D. Immobility – prolonged immobility from any cause
E. Severe Intra-abdominal Sepsis – mechanism unclear
F. Neuromuscular and Muscular Disorders
   a. Muscular Dystrophies
   b. Myotonia
G. Upper Neuron Lesions – various lesions
H. Other Neurological Disorders – case reports suggest it should be avoided in:
   a. Friedreich's Ataxia
   b. Polyneuritis
   c. Familial Periodic Paralysis

with use of succinylcholine is very extensive and far beyond the scope of this review.[10–12] Prior to using succinylcholine, one should review and know the many contraindications and complications associated with its use. Although the other relaxants have fewer contraindications, unfortunately their effects are more prolonged than succinylcholine and they cannot be acutely reversed if the intubation attempts are unsuccessful (reversal could only be attempted after at least 20 minutes). Thus, if the other muscle relaxants are used, a patient will be paralyzed and unable to breathe thus necessitating assistance for ventilation and oxygenation.

After a patient is intubated, the most common problem is hypotension. Although excessive drug administration can cause this, there are several other reasons for the problem. The typical patient has gone from negative pressure ventilation, which augments venous return, to positive pressure ventilation, which does the opposite. A patient's sympathetic output will often decrease once intubation and institution of positive pressure ventilation have relieved the respiratory distress. The loss of this sympathetic output can contribute to a fall in the patient's blood pressure. The fall in the pressure can be minimized by giving a fluid bolus prior to intubation or by stopping medications that are lowering the blood pressure (a common example is intravenous or topical nitroglycerine). Despite these preventative measures, the blood pressure can still fall. The two "rescue" drugs most commonly given to temporarily restore the blood pressure are boluses of ephedrine (5–15 mg) and phenylephrine (50–200 mcg). These drugs are temporary measures and if the low blood pressure persists it must be dealt with.

● Specific Drugs

A. Midazolam

Although there are many different benzodiazepines, midazolam is the one best suited for airway issues. Unlike most of the other benzodiazepines (e.g., diazepam, lorazepam), midazolam has rapid onset but relatively short duration of effect.[18,19] Benzodiazepines are useful because of their amnestic and anesthetic effects and relatively minimal adverse cardiovascular and respiratory effects. When used alone, anesthesia can be induced with 0.1–0.2 mg/kg but lower doses are given if used in conjunction with opioids or other induction drugs. However, midazolam is more commonly administered in 0.5–1.0 mg aliquots and titrated to achieve the desired effects. Midazolam produces a dose related depression of the respiratory drive, which is potentiated if opiates are used. Likewise, the slight reduction it causes in arterial blood pressure is markedly potentiated if combined with opiates.[17]

B. Propofol

This is an anesthetic induction drug that is very useful for airway management. Although its precise mechanism of action is not completely understood, it is an excellent anesthetic and sedative drug.[21,22] The duration of effect is patient and dose dependent but usually averages around 5–10 minutes. The induction of anesthesia dose is 1–2.5 mg/kg intravenously but considerably less for elderly and critically ill patients. Propofol can be given in 10–30 mg boluses and titrated to effect. Unfortunately, it can cause more pronounced adverse cardiovascular effects than benzodiazepines or the other anesthetic drugs. Hypotension appears to be due to both vasodilation and myocardial depression. Propofol will block the protective airway reflexes, is a profound respiratory depressant and will usually cause apnea.

C. Thiopental

Although used less frequently, this barbiturate anesthetic induction drug is still useful for airway management.[23] Classically, it is used in patients with intracranial pathology since it reduces ICP and may have cerebral protective effects. The duration of effect is typically less than 10 minutes for initial doses but duration can increase with repeated doses.[23] The dose to induce anesthesia is 3–5 mg/kg but lower doses are required in the elderly and in patients with coexisting pathology (e.g., hypovolemia).[15] Thiopental will cause respiratory depression and apnea. The hypotension that can occur is primarily due to venodilation but there is some myocardial depression. Rare complications include the onset of a porphyria crisis.

D. Ketamine

This is an anesthetic induction drug that is related to the hallucinogenic drug LSD. It produces a so-called state of "dissociative anesthesia" which resembles a cataleptic state. It causes intense amnesia and is unique in that it has analgesic effects. Unlike the benzodiazepines, narcotics or the other anesthetic drugs, it will increase the sympathetic output and thus is less likely to cause hypotension.[24] It has a rapid onset and a relatively short duration of effect (usually under 20 minutes). Induction of anesthesia is achieved with 0.5–2 mg/kg intravenously. Alternatively, it can be given in 10–25 mg aliquots and titrated to effect. Since hallucinations and delusions can occur with its use, concomitant administration of a low dose benzodiazepine is recommended since it reduces these adverse effects. Although higher doses will produce apnea, in low doses it tends not to produce significant respiratory depression and airway reflexes are preserved. Ketamine is an ideal drug for asthmatic patients since it causes bronchodilation.[25,26] It should not be used in patients with increased ICP since it can acutely raise the pressure thereby worsening the cranial pathology. Although it is the least likely drug to cause hypotension since it raises sympathetic output, it does have negative cardiac and vasodilatory effects. Thus, in patients who have already maximized their sympathetic output, ketamine may have adverse cardiovascular effects.[24]

E. Fentanyl

Although there are many different narcotics, fentanyl is the synthetic narcotic that is best suited for airway management. Unlike morphine or meperidine, it has a rapid onset and short duration of effect when initially given. It does not cause the histamine release or the direct vasodilation that can occur with morphine. The primary benefit of fentanyl is its analgesic effects although it has mild sedative effects as well. The reduced perception of noxious stimuli is not only a compassionate reason for its use but this also greatly reduces the potentially catastrophic autonomic reflex responses that are usually stimulated during airway management. As with all narcotics, fentanyl can cause hypotension, due to reduced output from the sympathetic nervous system, and bradycardia (the latter occurs with high doses). The hypotension is often more pronounced in patients with high underlying sympathetic tone or when there is co-administration of a benzodiazepine (especially midazolam). Respiratory depression and apnea are also more pronounced when benzodiazepines are used. Although anesthesia can be induced with fentanyl by itself in very high doses (over 15 mcg/kg), it is usually safer to give it in 25–50 mcg aliquots up to 3–5 mcg/kg in conjunction with other drugs to facilitate airway intubation.

F. Succinylcholine

Succinylcholine is a depolarizing muscle relaxant that is still widely used because of its rapid onset and usually short duration, despite its numerous adverse effects including death.[10–12] The drug initially causes depolarization of the neuromuscular junction, which is seen clinically as fasciculations.[12] After this, the receptors stop responding to acetylcholine because of desensitization induced by the succinylcholine. The receptors recover after approximately 5–20 minutes depending on the dose given and the presence or absence of various underlying conditions that interfere with the metabolism of succinylcholine (e.g., atypical cholinesterases). The usual dose given for intubation is 1.0 mg/kg intravenously, which is increased to 1.5 mg/kg if a defasciculating drug is also used (a very small dose of a non-depolarizing muscle relaxant given before succinylcholine to reduce fasciculations).[12] Repeated doses should be avoided for two reasons: First, prolonged paralysis can occur due to a poorly understood phenomenon called phase II block. Second, but more important, failure to intubate with the first dose would suggest that the intubation is difficult and is likely to fail again. As stated above, muscle paralysis should be avoided if intubation is unlikely to be successful.

An exhaustive review of the contraindications and complications for succinylcholine is beyond the scope of this text,[10–12] but we will list some of the most important ones: A lack of familiarity with the drug and a low likelihood of successful intubation should be considered absolute contraindications to the drug's use. Conditions from which life-threatening complications are likely to occur are also absolute contraindications. Atypical pseudocholinesterases are not a contraindication to succinylcholine, but these patients will have a greatly prolonged response to the drug (approximately 4–6 hours of muscle paralysis).

Renal failure, although commonly cited, is not a contraindication, but the presence of hyperkalemia is.[27] Aside from allergic reactions, some of the unique but important complications associated with succinylcholine include:

a. hyperkalemia – Normally, potassium levels increase by 0.5–1.0 mEq/L with the administration of succinylcholine and this persists for about 10–15 minutes.[12,27] Patients with pre-existing hyperkalemia may be pushed to a level that causes cardiac complications. Marked rises of 5–7 mEq/L in potassium levels can, however, occur in patients with various lesions and diseases that have caused a proliferation of extra-junctional receptors. Table 7.6 lists some of the more common disorders, which include various neurologic disorders, crush trauma, burns and patients who have been immobile for a prolonged period of time. If a patient has a chronic neurologic problem, it is often safer to avoid succinylcholine rather than risk precipitating life-threatening hyperkalemia. Treatment for this complication is the same as for non-succinylcholine-related hyperkalemia.

b. cardiovascular effects – This drug has acetylcholine-like effects and thus can cause sinus bradycardia and even asystole, which is more common in children or if a second dose is given.[12]

c. increase in intracranial pressure – A dose of succinylcholine may increase the pressure up to 9 mm Hg. The rise can be attenuated by gentle hyperventilation or by administration of a defasciculating dose of a non-depolarizing muscle relaxant (e.g., rocuronium 5 mg). Although somewhat controversial, succinylcholine can be safely used in patients with intracranial pathology.[28] A cough, which is prevented with succinylcholine, can increase the ICP by over 50 mm Hg and thus has substantially more detrimental effects than the small rise due to the administration of the drug.

d. myotonic contractures – Patients with myotonia can develop life-threatening muscle contractures from succinylcholine. If this occurs, non-depolarizing muscle relaxants will not be beneficial. Procainamide and dantrolene have been used with variable success, as has direct injection of lidocaine into the muscle bellies of the contracted muscles.

e. malignant hyperthermia – This life-threatening problem can be triggered by the administration of succinylcholine. Management is complex and is clearly beyond the scope of this review but must include the administration of dantrolene.

G. Rocuronium

Rocuronium is a non-depolarizing muscle relaxant. Paralysis from this type of muscle relaxant is due to competitive antagonism at the neuromuscular junction. The advantage of non-depolarizing drugs is that they do not cause the hyperkalemia and the other unusual problems that occur with succinylcholine. The primary disadvantage is their longer duration of effect. Although these drugs can be reversed, this can only be done once some of the drug has been metabolized (i.e., after 20 minutes). The specific advantages of rocuronium are its quicker onset time and minimal cardiac effects. The dose for intubation is 0.6–1.2 mg/kg with the higher dose giving a more rapid onset time (at the expense of having a more prolonged duration).

● Conclusions

Medications clearly can make airway management considerably easier but they may do so at the expense of making the situation worse. Since there is no perfect drug or recipe, the physician will always have to make a decision based on the specific details of the situation and the patient's condition. Regardless of what drugs are selected, you should always adhere to the two guiding principles: Never use a drug that is recommended for a certain situation if you have no knowledge of that drug. Always be prepared to deal with a problem or complication that may arise once a drug is given.

Key Points

- Have a thorough knowledge of the medications you use.
- Titrate a drug in slowly since additional doses can be given if necessary.
- Medications are required for physiologic, technical and psychological reasons.

- Numerous factors influence drug dosing including physiology, volume status and the goals of the medications.
- The goals of the medications are the A's and R's.

References

1. Flacke JW, Flacke WE, Williams GD: Acute pulmonary edema following naloxone reversal of high-dose morphine anesthesia. *Anesthesiology* 1977;47:376–8.
2. Michaelis LL, Hickey PR, Clark TA, Dixon WM: Ventricular irritability associated with the use of naloxone. *Ann Thorac Surg* 1974;18:608–14.
3. Puri GD, Marudhachalam KS, Chari P, Suri RK: The effect of magnesium sulphate on hemodynamics and its efficacy in attenuating the response to endotracheal intubation in patients with coronary artery disease. *Anesth Analg* 1998;87:808–11.
4. Roy WL, Edelist G, Gilbert B: Myocardial ischemia during non-cardiac surgical procedures in patients with coronary artery disease. *Anesthesiology* 1979;51:393–7.
5. Spiekermann BF, Stone DJ, Bogdonoff DL, Yemen TA: Airway management in neuroanaesthesia. *Can J Anaesth* 1996;43:820–34.
6. Gal TJ: Bronchial hyperresponsiveness and anesthesia: Physiologic and therapeutic perspectives. *Anesth Analg* 1994;78:559–73.
7. Dronen S, Merigian KS, Hedges JR, et al: A comparison of blind nasotracheal intubation and succinylcholine-assisted intubation in the poisoned patient. *Ann Emerg Med* 1987;16:6502.
8. Ligier B, Bushman TG, Breslow MJ, Deutschman CS: The role of anesthetic induction agents and neuromuscular blockade in the endotracheal intubation of trauma victims. *Surg Gyn Ob* 1991;173:477–81.
9. Knopp RK: Rapid sequence intubation revisited. *Ann Emerg Med* 1998;31:398–400.
10. Book WJ, Abel M, Eisenkraft JB: Adverse effects of depolarising neuromuscular blocking agents: Incidence, prevention and management. *Drug Saf* 1994;10:331–49.
11. Gronert GA, Theye RA: Pathophysiology of hyperkalemia induced by succinylcholine. *Anesthesiology* 1975;43:89–99.
12. Stoelting RK: Chapter 8. Neuromuscular blocking drugs. p.172–225. In *Pharmacology and physiology in anesthetic practice*. 2nd ed. JB Lippincott, Philadelphia, 1991.
13. Vuyk J: Pharmacodynamics in the elderly. *Best Pract Res Clin Anaesthesiol* 2003;17:207–18.
14. Craig DB, McLeskey CH, Mitenko PA, et al: Geriatric anesthesia. *Can J Anaesth* 1987;34:156–67.
15. Lewis KP, Stanley GD: Pharmacology. *Int Anesthesiol Clin* 1999;37:73–86.
16. Stoelting RK, Dierdorf SF: Chapter 20. Renal disease. In *Anesthesia and co-existing disease*. 3rd ed. Churchill Livingstone, New York, 1993.
17. Tomicheck RC, Rosow CE, Philbin DM, et al: Diazepam-fentanyl interaction: Hemodynamic and hormonal effects in coronary artery surgery. *Anesth Analg* 1983;62:881–4.
18. Nordt SP, Clark RF: Midazolam: A review of therapeutic uses and toxicity. *J Emerg Med* 1997;15:357–65.
19. Khanderia U, Pandit SK: Use of midazolam hydrochloride in anesthesia. *Clin Pharm* 1987;6:533–47.
20. Robinson N, Clancy M: In patients with head injury undergoing rapid sequence intubation, does pretreatment with intravenous lignocaine/lidocaine lead to an improved neurological outcome? A review of the literature. *Emerg Med J* 2001;18:453–7.
21. Bryson HM, Fulton BR, Faulds D: Propofol: an update of its use in anaesthesia and conscious sedation. *Drugs* 1995;50:513–59.
22. Smith I, White PF, Nathanson M, Gouldson R: Propofol: An update on its clinical use. *Anesthesiology* 1994;81:1005–43.

23. Stoelting RK: Chapter 4. Barbiturates. p.102–17. In *Pharmacology and physiology in anesthetic practice.* 2nd ed. JB Lippincott, Philadelphia, 1991.

24. Reich DL, Silvay G: Ketamine: An update on the first twenty-five years of clinical experience. *Can J Anaesth* 1989;36:186–97.

25. L'Hommedieu CS, Arens JJ: The use of ketamine for the emergency intubation of patients with status asthmaticus. *Ann Emerg Med* 1987;16:568–71.

26. Beveridge RC, Grunfeld AF, Hodder RV, Verbeek PR: Guidelines for the emergency management of asthma in adults. CAEP/CTS Asthma Advisory Committee. Canadian Association of Emergency Physicians and the Canadian Thoracic Society. *CMAJ* 1996;155:25–37.

27. Thapa S, Brull SJ: Succinylcholine-induced hyperkalemia in patients with renal failure: An old question revisited. *Anesth Analg* 2000;91:237–41.

28. Clancy M, Halford S, Walls R, Murphy M: In patients with head injuries who undergo rapid sequence intubation using succinylcholine, does pretreatment with a competitive neuromuscular blocking agent improve outcome? A literature review. *Emerg Med J* 2001;18:373–5.

RAPID SEQUENCE INTUBATION

MICHELLE CHIU AND
DAVE NEILIPOVITZ

A 73-year-old male has come into your emergency room with an upper gastrointestinal bleed. He is pale and cool with vital signs of HR 130, BP 85/40, RR 24 and SpO$_2$ 85%. He is vomiting bright red blood and is disoriented and uncooperative. Over the next few minutes, as you apply 100% O$_2$ and begin to fluid resuscitate him, he progressively becomes more hypoxemic and obtunded and you are concerned about ongoing aspiration. What do you do?

The patient in this scenario presents the physician with many conflicting problems: The patient is hemodynamically unstable and needs further fluid resuscitation. The patient, however, may aspirate and suffer adverse pulmonary consequences if his airway is not secured immediately. The high likelihood of impending aspiration drastically decreases the time available to adequately resuscitate him. The urgency also reduces the time available to gently sedate and topicalize the airway, never mind the unlikelihood of being able to effectively topicalize his airway due to the ongoing hematemesis. The technique of rapid sequence intubation (RSI) has been advocated for a patient who requires endotracheal intubation but who is at high risk for aspiration of gastric contents. The goal of this chapter is to present the technique of RSI and discuss the advantages and disadvantages of this approach to airway management.

● Overview

The primary goal of the RSI technique is to provide optimal intubating conditions as quickly as possible. In brief, it involves pre-oxygenation of the patient, followed by rapid administration of predetermined doses of drugs and the application of cricoid pressure prior to intubation (Table 8.1). The logic underlying RSI is to minimize the duration of time between the patient's loss of consciousness and the inflation of the cuff of an endotracheal tube in the trachea. The

Table 8.1 – Overview of RSI

1. Preparation for Intubation
2. Pre-oxygenation
3. Induction Drug Administration
4. Application of Cricoid Pressure
5. Paralyzing Drug Administration
6. Endotracheal Tube Insertion
7. Inflation of Cuff on Tube
8. Confirmation of Tube Placement
9. Release of Cricoid Pressure

premise is that during the time when the patient is unconscious and airway reflexes are lost, the patient is at the highest risk for aspiration of gastric contents. In general, RSI is the preferred method for securing a patient's airway in emergency situations or when a patient is at a very high risk for regurgitation and aspiration.[1–3] The use of RSI is also recommended to secure the airway of a patient with increased intracranial pressure (ICP).[4] RSI is preferred because disastrous elevations in the ICP associated with laryngoscopy are mitigated by the induction drugs, and the patient is unlikely to cough due to the paralyzing agents. Although the technique offers considerable advantages to airway management, the potential for disastrous and irreparable complications are inherent in its use.

The exact origin of RSI is unclear but is most likely attributable to Morton and Wylie in 1951.[5] The technique they described is very similar to the modern day method with the exception that cricoid pressure[6] was not included. Morton and Wylie stated that the technique provided for "a pleasant induction and facilitates quick and easy intubation." They recommended, however, that the use of this approach be restricted and that it should not be attempted by inexperienced physicians because of the greater likelihood of complications associated with its use. The authors cautioned that it was only suitable for healthy patients as the rapid administration of predetermined doses of the induction drugs could cause catastrophic circulatory problems. Indeed, the inherent hazards of RSI were reflected in the colloquial synonym that was often used to describe the method: "crash induction." Numerous reports followed that described deaths that were attributed to this technique and suggested caution for its widespread use along with its potential limitations.[7–9]

The use of RSI was primarily restricted to anesthesiologists until the 1980s. Prior to this time, emergency intubation in a spontaneously breathing patient by non-anesthesiologists was usually performed by awake nasotracheal intubation.[10] The role of a modified RSI for emergency patients was periodically suggested but the method was restricted to experienced anesthesiologists.[11] By the late 1980s and early 1990s, a shift from nasotracheal intubation to RSI for emergency airway management by non-anesthesiologists had occurred.[12] The reasons for this are numerous but primarily rest on the fact that this technique has a higher success rate and potentially fewer complications compared to nasotracheal intubation.[13,14] Illustrative of this paradigm shift is the fact that RSI is supported in the 1997 Advanced Trauma Life Support (ATLS) manual when previously in 1993 it was not even discussed.[15] The RSI approach to airway management is now practiced to some extent in the majority of emergency rooms and its use is steadily increasing. A thorough understanding of the advantages and limitations of the technique are critical if this increased use is to improve patient care.

● Cricoid Pressure (Sellick's Manoeuvre)

The use of cricoid pressure, also referred to as Sellick's manoeuvre, in order to prevent the passive regurgitation of gastric contents during tracheal intubation was reintroduced to modern airway management by Brian Sellick in 1961.[6] A historical review of cricoid pressure by several authors, including Sellick, credited the technique to authors in the late 1700s.[24] The manoeuvre was used to prevent gastric distension during inflation of the lungs of patients recovering from near drownings. Indeed, the landmark article from Sellick also suggested that the manoeuvre could be used to prevent gastric inflation during the application of positive pressure mask ventilation.[6] Surprisingly, despite its popularity and recommended use,[25–27] the efficacy and effectiveness of cricoid pressure in preventing aspiration has remained relatively unproven.[28] Its widespread use has spawned debate and the exact role of cricoid pressure in airway management is still under question.[29–31] The current knowledge of the effectiveness of cricoid pressure in preventing aspiration is limited and further studies are needed to definitively establish its safety profile and efficacy.[28,31] Despite this lack of evidence, the manoeuvre is generally accepted as part of the RSI technique. The original description by Sellick remains the standard for performance of the manoeuvre.[6] The cricoid cartilage is used because it is the only complete cartilage ring in the larynx and trachea. The cricoid cartilage is identified in a supine patient. Sellick recommended that a patient's head and neck be fully extended as this stretches the esophagus and prevents its lateral displacement when pressure is applied. Unfortunately, this worsens laryngoscopic view and thus the ideal sniff position is typically recommended.[28] The thyroid cartilage is identified and palpated. Immediately below the thyroid cartilage is the cricothyroid ligament. The next palpated structure is the cricoid cartilage ring (Figure 8.1). To apply cricoid pressure, the assistant's thumb and index finger are placed on the cricoid cartilage and it is pressed posteriorly, thereby obliterating the esophageal lumen at the level of the fifth cervical vertebra. The recommended amount of pressure that is traditionally accepted is at least 30 newtons (N), which is approximately 6.7 pounds of force.[28,32] Unfortunately, this amount of pressure is considerably higher than what most assistants apply when tested.[32] When applied properly, cadaveric studies demonstrate it could withstand regurgitation pressures of at least 50 cm H_2O and up to 100 cm H_2O in certain individuals.[33,34]

The goal of cricoid pressure is to prevent passive regurgitation and is contraindicated in the actively vomiting patient.[6] If a patient actively vomits during intubation, standard practice recommends cricoid pressure be released and the patient turned on their side. The release of cricoid pressure is recommended to reduce the risk of esophageal rupture, as deaths from this complication have been reported.[28,35] Sellick has suggested that this complication would not happen if the proper sequence occurs with unconsciousness, paralysis and cricoid pressure occurring simultaneously.[36]

The use of cricoid pressure is a controversial manoeuvre in the patient with a C-spine injury as theoretically it could exacerbate pre-existing spinal cord injury.[28] The use of the manoeuvre is also contraindicated when a laryngeal fracture is suspected as its application may result in further disruption of the tissues and cause complete airway obstruction. The presence of a Zenker's diverticulum is another contraindication to cricoid pressure as the manoeuvre may expel its contents and cause aspiration. A two-handed modification of Sellick's original description has been described whereby the second hand is placed behind a patient's neck to apply counter pressure.[28,37] The suggested advantage is that laryngoscopic view is improved although there is little evidence to support this practice.[28]

The timing of application of cricoid pressure is important but somewhat controversial.[28] Sellick's

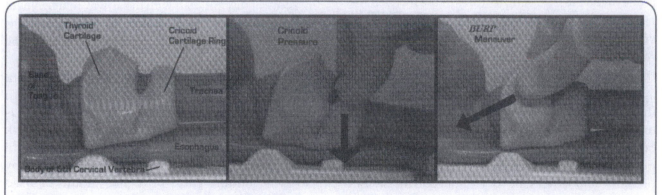

Figure 8.1 – Technique of Cricoid Pressure

Figure 8.1 shows a model of the neck, including the thyroid and cricoid cartilages. The middle picture demonstrates cricoid pressure or Sellick's manoeuvre, which is performed to decrease the risk for passive gastric regurgitation. Pressure from the thumb and index finger is exerted posteriorly towards the fifth cervical vertebra. The BURP manoeuvre is designed to improve view during laryngoscopy and is performed by applying pressure to the thyroid cartilage in a cephalad manner.

original description suggested it should be applied to an awake patient with the pressure increasing simultaneously with the injection of the induction drug.[6] Cricoid pressure when applied correctly is however often painful and can trigger coughing, worsen spontaneous breathing and even induce vomiting. A reasonable compromise is to have the assistant identify and place their fingers in the proper position on the awake patient. A very light amount of pressure, no more than 20 N, can usually be applied and increased simultaneously with the achievement of unconsciousness.[28] What to do with an in situ nasogastric tube is controversial although it can usually be left in place during application of cricoid pressure with the proviso that its lumen remain open to atmosphere.[28]

Cricoid pressure should be released once correct endotracheal tube placement has been confirmed. A very common mistake is that the assistant releases cricoid pressure after the laryngoscope has been withdrawn but before tube placement has been confirmed. The risk of premature removal is that if esophageal placement occurred, when the stomach is mistakenly inflated, the patient is at even greater risk for regurgitation. If cricoid pressure is maintained in this situation, it can theoretically decrease the risk of aspiration. Thus, the assistant should maintain the pressure until told that it is safe to discontinue its application.

The impact of cricoid pressure on laryngoscopy is one of the most limiting features of the manoeuvre. Despite a common misconception to the contrary, cricoid pressure can make airway management considerably more difficult. Although some attribute the distortion of the upper airway to improper application of the cricoid pressure, the exact impact of this manoeuvre on airway management is presently unclear.[28] It is important to make the clear distinction between cricoid pressure and BURP (back-up-right pressure) and other variants of external laryngeal pressure manoeuvres. BURP is applied to the thyroid cartilage to assist visualization of the larynx during intubation and does not compress the esophagus, thereby providing no protection against aspiration. Cricoid pressure and BURP cannot be applied simultaneously. Thus, if BURP is deemed necessary for intubating the patient, cricoid pressure must be removed thereby exposing the patient to potential aspiration.

● Considerations

Although the patient in the case scenario would likely benefit from RSI to secure his airway, several considerations must be addressed prior to using it in this or any other patient. One must decide whether an RSI approach to airway management is appropriate and determine that there are no contraindications to its use. Technically, there are no *absolute* contraindications to RSI aside from physician inexperience with its use and inadequate airway intubation skills. The *relative* contraindications to RSI include potentially difficult intubation, difficult bag-mask ventilation and anticipated adverse hemodynamics.

A patient with a potentially difficult airway may be intubatable, but failure to intubate is not acceptable. Inability to secure the airway in a paralyzed patient will be a life-threatening situation. Thus, if a patient's airway appears to be difficult to intubate, the best strategy may be to manage a patient conservatively and not to proceed with RSI. A conservative approach is especially appropriate if one is not familiar with advanced techniques of airway management. In this case, call for help, continue to give 100% oxygen and proceed with patient resuscitation. If the patient is actively vomiting and there is no concern of possible cervical spine injury, turn the patient on their left side in a head-down position and apply suction to the oropharynx to evacuate blood or vomit. While applying 100% oxygen with assistance from a bag-mask assembly, proceed with the airway management strategy that you are most familiar with. Certainly, an awake intubation with topicalization should be considered.

The decision to use the RSI technique in a patient who has characteristics that would make them a potentially difficult mask ventilation (Chapter 9) is controversial. The obvious reason is that bag-mask ventilation is typically the initial rescue method for a patient who was unsuccessfully intubated by a RSI technique. Thus, prudence should be used before using RSI in this patient group. Finally, since the use of predetermined drug doses can cause severe myocardial depression and vasodilation, any medical condition that would not tolerate this hemodynamic compromise (e.g., aortic stenosis) is a relative contraindication. It is still possible to do an RSI in these patients; however, extensive knowledge of the potential side effects of the drugs used in this technique as well as the drugs used to support the cardiovascular system is mandatory. Thus, if the patient's airway does not have signs of difficulty (Chapter 5), nor are there any other relative contraindications, then this is a case for RSI.

● Technique of Rapid Sequence Intubation

Once the decision to use a RSI has been made, an orderly approach to the technique is essential (Figure 8.2). The first step, as always, is to carefully assess the airway and formulate an approach to securing the patient's airway. The next step in the RSI approach, as with all strategies for airway management, is preparation for intubation. The necessary preparation of the airway equipment is crucial to avoid problems (Table 8.2). A bag and mask device along with an oxygen source is essential. A good selection of airways and a functioning laryngoscope with a proper sized blade should be prepared. An endotracheal tube with a stylet in place is required. At least one suction device should be readily available but two or more suction devices is preferable especially in a patient with massive upper gastrointestinal bleeds. Ideally, several monitors will be applied to the patient before proceeding with RSI. A pulse oximeter to measure oxygen saturation and a device to measure blood pressure are invaluable. A device to detect expired carbon dioxide is extremely useful to confirm the position of the endotracheal tube. The presence of ECGs can also be helpful.

The preparation of drugs for facilitating intubation and treating complications is required before any airway management strategy (Chapter 7). In the RSI approach, unlike other strategies, predetermined doses of drugs are given rather than titrating the drug to desired effect. The safer adage of "you can always give more but you can't take it back" is eschewed in favour of speed. Indeed, this is a major advantage and disadvantage of the RSI approach. By predetermining the doses of drugs and administering them quickly, optimal intubating conditions are achieved sooner. But obviously this approach can lead to both under dosing and more commonly overdosing of the intubating drugs. Thus, the respective complications of these dosing errors are more likely in the RSI approach. Accordingly, a thorough knowledge of the drugs and the impact of

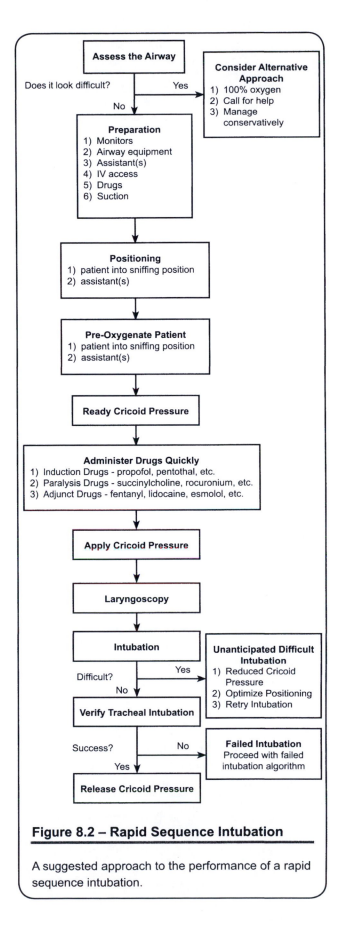

Figure 8.2 – Rapid Sequence Intubation

A suggested approach to the performance of a rapid sequence intubation.

Table 8.2 – Airway Equipment to Prepare

1. Reliable Oxygen Source
2. Ambu® Bag
3. Face Masks (appropriate sizes)
4. Oral and Nasal Airways
5. Endotracheal Tube (appropriate sizes)
6. Metal Stylet
7. Suction Device
8. Rescue Airway Devices (e.g., Combitube®, etc.)
9. Syringe (to inflate endotracheal tube)

patient pathology on the required doses is mandatory if this approach is to be used.

The selection of drugs is a reflection of the goals one is hoping to achieve, namely anesthesia and muscle relaxation (Chapter 7). Normally, only two drugs are given, which include an induction agent and a muscle relaxant. However, if an important requirement for the intubation includes attenuation of autonomic reflexes, such as in a patient with increased ICP, additional medications to further attenuate the hemodynamic response to intubation should be used. These medications must have a rapid onset and short duration, so as to limit the hemodynamic effects of the drugs to the time of laryngoscopy and tube insertion. Typically these agents must be given in advance of other medications to allow them to be effective for the time of intubation. Esmolol, a short acting beta blocker, at a dose of 0.25–0.5 mg/kg IV can be given to slow the heart rate and attenuate any rise in blood pressure during intubation. Lidocaine 1 mg/kg IV has classically been recommended for the intubation of a patient with increased ICP. It has weak general anesthetic properties that can deepen the plane of anesthesia caused by other induction drugs thereby blunting the response to laryngoscopy. Lidocaine by itself is unable to induce a state of anesthesia and thus is limited to use as an adjunct drug. Although the merits of this drug have been challenged,[38] often it is given an insufficient amount of time to become effective as it requires at least 90 seconds to begin to work. Fentanyl, a synthetic narcotic, at a dose of 25–200 mcg has analgesic properties and also acts synergistically with the induction drug.

The induction drugs used in RSI also have a rapid onset and limited duration of action. The agents most commonly used in RSI are propofol (1.0–2.0 mg/kg

IV) and thiopental (3.0–5.0 mg/kg IV). Both propofol and thiopental can cause vasodilation and can result in profound hypotension at these doses. If the patient is already hypotensive, consider the use of ketamine (1.0–2.0 mg/kg IV) or etomidate (0.2–0.4 mg/kg IV). Ketamine indirectly increases the sympathetic tone thereby counterbalancing its direct myocardial depression and vasodilation. A patient, however, who has maximized their sympathetic output, can still experience deleterious hemodynamic effects due to ketamine use. Its use in the patient with increased ICP is controversial because of remote studies linking the use of ketamine with a rise in ICP. Etomidate is not approved for use in Canada but can be obtained by special request. It is said to have minimal hemodynamic effects but has a high rate of nausea and emesis associated with its use and causes adrenal suppression.[39] The use of midazolam (0.1–0.2 mg/kg IV) as an induction drug for RSI has been advocated[40] although its onset is considerably slower and it has prolonged effects,[40–41] causes significant hypotension[42] and is often used incorrectly.[43]

Integral to the RSI approach is the pharmacologic-induced muscle paralysis from the use of muscle relaxants. The use of muscle relaxants is a major reason that the RSI technique can potentially severely injure or even kill a patient. Although paralysis improves intubating conditions, once paralyzed, the patient is solely dependent on others to maintain the airway and to breath for them. Thus, in the setting of pharmacologic-induced paralysis, inability to intubate, bag-mask ventilate, or secure some form of an airway will kill the patient. Typically, the classic paralytic drug of choice for a RSI is succinylcholine (1.0–1.5 mg/kg IV) due to its rapid onset and usually brief duration of action (5–10 minutes). Unfortunately, succinylcholine has numerous contraindications to its use, including some with life-threatening consequences. An exhaustive review of this drug is beyond the scope of this text, but all the issues with this drug must be known and understood prior to its use. Further, although its effect is of relatively short duration, this can be sufficiently long to cause life-threatening hypoxemia and related complications. If contraindications to the use of succinylcholine exist, a high dose of a non-depolarizing muscle relaxant, such as rocuronium (1.2 mg/kg IV) can be used. Unfortunately, these longer acting drugs will result in paralysis for at least one hour. Although reversal drugs for non-depolarizing muscle relaxants exist, these drugs will be ineffective until most of the effects of the relaxant drug have worn off.

As with any airway management strategy, rescue drugs should be prepared prior to intubation. Many patients are hemodynamically unstable and will not tolerate large doses of sedative or induction drugs for intubation. The subsequent fall in blood pressure must be anticipated and vasopressors should be immediately available to treat the hypotension. Ephedrine (5–10 mg IV) primarily has α_1 agonist properties that cause vasoconstriction but also has β_1 agonist effects that will increase myocardial contractility and the heart rate. Phenylephrine (50–100 mcg IV) has primarily α_1 agonist activity that again will increase the blood pressure via vasoconstriction. Either of these drugs or a related agent should be drawn up before proceeding with an RSI approach to airway management.

Once the equipment and drugs are prepared, the next step is to fully prepare the patient and the assistants who are helping to intubate them. A reliable intravenous access, preferably of large calibre, must be obtained. Place the patient into the best possible sniff position (Chapter 5). Poor position is the most common cause of difficulties during intubation. Remember, the first attempt at intubation should be the best and thus conditions must be optimized prior to administering the drugs. The assistant should be positioned to the right of the patient so as to be able to apply cricoid pressure without impairing your ability to manipulate the laryngoscope. As discussed above, it is important to explain to the assistant to apply cricoid pressure only after the patient is asleep, since its use in the awake patient can stimulate coughing and the gag reflex. Remind the assistant to not release cricoid pressure until tracheal intubation has been confirmed and you have told them to do so. A second assistant is required if in-line stabilization of the head is being employed due to possible cervical spine injury.

Once you have ensured that everything has been prepared and the assistants are ready, begin to pre-oxygenate the patient with 100% oxygen. Typically, the oxygen is administered by a bag-mask assembly for at least three minutes of tidal volume breathing. Alternatively, if the patient is fully co-operative, three vital capacity breaths can usually be sufficient. The process can be sped up if the patient was breathing 100% oxygen by mask during equipment and drug preparation. The induction and paralysis drugs are rapidly administered with the simultaneous application of full cricoid pressure by the assistant as soon as the patient loses consciousness. Classically, the patient is usually not manually ventilated with the bag and mask apparatus in order to minimize insufflation of the stomach, which might increase the risk of regurgitation and aspiration. This practice is however controversial, as others, including the original description by Sellick, advocate gentle manual ventilation.[6] Depending on the patient's physiology and the choice and dose of the drugs given, laryngoscopy is usually performed at 60–90 seconds after the drugs have been given. Intubate the trachea with the endotracheal tube and inflate the cuff of the tube. Verify that correct tracheal intubation has been achieved (Chapter 5). Do not allow the assistant to release cricoid pressure until correct tube placement has been confirmed. Once position is verified, release the cricoid pressure and secure the endotracheal tube while beginning to ventilate the patient. Ensure that no complications or deterioration in the patient's condition has occurred by repeating the initial assessment. If complications have occurred, treat accordingly.

● Problem Solving

Inability to successfully intubate a patient after using the RSI approach is an emergency situation. If the intubation is unexpectedly difficult, first check to see if the assistant has unintentionally deviated the airway by pushing the cricoid cartilage to the left or right. Correct the hand position to see if this improves visualization of the larynx. If this does not improve the situation, have your assistant release cricoid pressure briefly to see if you can obtain *any* view of the larynx.[28] Too much cricoid pressure may cause airway obstruction. This situation can also manifest as inability to advance the endotracheal tube past the glottic inlet. Although releasing cricoid pressure is controversial as it may increase the risk for aspiration, often it allows for successful tube placement. If intubation is still unsuccessful despite releasing cricoid pressure, the pressure should be reapplied. The situation should now be considered to be a failed intubation situation and thus one must proceed with alternate plans for managing the airway.

In a failed intubation situation, it is critical to avoid repeated attempts at laryngoscopy as this will cause soft tissue trauma. As the swelling worsens during repeated attempts, this will result in further airway compromise and can make intubation impossible. Always call for help. The assistant should maintain cricoid pressure while you attempt to gently bag-mask ventilate the patient. If you can achieve adequate ventilation, you will be able to avoid hypoxemia while waiting for the patient to wake up. Once awake, securing the patient's airway can proceed with an alternative technique. Most commonly, the alternative technique is to apply topical anesthetics to the airway and proceed with awake intubation. During bag-mask ventilation, it is essential that cricoid pressure be maintained to minimize gastric insufflation. Ideally the inflation pressures should be kept less than 20 cm H_2O to further minimize gastric inflation.

The situation of being unable to either intubate or bag-mask ventilate the patient is a medical emergency (Chapter 9). The primary goal in this situation is to maintain patient oxygenation. Although each situation is unique, the use of a rescue device such as the laryngeal mask airway (LMA™) or the Combitube® is usually indicated. The LMA™ can usually be inserted and used with continued cricoid pressure.[28] Sometimes however, LMA™ insertion is difficult, which warrants transient release of cricoid pressure until it is correctly positioned at which point it should be reapplied. The Combitube®, by the nature of the device, typically enters the esophagus, which requires the release of cricoid pressure for its safe insertion. Failure of the rescue device to maintain oxygenation is an indication for more invasive techniques of airway management including a surgical airway.

● Controversies

The major controversy with RSI is whether it is a safe technique for airway management by physicians with limited experience. Who should or should not use the technique is a subject of heated debate that is not likely to have an agreed upon solution in the near future. The evidence clearly suggests that the use of the technique, most likely due to the use of paralytic drugs, makes intubation easier thereby increasing the success rate for tube placement. Although rates vary depending on the physician background, in non-anesthesiologists the reported success rates are around 97%. Unfortunately, regardless of which physician or patient population is studied, no study has yet to clearly demonstrate that RSI or cricoid pressure improves or worsens patient outcome. The theoretical concerns surrounding the use of paralytics and un-titrated induction drugs remain but complication rates are relatively unknown.

The use of RSI has been advocated for paramedics in out-of-hospital resuscitation situations.[16–18] Unfortunately, these recommendations now must be tempered with the evidence that the use of RSI has paradoxically increased mortality.[19] The San Diego Paramedic RSI Trial clearly demonstrated an increase in mortality and decrease in good outcomes when patients underwent RSI by paramedics. The reasons proposed for the increase in mortality included potential delays in transport due to its performance, significant hypoxemia during intubation,[20] inadvertent hyperventilation and other possible ill-defined mechanisms. Surprisingly, the initial studies that advocated the use of RSI often had a near absence of significant complications.[21] The validity of the self-reporting nature of these studies has now been questioned, especially in light of a sub-study from the San Diego trial. The investigators reported a high discordance between the actual incidence of complications as identified by monitors and the perceived events as reported by the paramedics.[20] Indeed, the whole premise of out-of-hospital RSI has been questioned.[21,22] Further, examination of some of the studies that advocated the use of RSI could question their recommendations. Is an 84% intubation success rate[16] high enough to justify the use of a paralyzing drug and induction drugs?

The questions of who should use the RSI technique and when it should or should not be used remain unanswered. The San Diego study[19] would suggest that widespread dissemination of the RSI technique should be tempered until evidence demonstrates benefit. Further, the definition of what constitutes airway management success must be standardized. Possibly, success should no longer be simply the rate of successful intubation but must focus on mortality outcomes as well.[23] Clearly, future studies are warranted to help answer these and other questions surrounding the use of RSI for emergency airway management.

Case Scenario

Let's go back to the case at the beginning of this chapter to illustrate these principles.

* * * * *

As the nurses draw up medications, you begin to assemble your airway equipment. You examine the patient's airway. He is thin, edentulous, has a normal thyromental distance and you are sure you can secure his airway. The patient is on a cardiac monitor, which displays vital signs of HR 135, BP 80/40, RR 24 and SpO_2 83%. The patient is receiving 2L normal saline (NS) under pressure through two large bore IVs and is breathing 100% oxygen by a non-rebreather mask. You replace the non-rebreather mask with a bag-mask assembly in an attempt to raise his saturation. Unfortunately, he requires frequent suctioning of his oropharynx as he is still actively vomiting. While you are pre-oxygenating the patient, ensure that all your assistants, airway equipment and all rescue devices are ready. Importantly, you ensure that there is an extra suction available. The nurse has prepared ketamine, succinylcholine and phenylephrine.

You position the patient in an optimal sniff position and direct an assistant to correctly apply cricoid pressure. Meanwhile, the patient's condition has improved somewhat—HR 125, BP 87/43, RR 22 and SpO_2 90%—but you are still suctioning copious amounts of blood from the patient's mouth. You administer 1.5 mg/kg ketamine immediately followed by 1.0 mg/kg succinylcholine as the assistant applies cricoid pressure. After suctioning the oropharynx, your laryngoscopy reveals a grade 1 larynx and you visualize the endotracheal tube entering the trachea. The cuff is inflated and you ventilate the patient with the ambubag. The presence of end tidal CO_2 confirms tube placement and thus you instruct the assistant to release the cricoid pressure. You notice the patient's blood pressure has dropped to 75/36 and you administer 100 mcg of phenylephrine. As the assistant helps you secure the endotracheal tube, the patient is connected to the ventilator and you continue to further resuscitate the patient.

Key Points

- The purpose of RSI is to provide optimal intubating conditions as quickly as possible.
- Preparation of all equipment, drugs, assistants and patient is fundamental for success.
- The relative contraindications to RSI include difficult airway, difficult bag-mask ventilation and severely abnormal hemodynamics.

- Predetermined drug doses are administered to hasten onset but this creates an increased risk of complications.
- Ensure that the assistant understands when and how to apply cricoid pressure, including when it is safe to release.
- There is currently no evidence that RSI improves outcomes.

References

1. Walls RM: Rapid-sequence intubation comes of age. *Ann Emerg Med* 1996;28:79–81.
2. Dunham CM, Barraco RD, Clark DE, et al: Guidelines for emergency tracheal intubation immediately after traumatic injury. *J Trauma* 2003;55:162–79.
3. Wang HE, O'Connor RE, Domeier RM: Position paper: National Association of EMS Physicians: Prehospital rapid-sequence intubation. *Prehosp Emerg Care* 2001;5:40–8.
4. Procaccio F, Stocchetti N, Citerio G, et al: Guidelines for the treatment of adults with severe head trauma (part I): Initial assessment; evaluation and pre-hospital treatment; current criteria for hospital admission; systemic and cerebral monitoring. *J Neurosurg Sci* 2000;44:1–10.

5. Morton HJV, Wylie WD: Anaesthetic deaths due to regurgitation or vomiting. *Anaesthesia* 1951;6:190–201,205.

6. Sellick BA: Cricoid pressure to control regurgitation of stomach contents during induction of anaesthesia. *Lancet* 1961;2:404–6.

7. Woodbridge PD: "Crash induction" for tracheal intubation. *JAMA* 1967;202:845.

8. Marx GF, Steen SN, Berenyi KJ, et al: Hazards of "crash" induction-intubation technic. *N Y State J Med* 1968;68:1957–8.

9. Barr AM, Thornley BA: Thiopentone and suxamethonium crash induction: An assessment of the potential hazards. *Anaesthesia* 1976;31:23–9.

10. Tintinnali JE, Claffery J: Complications of nasotracheal intubation. *Ann Emerg Med* 1981;10:142–4.

11. Ligier B, Buchman TG, Breslow MJ, Deutschman CS: The role of anesthetic induction agents and neuromuscular blockade in the endotracheal intubation of trauma victims. *Surg Gyn Obs* 1991;173:477–81.

12. Knopp RK: Rapid sequence intubation revisited. *Ann Emerg Med* 1998;31:398–400.

13. Dronen S, Merigian KS, Hedges JR, et al: A comparison of blind nasotracheal intubation and succinylcholine-assisted intubation in the poisoned patient. *Ann Emerg Med* 1987;16:650–2.

14. Dufour DG, Larose DL, Clement SC: Rapid sequence intubation in the emergency department. *J Emerg Med* 1995;13:705–10.

15. American College of Surgeons Committee on Trauma: *ATLS Instructor Manual.* American College of Surgeons, Chicago, 1997:57.

16. Ochs M, Davis D, Hoyt D, et al: Paramedic-performed rapid sequence intubation of patients with severe head injuries. *Ann Emerg Med* 2002;40:159–167.

17. Bernard S, Smith K, Foster S, et al: The use of rapid sequence intubation by ambulance paramedics for patients with severe head injury. *Emerg Med* 2002;14:406–11.

18. Swanson ER, Fosnocht DE: Effect of an airway education program on prehospital intubation. *Air Med J* 2002;21:28–31.

19. Davis DP, Hoyt DB, Ochs M, et al: The effect of paramedic rapid sequence intubation on outcome in patients with severe traumatic brain injury. *J Trauma* 2003;54:444–53.

20. Dunford JV, Davis DP, Ochs M, et al: Incidence of transient hypoxia and pulse rate reactivity during paramedic rapid sequence intubation. *Ann Emerg Med* 2003;42:721–8.

21. Spaite DW, Criss EA: Out-of-hospital rapid sequence intubation: Are we helping or hurting our patients? *Ann Emerg Med* 2003;42:729–30.

22. Wang HE, Yealy DM: Out-of-hospital rapid sequence intubation: Is this really the "success" we envisioned? *Ann Emerg Med* 2002;40:168–71.

23. Neilipovitz DT: Rapid sequence intubation: How do we define success? *Can J Anesth* 2004;51:857–8.

24. Salem MR, Sellick BA, Elam JO: The historical background of cricoid pressure in anesthesia and resuscitation. *Anesth Analg* 1974;53:230–2.

25. Schwartz DE, Matthay MA, Cohen NH: Death and other complications of emergency airway management in critically ill adults. *Anesthesiology* 1995;82:367–76.

26. Standards and guidelines for cardiopulmonary resuscitation (CPR) and emergency cardiac care (ECC). *JAMA* 1985;255:2905–84.

27. Section 3: Adjuncts for oxygenation, ventilation, and airway control. *Circulation* 2000;102(suppl I): I95–I104.

28. Brimacombe JR, Berry AM: Cricoid pressure. *Can J Anaesth* 1997;44:414–25.

29. Kron SS: Questionable effectiveness of cricoid pressure in preventing aspiration. *Anesthesiology* 1995;83:431.

30. Schwartz DE, Cohen NH: In reply to Kron. *Anesthesiology* 1995;83:432.

31. Jackson SH: Efficacy and safety of cricoid pressure needs scientific validation. *Anesthesiology* 1996;84:751–2.

32. Wraight WJ, Chamney AR, Howells TH. The determination of an effective cricoid pressure. *Anaesthesia* 1983;38:461–6.

33. Fanning GL: The efficacy of cricoid pressure in preventing regurgitation of gastric contents. *Anesthesiology* 1970;32:553–5.

34. Salem MR, Wong AY, Fizzotti GF: Efficacy of cricoid pressure in preventing aspiration of gastric contents in paediatric patients. *Brit J Anaesth* 1972;44:401–4.

35. Ralph SJ, Wareham CA. Rupture of the oesophagus during cricoid pressure. *Anaesthesia* 1991;46:40–1.

36. Sellick BA: Rupture of the oesophagus following cricoid pressure? *Anaesthesia* 1982;37:213–4.

37. Crowley DS, Giesecke AH: Bimanual cricoid pressure. *Anaesthesia* 1990;45:588–9.

38. Robinson N, Clancy M: In patients with head injury undergoing rapid sequence intubation, does pretreatment with intravenous lignocaine/lidocaine lead to an improved neurological outcome? A review of the literature. *Emerg Med J* 2001;18:453–7.

39. Schenarts CL, Burton JH, Riker RR: Adrenocortical dysfunction following etomidate induction in emergency department patients. *Acad Emerg Med* 2001;8:1–7.

40. White PF: Comparative evaluation of intravenous agents for rapid sequence induction: Thiopental, ketamine, and midazolam. *Anesthesiology* 1982;57:279–84.

41. Sivilotti ML, Ducharme J: Randomized, double-blind study on sedatives and hemodynamics during rapid-sequence intubation in the emergency department: The SHRED Study. *Ann Emerg Med* 1998;31:313–24.

42. Davis DP, Kimbro TA, Vilke GM: The use of midazolam for prehospital rapid-sequence intubation may be associated with a dose-related increase in hypotension. *Prehosp Emerg Care* 2001;5:163–8.

43. Sagarin MJ, Barton ED, Sakles JC, et al: Underdosing of midazolam in emergency endotracheal intubation. *Acad Emerg Med* 2003;10:329–38.

CHAPTER 9

DIFFICULT MASK VENTILATION AND DIFFICULT INTUBATION

Chris Christodoulou

You are managing a 45-year-old woman who presented to hospital after an overdose of tricyclic antidepressants, alcohol and methanol. She is having repeated convulsions despite repeated doses of lorazepam. Her oxygen saturations are in the low 80s. You have attempted to intubate her using your best techniques but are unsuccessful. Help has been called but is over 20 minutes away. You try to assist her ventilation and oxygenation but are unable to effectively bag her as her saturations continue to fall. What do you do?

Airway management is usually the first fundamental act in the care of the critically ill patient. It is a process that represents a continuum of evaluation and concurrent management, in which the goal is to preserve oxygen delivery to end organ systems. The American Society of Anesthesiologists (ASA) Closed Claims Project of anesthesia related morbidity and mortality, has revealed a frighteningly high incidence of respiratory problems. Since the inception of the project, adverse respiratory events have constituted the single largest source of injury.[1] Respiratory related claims were associated with a high frequency of severe outcomes (85% death or brain damage) and costly payments (median $200 000). The mechanisms related to nearly 75% of these outcomes include inadequate ventilation (38%), difficult intubation (17%) and esophageal intubation (18%).

Esophageal intubation with resultant hypoxemia remains a prominent cause of morbidity and mortality in all areas where airway management is undertaken. The incidence of unrecognized esophageal intubation in Emergency Medicine literature has varied between 0% and 5.1%.[2] Recently, alarming evidence of misplaced endotracheal tubes is provided by Katz and Falk,[3] who report a 25% incidence of unrecognized esophageal intubation. These figures may only represent the tip of the iceberg as many cases may go unreported.

Obviously, failure to intubate a patient can have devastating consequences. The previous chapters described techniques and strategies to facilitate airway intubation. The present chapter will discuss two terrifying problems of airway management: difficult mask ventilation and difficult intubation. The goal is to both review the circumstances surrounding these issues and present an approach to deal with these life-threatening problems.

● Difficult Mask Ventilation

Difficult mask ventilation (DMV) describes the inability to obtain an adequate face mask seal to be able to effectively ventilate and oxygenate the patient. The reasons for having difficulty are numerous but are usually related to the presence of one or more of the various risk factors (Table 9.1).[4] The importance of the issue of DMV is magnified considerably by the fact that difficult intubation is more frequent in patients with DMV. For the majority of physicians, bag-mask ventilation is often a primary backup strategy when intubating attempts are unsuccessful. Patients who were judged to be a difficult intubation had a DMV rate of 30% whereas those who were not difficult had a rate of only 8%. The association between difficult intubation and DMV is a consistent finding in the literature.[5] Clearly, identifying patients with DMV is an important component of the difficult airway assessment (Table 9.2).

Early detection of DMV is vital but can be especially challenging when the patient is obese or there are few available monitors. Signs of inadequate

---

Table 9.1 – Factors Associated with Difficult Ventilation

1. Increased body mass index (BMI >26 kg/m²)
2. Age >55 years
3. Lack of teeth
4. History of snoring
5. Beards
6. Macroglossia
7. Decreased lung compliance
8. Facial deformities preventing adequate mask seal

Table 9.2 – Difficult Airway Assessment

1. Difficult mask ventilation?
2. Difficult airway intubation?
3. Difficulty with patient co-operation and consent?
4. Difficult surgical airway?

---

face mask ventilation include absent or inadequate chest movement with accompanying breath sounds that are undetectable or greatly diminished. Auscultation can also reveal the presence of severe airway obstruction (i.e., stridor) or gastric air entry. Occasionally, distension of the abdomen can be noted prior to development of gross cyanosis. Monitors, if present, can report decreasing or inadequate oxygen saturation (SpO_2) and the absence or decreased levels of exhaled carbon dioxide. Spirometer devices can also reveal the inadequate or even complete absence of measures of exhaled gas flow. Finally, hemodynamic and cardiac conduction changes associated with hypoxemia or hypercarbia are late and non-specific signs of DMV.

Since preventing problems is always easier than correcting problems, the first step involves identifying the patient who is at risk of DMV (Table 9.1). The largest prospective study looking at the prediction of DMV was undertaken by Langeron et al.[4] who assessed a total of 1502 patients. Mask ventilation was reported to be difficult in 75 cases or roughly 5% of all patients (95% confidence interval of 3.9–6.1%). A sobering finding is that anesthesiologists correctly anticipated DMV in only 13 patients or 17% of these cases. Independent risk factors for DMV include a body mass index > 26 kg/m², age older than 55 years, lack of teeth, history of snoring and the presence of a beard (Table 9.1). The presence of two or more risk factors correlated strongly with the potential for difficulties with bag-mask ventilation.

● Management Strategies

Although measures to avoid situations of DMV are important, the unfortunate reality is that this complication will still occur. An approach to this problem is crucial to avoid disastrous outcomes. Several techniques are available to help obtain airway patency and enhance the chances of success for face mask ventilation (FMV) in patients (Table 9.3). A prerequisite before commencing FMV is the choice of an appropriate size mask that will provide an adequate seal. Regardless of the actual type of mask used, it should cover the bridge of the nose down to the chin. Other prerequisites before FMV include the use of the highest possible concentration of oxygen at all times and checking airway equipment according to accepted standards prior to its use.

An important observation is that the optimal position for intubation (flexed neck of the sniff position) is not always the best position for ventilation. The flexed neck position in the absence of extension often brings the epiglottis in proximity with the posterior pharyngeal wall thus causing airway obstruction. Manoeuvres that help FMV by improving the patency of the upper airway include a head tilt, a chin lift and a jaw thrust. The insertion of oral airways, nasopharyngeal airways and even both together can improve FMV. An important technique that one should consider early is the two-person bag-mask ventilation technique. The first person holds the mask with both hands to obtain a good seal while the second person squeezes the bag to ventilate the patient. Once FMV is successfully undertaken, constant evaluation of airway patency should occur and corrective measures instituted if it is deemed to be inadequate.

Failure to obtain adequate FMV is obviously a life-threatening situation. A decision must be made quickly in the patient with DMV. Occasionally, a patient with DMV is actually an easy intubation and thus proceeding to intubation is appropriate.

Table 9.3 – Optimizing Face Mask Ventilation

1. Consider two person technique early
2. Head tilt
3. Chin lift
4. Jaw thrust
5. Insertion of an oral pharyngeal airway (e.g., Guedel airway)
6. Insertion of nasopharyngeal airways
7. Insertion of both oral and nasopharyngeal airways
8. Application of continuous positive airway pressure (CPAP)

Remember though, 30% of difficult intubations are also patients who have DMV and proceeding to intubation may not be a safe decision. The use of a rescue device to oxygenate patients such as a laryngeal mask airway (LMA™) or Combitube® can be a life-saving manoeuvre.

● Specific Scenarios

Beards
A simple method to obtain an adequate seal in these patients is to apply a large Tegaderm™ or OpSite® dressing over the patient's mouth.[6] A hole is made in the dressing over the mouth area to allow ventilation to occur.

Edentulous Patients
It is advisable to leave dentures in the mouth whilst performing FMV as this usually results in a more effective face mask seal.[4] The dentures can be removed just prior to intubation.

Continuous Positive Airway Pressure
This can be applied in situations where an anesthesia circuit and/or a ventilator are being used to deliver the ventilation. A level of 5–10 cm H_2O can be effective in improving airflow by minimizing airway obstruction from collapse of the pharyngeal tissues and tongue.

Cricoid Pressure
Cricoid pressure has been shown to reduce gastric insufflation when applied during FMV.[7] This is particularly important in patients who are at risk of passive gastric regurgitation and aspiration during prolonged ventilation. Care should be taken not to apply too much pressure as this has been associated with difficulty in ventilation.[8]

● Difficult Intubation

The definition of what constitutes a difficult intubation varies considerably. The definition put forth by the American Society of Anesthesiologists (ASA) Task Force on Management of the Difficult Airway[9] and the Canadian Consensus Group[10] define it as: "when an experienced laryngoscopist, using direct laryngoscopy, requires: 1) more than two attempts with the same blade; or 2) a change in blade or an adjunct to a direct laryngoscope (e.g., bougie); or 3) use of an alternative device or technique following failed intubation with direct laryngoscopy."[10]

The incidence of difficult direct laryngoscopy will vary depending on the population in question and the experience of the physician who is performing the intubation. Difficulties with laryngoscopy occur in 1.5–8.5% of general anesthetics with a similar incidence of difficult intubation.[11-13] The incidence of failed intubation has been reported to occur in 0.13–0.3% of general anesthetics (one to three times per 1000 attempts). The incidence of failed intubation in critical care settings is however not clearly established.

As with DMV, the best strategy is to identify patients who are difficult intubations before embarking on the securing of the airway thereby preventing numerous problems. Airway assessment, including the identification of a potentially difficult airway, must always be performed (Chapter 5). The TUMS algorithm describes the assessment of the teeth, uvula, mandible and cervical spine. Additional information to help develop a management strategy is provided from difficult airway assessment (Table 9.2).

● Management Strategies

Even if all patients who are difficult intubations are identified before embarking on airway management, an approach to securing their airways is still necessary. Further, unexpected difficult intubations will be encountered, which mandates that all physicians have an approach to these situations. The ASA Difficult Airway Algorithm may serve as a guide to aid experienced clinicians in making appropriate airway management decisions.[9] Unfortunately, the ASA Algorithm has numerous branches that makes it difficult to remember and has some specialized techniques that limit its applicability to general physicians. Thus, clinical experience and judgment are of paramount importance when difficult intubation scenarios are encountered. All physicians should therefore know their approach, or their algorithm, when dealing with this problem.

After the difficult airway assessment is complete, then consideration should be given to the relative merits and feasibility of basic management choices (Table 9.4). It is important to try not to limit the

Table 9.4 – Difficult Airway Management Options

A. Awake intubation vs. intubation attempts after induction of general anesthesia
B. Non-invasive technique vs. invasive technique for initial approach to intubation
C. Preservation vs. ablation of spontaneous ventilation

available options. For example, paralyzing a patient may make direct laryngoscopy easier but makes a situation considerably worse if intubation is unsuccessful. Paralysis removes several important airway management options but mandates that the physician control the airway since all spontaneous patient effort has been removed. Thus, each decision of the management strategy must be made wisely.

Regardless of the approach, several aspects are important to all strategies. In all cases, the first priority is to maintain an adequate level of oxygenation (Table 9.5). Ventilation is important but it is hypoxemia that causes irreparable harm and death. Call for assistance early if unanticipated difficulty in securing an airway occurs. Remember that help is often not immediately available and may take time to arrive. Call for help sooner rather than later. Expert assistance can be provided in various forms including other physicians (e.g., anesthetists) or other health care professionals (e.g., respiratory therapists).

Table 9.5 – Techniques to Maintain Oxygenation

1. Nasal cannulae at high flow (10 l/min)
2. Face mask (non rebreathe at 15 l/min)
3. Ambu® Bag with assisted ventilation
4. Supplemental O_2 via bronchoscope or indirect laryngoscope (e.g., Bullard) suction port
5. Via endotracheal tube with Ambu® Bag IPPV when using the LMA Fastrach™

n.b. Every effort should be made to maintain oxygenation during the entire airway management process.

Ideally, a difficult airway cart with various airway adjuncts should be available at all sites where airway management is to be undertaken. Ready access to equipment set up in a standardized and organized fashion will help minimize delays and complications during the management of patients who are a difficult intubation.

● Specific Airway Tools

As discussed in Chapter 5, the art of laryngoscopy is obviously best learned in elective situations such as the operating room, airway laboratory and simulation facilities. The Macintosh (curve) and Miller (straight) blades are the first and most essential airway intubation tools that practitioners should become competent in using. Blade selection is generally based on the type the physician is the most proficient with. However, a Macintosh blade is preferable when there is less upper airway space to pass the tube (e.g., small mouth) while the Miller blade is better for patients with a small mandibular space, large incisors or a long floppy epiglottis. An important first adjunct for a difficult intubation scenario is the use of a stylet, including the Eschmann bougie, with either the Macintosh or Miller blades.[14] A list of recommended airway adjuncts that should be part of a difficult airway cart has been published by both the ASA and the Canadian Task Force (Table 9.6).[9,10] Experience should guide the choice of airway tool in the different clinical scenarios encountered in clinical practice. Although a full discussion of these

devices is found in Chapter 6, certain aspects that are particularly useful will be highlighted here.

Airway tools that are recommended for cannot intubate and cannot ventilate (CICV) situations include the laryngeal mask airway (LMA™) devices (LMA North America, Inc., San Diego, CA), esophageal-tracheal Combitube® (Kendall-Sheridan Catheter Corp., Argyle, NY) and trans-tracheal jet ventilation (TTJV). The LMA™ devices and the Combitube® are supraglottic airway instruments that can provide effective ventilation in settings where FMV has failed.

Several different LMA™ devices are available including the LMA Classic™, LMA Fastrach™ and LMA ProSeal™. The LMA Fastrach™ is a unique device that allows for effective ventilation and can also serve as a conduit for intubation. The largest case series of difficult airways (254) managed with the LMA Fastrach™ was published by Ferson et al.[15] The patients all had a history of difficult intubation or were expected to be difficult based on the patient's underlying disease and physical findings. Study groups included patients with immobilized cervical spines, distorted airways and stereotactic head frames applied. The overall success rates for blind and fiberoptic-guided intubations through the LMA Fastrach™ were 96.5% and 100%, respectively. An extremely important finding in the study was the ability to effectively ventilate all patients with the LMA Fastrach™.

The LMA ProSeal™ is a new supraglottic airway device that allow for separation of the respiratory and gastrointestinal tracts. It has been used successfully in CICV situations.[16] A major advantage in these settings is the ability to effectively decompress the stomach, particularly when prolonged bag-mask ventilation has been used. Unlike the LMA Fastrach™, it does not provide a simple conduit for intubation, although this has been described using a Cook (Arndt) airway exchanger set.[17] The esophageal-tracheal Combitube® is placed blindly in the esophagus and ventilation is achieved via ports situated between an inflated distal esophageal balloon and a proximal pharyngeal balloon.[18] Ventilation pressures obtained with this device exceed those of the LMA™ devices. In addition the esophageal lumen allows for effective drainage of stomach contents. There have been no case reports of aspiration with a correctly positioned Combitube®. Intubation of the trachea can be readily achieved by deflating the pharyngeal balloon whilst maintaining

---

Table 9.6 – Airway Tools

1. Curved blade laryngoscopes (e.g., Macintosh blade)
2. Straight blade laryngoscopes (e.g., Miller blade)
3. Indirect laryngoscopes (e.g., Bullard laryngoscope)
4. LMA™ devices (LMA Classic™, LMA ProSeal™, LMA Fastrach™)
5. Esophageal tracheal (Combitube®)
6. Tracheal lighted stylets (Trachlight®)
7. Fiberoptic bronchoscope
8. Indirect laryngoscopes
9. Trans-tracheal jet ventilation

the distal esophageal balloon inflated. Aspiration can thus be effectively prevented. This device should not be inserted in awake patients with an active gag reflex as esophageal rupture has been reported.[19] The ease of use of this device coupled with its unique design characteristics should make it an essential tool on every difficult airway cart.

● Extubation Strategies

An often-neglected aspect of airway management is the issue of extubation. Unlike intubation, extubation is virtually always an elective procedure. Thus, the extubation strategy of any patient with a history of a difficult intubation should always be carefully planned and executed. Extubation represents a key time during which a failure to recognize potential difficulties can result in disastrous patient outcomes. Both the environment of extubation and the available personnel should be appropriate for possible reintubation.

A useful adjunct for airway extubation is the use of the various modern airway exchange catheters (Cook airway exchange catheters, Cook Critical Care, Bloomington, IN). These devices come in various sizes and serve as both intubation and ventilation conduits. The technique for extubating over an airway exchange catheter (AEC) is similar to that for exchanging an endotracheal tube. All preparations for intubating a difficult airway should be conducted prior to extubation. A patient is pre-oxygenated on 100% oxygen for at least five minutes. The AEC is passed through the existing tube. The tube is withdrawn with care taken not to dislodge the exchange catheter. The AEC must have a central lumen that allows for jet ventilation (i.e., oxygenation) should the patient run into trouble. The AEC is therefore used both to oxygenate the patient and to help reintubate the patient. The routine use of an AEC for the extubation of patients with known or anticipated difficult airways is strongly recommended.

● Patient Follow-Up

It is incumbent on any physician who instruments a patient's airway, to document firstly the ease of ventilation and the grade of laryngoscopy (direct and indirect laryngoscopy techniques) seen at intubation. Documentation provides all subsequent clinicians an opportunity to identify a *difficult mask ventilation* or *difficult intubation,* and to take appropriate steps in future to secure the airway in a safe manner. Patients should upon recovery from their illness or surgery be notified both verbally, and with written documentation of the difficulties encountered during airway management. Family physicians should also be notified so that appropriate arrangements can be ordered (i.e., MedicAlert® bracelets). Patient follow-up is an extremely important but often neglected issue in patient care.

● Conclusions

"You can always tell who's read it, and who's done it!" – Brian Sellick

The art of airway management is a fundamental thought process and skill that is central to the care of all critically ill patients. It can be highly stressful for both patient and physician alike. The many conflicts that arise between airway management interventions and medical or surgical disease processes (e.g., difficult airway in the patient with elevated intracranial pressure) are a constant challenge that serve to stimulate all clinicians to continually improve their airway management skills. Airway management is a team effort that requires leadership, knowledge and skill. It is important to remember, though, that a failure to oxygenate is far more serious than a failure to intubate.

Key Points

- Identification of potentially difficult mask ventilation and intubation is essential to minimize complications.

- Increased BMI, advanced age, lack of teeth, a history of snoring and a beard are major risk factors for difficult mask ventilation.

- A predetermined approach to failed mask ventilation or intubation is critical.
- The LMA™ and Combitube® are potentially life-saving airway devices in failed intubation patients.
- Extubation strategy is an often neglected yet crucial aspect of difficult mask ventilation or intubation patients.

References

1. Caplan RA, Posner KL, Ward RJ, Cheney FW: Adverse respiratory events in anesthesia: A closed claims analysis. *Anesthesiology* 1990;72:828–33.
2. Falk JL, Sayre MR: Confirmation of airway placement. *Prehosp Emerg Care* 1999;3:273–8.
3. Katz SH, Falk JL: Misplaced endotracheal tubes by paramedics in an urban emergency medical services system. *Ann Emerg Med* 2001;37:32–7.
4. Langeron O, Masso E, Huraux C, et al: Prediction of difficult mask ventilation. *Anesthesiology* 2000;92:1229–36.
5. Hawthorne L, Wilson R, Lyons G, Dresner M: Failed intubation revisited: 17-yr experience in a teaching maternity unit. *Br J Anaesth* 1996;76:680–4.
6. Johnson JO, Bradway JA, Blood T: A hairy situation. *Anesthesiology* 1999;91:595.
7. Lawes EG, Campbell I, Mercer D: Inflation pressure, gastric insufflation and rapid sequence induction. *Br J Anaesth* 1987;59:315–8.
8. Hocking G, Roberts FL, Thew ME: Airway obstruction with cricoid pressure and lateral tilt. *Anaesthesia* 2001;56:825–8.
9. Practice guidelines for management of the difficult airway: An updated report by the American Society of Anesthesiologists Task Force on Management of the Difficult Airway. *Anesthesiology* 2003;98:1269–77.
10. Crosby ET, Cooper RM, Douglas MJ, et al: The unanticipated difficult airway with recommendations for management. *Can J Anaesth* 1998;45:757–76.
11. Rose DK, Cohen MM: The airway: Problems and predictions in 18 500 patients. *Can J Anaesth* 1994;41:372–83.
12. Rocke DA, Murray WB, Rout CC, Gouws E: Relative risk analysis of factors associated with difficult intubation in obstetric anesthesia. *Anesthesiology* 1992;77:67–73.
13. Rose DK, Cohen MM: The incidence of airway problems depends on the definition used. *Can J Anaesth* 1996;43:30–4.
14. Nolan JP, Wilson ME: An evaluation of the gum elastic bougie: Intubation times and incidence of sore throat. *Anaesthesia* 1992;47:878–81.
15. Ferson DZ, Rosenblatt WH, Johansen MJ, et al: Use of the intubating LMA-Fastrach in 254 patients with difficult-to-manage airways. *Anesthesiology* 2001;95:1175–81.
16. Rosenblatt WH: The use of the LMA-ProSeal™ in airway resuscitation. *Anesth Analg* 2003;97:1773–5.
17. Matioc A, Arndt GA: Intubation using the ProSeal laryngeal mask airway and a Cook airway exchange catheter set. *Can J Anaesth* 2001;48:932.
18. Urtubia RM, Aguila CM, Cumsille MA: Combitube®: A study for proper use. *Anesth Analg* 2000;90:958–62.
19. Klein H, Williamson M, Sue-Ling HM, et al: Esophageal rupture associated with the use of the Combitube®. *Anesth Analg* 1997;85:937–9.

SECTION III

RESPIRATORY MANAGEMENT

Objectives

1. Recognize and manage the patient with acute respiratory failure.
2. Learn respiratory mechanics including static/dynamic compliance and resistance.
3. Develop a working knowledge of non-invasive ventilation.
4. Describe volume and pressure controlled ventilation and pressure support ventilation.
5. Learn the pathophysiology and causes of hypoxemia and hypercapnia.
6. Discuss the principle of permissive hypercapnia and lung protective ventilation.
7. Explore the subject of PEEP, including its use, risks and relative contraindications.
8. Develop an approach to the management of refractory hypoxemia.
9. Understand oxygen content of blood and its relationship to oxygen saturation.

CHAPTER 10

PHYSIOLOGY OF GAS EXCHANGE

Pierre Cardinal,
Lois Champion, and
Richard Hodder

A 75-year-old woman has presented to you complaining of shortness of breath, which has worsened over the last week. She is clearly dyspneic with a respiratory rate of 30 and pulse oximeter reading of 82%. She has been a heavy smoker for over 50 years but has been reasonably well otherwise. Although oxygen is given by mask, her oxygenation fails to improve. Why is she not improving?

Oxygen is obviously essential for survival. Problems with oxygenation are however quite common but have numerous possible etiologies. In this chapter, we will briefly review how oxygen is transported to the cells. We will also discuss hypoxia and hypoxemia along with mechanisms that lead to them. We will explore the relationship between the partial pressure of oxygen and the hemoglobin saturation along with the impact each has on the oxygen content of blood. Finally, we will also review the mechanisms leading to hypercapnia (high $PaCO_2$) including the different components of the minute ventilation.

● Oxygenation

Hypoxia kills. *Hypoxia* refers to the lack of O_2 at the cellular level while *hypoxemia* refers to a low partial pressure of O_2 in the blood (PaO_2). Lack of oxygen at the cellular level results in anaerobic metabolism and lactic acidosis, and if severe and prolonged, to cellular, tissue, and organ death, culminating eventually in the death of the person. Hypoxia can result from several causes, including (1) low PaO_2; (2) anemia (but anemia will not cause hypoxemia) or abnormal hemoglobin; (3) low cardiac output states; and (4) an inability of cells to utilize oxygen that is delivered, such as in cyanide toxicity (Table 10.1). It is important to understand the mechanisms that lead to hypoxia since our therapeutic interventions are specifically designed to correct these mechanisms.

Table 10.1 – Different Causes of Hypoxia

1. Hypoxemia hypoxia – low PaO_2
2. Anemic hypoxia – low or abnormal hemoglobin
3. Distributive hypoxia – poor cardiac output or impaired perfusion
4. Metabolic or toxic hypoxia – cells unable to utilize oxygen

Some useful equations relating to gas exchange and oxygen delivery are listed in Table 10.2.

Arterial oxygen content (CaO_2) refers to the amount of oxygen contained in blood. Most of the O_2 carried in the blood is reversibly attached to hemoglobin (Hb). A much lower fraction of O_2 is carried in its dissolved form, which explains why the arterial oxyhemoglobin saturation (SaO_2) gives us much more meaningful information on the state of arterial oxygenation than does the PaO_2. Note that real-time measurements of SaO_2 are readily available with pulse oximetry (often designated as SpO_2), but the SaO_2 does not tell us anything about the adequacy of alveolar ventilation, which is best followed by the $PaCO_2$ (see below). In order for arterial O_2 to be useful, it must be delivered to the tissues and this depends on the adequacy of cardiac output (CO). Finally, delivered O_2 must be utilized by the tissues and cells and so the concept of O_2 uptake must be considered, as this can be abnormal in certain disease states (e.g., sepsis, cyanide poisoning, etc.).

The relation between the SaO_2 and PaO_2 is expressed graphically by the oxyhemoglobin dissociation curve (Figure 10.1). The sigmoid shape of the curve reflects how O_2 is progressively bound to the Hb molecule and is very well suited to facilitate oxygen loading (in the lungs where O_2 pressures are hopefully high) and unloading in the systemic capillaries (where O_2 pressures are low). The steep part of the O_2 dissociation curve (the so-called "slippery slope") implies that minor falls in PaO_2 may dramatically reduce the O_2 saturation and arterial O_2 content, which may result in tissue hypoxia (physiologic defence mechanisms that help to combat this include increased cardiac output and increased O_2 uptake in the tissues). Similarly, the upper flat part of the curve has therapeutic implications because a

Table 10.2 – Important Equations for Gas Exchange

CaO_2 = Arterial oxygen content (O_2 bound to hemoglobin + dissolved O_2)
= $(SaO_2 \times Hgb \times 1.34) + (PaO_2 \times .0031)$

O_2 Delivery = $CaO_2 \times CO$

$P(A–a)O_2$ Difference (Alveolar to arterial oxygen gradient)
P_AO_2 = $FiO_2 [PB – PH_2O] – [PaCO_2 / RQ]$
= $[713 \times FiO_2] – [1.25 \times PaCO_2]$

Assuming: PB is 1 atmosphere pressure or 760 mm Hg
PH_2O is 47 mm Hg (fully saturated air)
RQ is the respiratory quotient and is 0.8

$P(A–a)O_2 = P_AO_2 – PaO_2$

$PaCO_2$ = K × CO_2 production / alveolar ventilation
= $K \times VCO_2 / [RR \times (V_T – V_D)]$

SaO_2 = arterial oxygen saturation; K is a constant; RR = respiratory rate; V_T = tidal volume; V_D = dead space volume; VCO_2 = CO_2 production

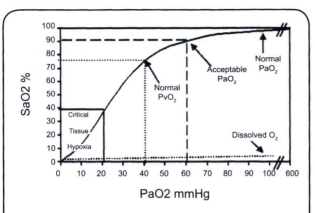

Figure 10.1 – Oxyhemoglobin Dissociation Curve

The oxyhemoglobin dissociation curve demonstrates that the vast amount of oxygen in the blood bound to the hemoglobin form as opposed to dissolved in solution. Several important points on the curve should be observed: At a PaO_2 of 60, the oxygen saturation is 90%. Above a saturation of 90% there is little increase in arterial oxygen content. A PaO_2 of 40 mm Hg is the normal mixed venous PO_2 and it corresponds to a saturation of ~75% (SvO_2). The PaO_2 of 27 mm Hg corresponds to an SaO_2 of 50% and is known as the P50. Above a PaO_2 of 80 mm Hg, a large change in PaO_2 will produce only a small change in SaO_2. A normal PaO_2/FiO_2 ratio is ~ 450–500 mm Hg at one atmosphere whereas a P/F ratio below 200 indicates severe hypoxemia.

large increase in PaO_2 will have little effect on arterial O_2 content (at least at one atmosphere pressure).

One way of following the efficiency of gas exchange is to calculate the alveolar-to-arterial oxygen ($PAO_2 - PaO_2$) gradient (or simply called the A–a gradient) (Table 10.2). The normal value for the A–a gradient is 5–10 mm Hg. In general, a "wide" A–a gradient signifies lung pathology that creates problems with gas exchange, whereas a normal gradient implies healthy lungs. However, this index is cumbersome to use, which limits its utility. Further, normal values when breathing supplemental oxygen are not known with certainty, thereby further limiting its clinical usefulness in patients breathing extra oxygen. Another, simpler way of following changes in arterial oxygenation is to calculate the P/F ratio. The P/F ratio is PaO_2 / FiO_2 with the FiO_2 representing

the fraction of inspired oxygen. At one atmosphere pressure and breathing normal air ($FiO_2 = 0.21$), the P/F ratio for a non-intubated, healthy young person is in the 450–500 mm Hg range. Intuitively it is clear that a low P/F ratio indicates a problem with gas exchange, because it suggests that the PaO_2 is low despite a high FiO_2. You should be aware that the P/F ratio tells us nothing about alveolar ventilation and that in ventilated patients, the ratio will also be dependent upon the level of applied positive end expiratory pressure (PEEP), or continuous positive airway pressure (CPAP). For the purpose of research, the P/F ratio is often used to define acute respiratory distress syndrome (ARDS) and is a P/F 200 mm Hg with PEEP of 5 cm H_2O and acute lung injury (ALI) is a P/F 300 mm Hg with PEEP 5 cm H_2O.

● Physiologic Mechanisms of Hypoxemia

In the critically ill, hypoxemia is most commonly due to ventilation-perfusion (V/Q) mismatch and/or intrapulmonary shunt. However, it is important to understand and appreciate the different mechanisms that can contribute to a patient's hypoxemia. The six physiologic mechanisms that result in hypoxemia are:

1. Low Inspired Partial Pressure of O_2 (PiO_2) – This results from high altitude or disconnection of oxygen tubing. Note that even at high altitude, the FiO_2 remains the same at sea level (i.e., 0.21 if breathing air). For example at the top of Mount Everest, the FiO_2 is still 0.21, but due to low barometric pressure and despite hyperventilation to a $PaCO_2$ of 12 mm Hg, the measured PaO_2 may be as low as 30 mm Hg.

2. Hypoventilation – This can cause hypoxemia, as can be seen from an analysis of the ($PAO_2 - PaO_2$) equation. However if the patient is receiving supplemental oxygen (e.g., by mask or nasal prongs), oxygen saturation may be maintained despite significant hypoventilation, at least initially. The degree of hypoventilation is best measured by the $PaCO_2$ level.

3. Ventilation-Perfusion (V/Q) Mismatch – Ventilation-perfusion (V/Q) mismatch refers to inappropriately low ventilation relative to perfusion

(Figure 10.2). Generally the overall ventilation and perfusion of the lungs are well-matched (V/Q ~ 1). Hypoxemia that results from V/Q mismatch will usually respond to an increase in FiO_2.

4. Shunting – This is an extreme form of V/Q mismatch (Figure 10.2). Shunts are either intrapulmonary or intracardiac. An intrapulmonary shunt develops when alveoli that are perfused are not ventilated (V/Q = 0). The venous blood flows through non-ventilated alveoli and enters the systemic circulation (via the pulmonary veins) with the local PO_2 unchanged in lung units with the shunt. Note that with a true shunt, there can be little effect on PaO_2 from an increase in FiO_2. The oxygen content of blood leaving the healthy alveoli hardly increases as the FiO_2 is increased from air to 100% because of the shape of the oxyhemoglobin dissociation curve (Figure 10.1). The curve demonstrates that even at a PaO_2 of 1 atmosphere (760 mm Hg), the arterial O_2 content will increase by at most one volume percent. Thus, the healthy alveoli can never compensate for the sick ones. Simply increasing the FiO_2 is insufficient to affect the desaturated blood that comes from the shunt alveoli. The lower saturated blood will mix with the fully saturated blood from the healthy units but the end result is still that of blood with a poor overall saturation. It is not uncommon to see shunt fractions of 50% or more in severe lung disease and in this setting oxygenation can only be improved if therapy results in recruitment of shunt units (i.e., the V/Q improves). Intracardiac shunts (right-to-left shunts) can also lead to hypoxemia. While shunting could result from multiple congenital cardiac defects, the most common cause of intracardiac shunting in the adult critically ill patient is shunting through a patent foramen ovale in the presence of pulmonary hypertension.

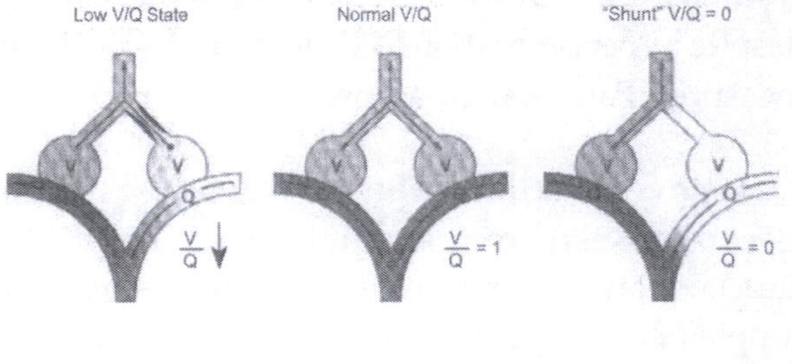

5. Low Mixed Venous Oxygen Saturation (SvO_2) – This can result from either a low cardiac output or an increased O_2 consumption. A low cardiac output will lower the SvO_2 because the tissues compensate by increasing their O_2 extraction. Normally, a low SvO_2 does not lead to significant hypoxemia in the presence of normal lungs. However, in the presence of a large shunt, any reduction in the O_2 content of the shunted blood will further lower the PaO_2. For example, in a patient with a shunt fraction of 50%, if the SvO_2 was 70%, the final saturation of the blood would be approximately 85% (the shunted half of the blood would have a saturation of 70% the other half would be 100% and thus the final average would be 85%). If the SvO_2 were to decrease to 40%, the final saturation of the blood returning to the left side of the heart would now be 70%. In this setting, an improvement in cardiac output or a decrease in O_2 consumption may lead to a significant increase in PaO_2.

6. Diffusion Abnormality – This can theoretically contribute to hypoxemia, particularly during exercise. It is probably a contributing factor for hypoxemia in diffuse lung disease. However, it is not practical to measure diffusion in the critically ill and it is simply assumed that diffusion improves as the underlying disease responds to treatment.

● **Ventilation**

The best measure of ventilation is the $PaCO_2$. The level of CO_2 in the blood, however, does not only depend upon ventilation but also on CO_2 production. However, high CO_2 production will not lead to clinically significant hypercapnia in the absence of some impairment of alveolar ventilation (Table 10.2).

1. Alveolar Ventilation – This is essentially that portion of the inspired air that comes into contact with alveoli and blood flow and thus contributes to gas exchange.

Figure 10.2 – Ventilation-Perfusion Relationships

Figure 10.2 shows the range of ventilation to perfusion (V/Q) matching in the lung, from dead space ventilation (Q approaches zero) to a shunt (V approaches zero).

2. Dead Space Ventilation – This is also called "wasted" ventilation, in that the air flows in and out of the lungs but never comes in contact with pulmonary blood flow and thus does not contribute to gas exchange. The normal dead space to tidal volume ratio (known as VD/VT) is approximately 0.3. The physiologic dead space consists of both the anatomic dead space and alveolar dead space.

i. anatomic dead space – This consists of the volume of air occupying the mouth, pharynx, trachea and all the way down to the respiratory bronchioles. Its normal volume is approximately 150 ml.

ii. alveolar dead space – This consists of alveoli that are ventilated but not perfused and therefore do not contribute to gas exchange. Normal lungs have very little alveolar dead space. Patients with lung disease (e.g., emphysema) may have a large alveolar dead space and these patients will require a high minute ventilation to maintain a normal $PaCO_2$. Pulmonary embolism is a cause of alveolar dead space where the V/Q = infinity (Figure 10.2). In practice, however, massive occlusion of the pulmonary vasculature by pulmonary emboli is required to result in significant hypercapnia (Q reduced by at least 70%). In fact, most pulmonary emboli are associated with an increased drive to breathe, which may result in hypocapnia as patients often overcompensate for the increased dead space.

iii. total dead space – In mechanically ventilated patients, this consists of the sum of anatomic, alveolar and equipment dead spaces (Figure 10.3). The equipment dead space in ventilated patients is due to tubing and connectors and is usually very small. The dead space of an endotracheal tube is actually less than the normal anatomic dead space of the nose and pharynx.

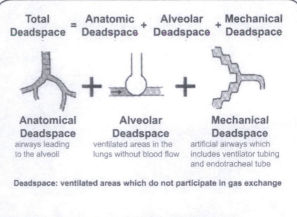

Figure 10.3 – Dead Space Ventilation

Figure 10.3 illustrates the various forms of dead space ventilation. The total amount is the sum of both anatomical dead space (conducting airways that do not participate in gas exchange), alveolar dead space (ventilated alveoli that are not perfused) and finally the volume lost to the ventilator tubing and endotracheal tube.

● Minute Ventilation (MV)

The minute ventilation refers to the total amount of gas inhaled (in litres) per minute and represents the sum of the alveolar ventilation and dead space ventilation. It is the product of the respiratory rate and tidal volume. The normal minute ventilation is approximately 6–8 l/min. A high minute ventilation has many potential causes including pain, anxiety, increased metabolic drive to breathe (e.g., pregnancy), hypoxemia, lung disease itself associated with high dead space ventilation (e.g., pulmonary edema, pulmonary fibrosis, ARDS, pulmonary embolism, COPD, etc.) and states where there is a high CO_2 production (e.g., sepsis, fever, thyrotoxicosis, etc.).

Key Points

- Oxygen content is primarily a reflection of oxygen bound to hemoglobin.
- Oxygen delivery is the product of oxygen content and the cardiac output.
- The most important causes of hypoxemia are V/Q mismatch and shunting.

- $PaCO_2$ is the best indication of the adequacy of alveolar ventilation.
- Physiologic dead space consists of both anatomic and alveolar dead space.
- A reasonable and safe oxygenation goal is an SaO_2 of 88%.
- Modest hypercapnia is generally well-tolerated.

CHAPTER 11

EARLY MANAGEMENT OF RESPIRATORY FAILURE

RICHARD HODDER,
PIERRE CARDINAL, AND
LOIS CHAMPION

While in the emergency department (ED) assessing an intubated patient with a sedative overdose prior to transfer to the ICU, you are asked to see another patient who is not doing well. Mr. Puffer is a 63-year-old heavy smoker with known COPD who visits the ED two or three times a year with a COPD exacerbation. His last admission to hospital was two months ago, during which he was successfully managed on the ward and discharged home after five days. He has known coronary artery disease as he had an MI three years ago but does not have angina. The rest of his past history is unremarkable. He takes salbutamol, ipratropium and budesonide inhalers, atenolol, and enteric-coated aspirin. He has not been on oral corticosteroids since his last admission and is not on long-term oxygen therapy. Prior to discharge from hospital two months ago, his pulmonary function tests were: FVC 68% predicted, FEV1 35% predicted, FEV1/FVC 0.40, PaO_2 78 mm Hg breathing air, $PaCO_2$ 47 mm Hg, pH 7.39, and a hemoglobin level of 124 g/L.

For the past week, Mr. Puffer has had an increase in his usual cough and mucoid phlegm, and he has been getting more breathless with his usual activities. Yesterday the phlegm turned yellow and was stickier and more difficult to cough up. He started taking some amoxicillin left over from his last admission, but last night could not sleep because of breathlessness. This morning he called 911 and came to the ED. During the ambulance ride he was put on oxygen at 2 l/min and upon arrival this was continued. He underwent a chest radiograph, received 8 puffs each of salbutamol and ipratropium, and was started on IV cefuroxime and dexamethasone. An arterial stab was attempted, but it was presumed venous, as the results were: pH 7.23, $PaCO_2$ 69, PaO_2 45, SaO_2 76%.

When you examine Mr. Puffer, you note that he is drowsy, but able to carry on an accurate conversation punctuated with pauses for breath. He says that he is very breathless and a bit frightened. He cannot get comfortable and is sitting upright on the stretcher. His respiratory rate is 30 bpm, his heart rate is irregular *between 119–130 bpm. The remainder of his vital signs include a BP of 165/60, temperature of 36.7°C and an oxygen saturation (Sao_2) of 85% on O_2 at 2 l/min via nasal cannulae. The ECG monitor shows atrial fibrillation but there are no obvious signs of ischemia. He is a thin man and is using both his accessory inspiratory neck muscles and his abdominal expiratory muscles with each breath. There is indrawing in the supraclavicular region and his costal margins move inward during inspiration (Hoover's sign). Inspiratory breath sounds can be heard throughout the lung fields, but almost no sounds can be heard over the lung fields during exhalation except perhaps an intermittent, faint, high-pitched wheeze. While listening over the trachea however, expiratory breath sounds can be heard and they persist right up until the next inspiration. Heart tones are faint but normal. There is neither central nor peripheral cyanosis.*

The patient, Mr. Puffer, certainly appears to be quite sick. Several questions about what to do for him are apparent. Does Mr. Puffer have acute respiratory failure? What are your immediate concerns? What are your initial management goals and how will you accomplish them? The goal of this chapter is to use this case is to illustrate an approach to a patient in respiratory failure.

● Respiratory Failure

Acute respiratory failure may be simply defined as "any impairment of O_2 uptake or CO_2 elimination or both that is severe enough to be a threat to life." This definition implies that the delivery of oxygen to the tissues is an important factor and emphasizes the important interrelationship of the pulmonary and cardiac systems (Equation 11.1). Although this definition describes a fundamental concept, it is not likely to be very helpful at the bedside, where we

Equation 11.1

Oxygen Delivery = Cardiac Output × [(1.34 × Hgb × SaO_2) + (0.0031 × PaO_2)]

are concerned primarily with treating our patients' symptoms and ensuring their safety and not with labelling them as being either in or out of "respiratory failure." Nevertheless, it is important to have an understanding of what constitutes a dangerous gas exchange abnormality, so we can act to prevent or correct it.

What then is a dangerous level of hypoxia or hypoxemia, and what is a dangerous level of hypercapnia? The answer, as is often the case, is not always clear, and so a logical (albeit unhelpful) response is: "it depends" (Text Box 11.1). While most people would not be at immediate risk of dying with a Pao_2 of 50 mm Hg, this level of hypoxemia might be very dangerous in a patient whose oxygen delivery is already compromised. Such a patient might be severely anemic or hypotensive or have acute coronary insufficiency or heart failure. Similarly, in a young person obtunded from a sedative overdose, a $PaCO_2$ of 70 mm Hg and a pH of 7.16 are unlikely to be life-threatening.[15,17] Other factors, such as the attendant hypoxemia, hypotension and inability to protect the airway, rather than the hypercarbia, are most likely to threaten the life of such a patient, and it is these issues that would require prompt attention.

Although blood gases should never be interpreted in isolation, since they must be assessed in the context of the patient's clinical situation, there are clearly thresholds of blood gas derangement that should be considered warning signs and should not go unheeded. Hypoxemia as defined by an acute fall in PaO_2 to less than 50–55 mm Hg, or an SaO_2 less than 85–88% is important, because it defines a significant loss of homeostasis and defines a status of minimal oxygenation reserve for the patient. Similarly, an acute rise in $PaCO_2$ causing a fall in pH to less than 7.20–7.30 cannot be ignored, because it also indicates a potentially dangerous loss of ventilatory reserve and capacity, and equally importantly, probably a fatiguing patient. Patients with these degrees of blood gas derangement need to be watched closely and managed aggressively, lest they suddenly lose their remaining reserves and plummet into cardiorespiratory collapse.

● Classifying Respiratory Failure

Traditionally, respiratory failure is divided into a primary failure to oxygenate, so-called hypoxemic

What is a dangerous PaO_2, SaO_2?

If the atmospheric pressure was suddenly reduced so that your PaO_2 fell to 50 mm Hg (SaO_2 85%), all other things being equal, you would not be in danger (except perhaps from whatever caused the precipitous fall in atmospheric pressure!). Even with an SaO_2 of 85%, you still have a reasonable arterial oxygen content to go along with your normal cardiac output and oxygen uptake. You might even scarcely notice the hypoxemia, apart from some mild breathlessness secondary to hypoxic drive–induced tachypnea. Consider also the extreme blood gas abnormalities experienced by those remarkable individuals who can climb Mt Everest[1] without supplemental oxygen (e.g., PaO_2 30 mm Hg, $PaCO_2$ 12 mm Hg, pH 7.57). The pathogenesis of the acute mountain sickness that these individuals may experience is not clear, but is thought to reflect neuroendocrine effects of hypobarism and the consequences of extreme hypocarbia, rather than hypoxemia.[2] Even patients with COPD have been observed to have no symptoms or complications attributable to hypoxemia at levels of PaO_2 of 45–55 mm Hg when travelling in commercial aircraft pressurized to approximately 8000 ft (2438 m).[3-4]

Warning blood gas thresholds – (Oxygenation)

SaO_2 <85–88%, or PaO_2 <50–55 mm Hg (regardless of FiO_2)

What is a dangerous $PaCO_2$ or pH?

The presence of acidemia, whether respiratory or metabolic, indicates a loss of physiologic homeostasis and the presence of disease or dysfunction, and may even be predictive of death in certain situations such as cardiac arrest[5] and sepsis.[6] However these data indicate an association rather than a cause and effect relationship. Indeed, the systemic consequences of respiratory acidosis are relatively benign, even if the pH falls to 7.15, with the typical patient experiencing either no change or only slight increases in cardiac output and systemic blood pressure.[7-8] The safety of hypercapnic acidosis is fairly well documented in the critical care literature,[9-12] even with pH levels well below 7.20. It is interesting to note that the time-honoured concept of so-called "CO_2 narcosis" has been challenged.[13-14,16] Although CO_2 has anesthetic properties, it requires extreme levels, far above what is common clinically. When hypercapnia is observed in a drowsy patient, it is usually seen in the context of concomitant hypoxemia and patient fatigue from prolonged periods of high work of breathing, so that there are multifactorial causes for the observed altered level of consciousness. Thus although acidosis is common in critical illness, it is more of a marker of disease and of severity, than a cause of morbidity itself. It is the cause of the underlying disease, rather than the acidosis that is more likely to be the determining factor in outcome.[15]

Warning blood gas thresholds – (Ventilation)

Any rise in PCO_2 associated with a pH <7.20–7.30

---

failure, or a primary failure to ventilate, so-called hypercapnic or hypoventilatory failure (Figure 11.1). Examples of primarily hypoxemic failure include severe pneumonia, pulmonary edema and acute respiratory distress syndrome (ARDS). Quite often, early on in the course of hypoxemic failure, there is a high drive to breathe due to the stimulation from hypoxemia, various lung and airway receptors and the disease process itself. The increased respiratory drive allows the spared and relatively healthy lung regions to actually support alveolar hyperventilation and produce an initial hypocapnic respiratory alkalosis, despite significant hypoxemia. However, as the disease process advances and fewer normal lung regions remain, or if there is concurrent CNS depression or respiratory muscles fatigue due to the increased ventilatory loads, alveolar hypoventilation may supervene and the $PaCO_2$ begins to rise and cause secondary hypercapnia. This is a reason why a normal or rising $PaCO_2$ is a cause for concern, as it indicates

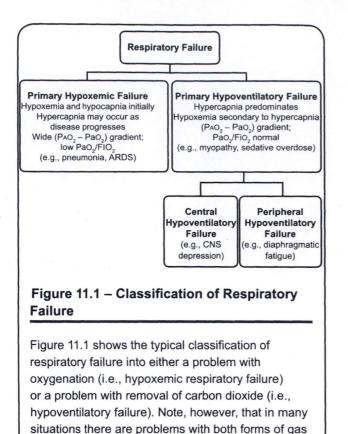

Figure 11.1 – Classification of Respiratory Failure

Figure 11.1 shows the typical classification of respiratory failure into either a problem with oxygenation (i.e., hypoxemic respiratory failure) or a problem with removal of carbon dioxide (i.e., hypoventilatory failure). Note, however, that in many situations there are problems with both forms of gas exchange.

the patient's loss of ventilatory reserve. In primary hypoxemic failure, the ($P_{A}O_2 - PaO_2$) gradient or the PaO_2/FiO_2 is abnormal, both indicating that the lungs are sick.

Primary hypercapnic respiratory failure can be further subdivided into failure of the respiratory centres (central failure), or failure of the ventilatory pump (peripheral failure). The ventilatory pump consists of the chest wall, diaphragm and accessory muscles of breathing. Patients with peripheral failure of the ventilatory pump often work very hard to breathe (e.g., in kyphoscoliosis, myopathy or acute COPD), but cannot breathe effectively and so develop hypercapnia. Ventilatory pump failure also commonly occurs if primary hypoxemic failure is sustained and the diaphragm begins to fail due to high breathing loads. Patients with central respiratory failure usually show no signs of distress and have a decreased respiratory rate (e.g., with narcotic or sedative overdoses, brain tumor, etc.). These patients may have healthy lungs, and hypoxemia is secondary to the hypercapnia, as evidenced by a normal ($P_{A}O_2 - PaO_2$) gradient, or normal PaO_2/FiO_2 ratio.

The classification of acute respiratory failure (Figure 11.1), although artificial, is nonetheless useful in that it allows one to conveniently divide patients into well-defined categories. These categories of respiratory failure help to narrow the differential diagnosis and facilitate further investigations and therapy. There are, however, limitations to this approach and patients often present with a mixed picture characterized by both hypoxemic and hypocapnic respiratory failure (e.g., acute COPD exacerbation in a patient with chronic hypercapnia). In addition, this classification is based on arterial blood gases (ABG). Unfortunately, as discussed below, obtaining an ABG should not be a primary preoccupation in the early management of the patient with possible respiratory failure. A more rational and efficient approach to the patient with suspected respiratory failure relies mostly on clinical examination and other tests such as oximetry, which are readily available at the bedside. Once the patient has been stabilized, therapy should be refined to treat and prevent potential complications of respiratory failure, and of course to treat the underlying cause.

● Recognizing Respiratory Failure

We have chosen to define and to classify acute respiratory failure in terms of blood gas and SaO_2 criteria. Therefore, to confirm the presence of respiratory failure, this data must be obtained, but it does not follow that an arterial puncture is immediately necessary for this purpose. An analysis of the oxygenation and acid-base status of any patient can be quickly obtained from the SaO_2 (sometimes referred to as SpO_2) reading of a pulse oximeter and from a venous blood gas sample (Text Box 11.2).

While it may be easy to establish a diagnosis once all investigations are available, testing takes time and therapy cannot be unduly delayed. Even without gas exchange data, a thoughtful clinical examination should raise the possibility of respiratory failure. The signs and symptoms of respiratory failure (i.e., dangerous gas exchange abnormalities) are non-specific (and often non-respiratory) and mainly reflect end organ dysfunction of the neurologic and cardiovascular systems (Table 11.1).

Signs and symptoms specific to the respiratory system (e.g., wheeze, breathlessness, cough), while indicative of significant lung disease, do not

Oximetry

Oximetry offers a quick, non-invasive, real-time indication of oxygenation status, provided a few caveats are recognized. Old style oximeters could be fooled by nail polish and tended to indicate a falsely reassuring SpO_2 of 85% if not attached to the patient. These deficiencies have largely been eliminated by the development of pulse oximeters that require pulsatile blood flow to function properly. They can thus give false results if applied to extremities (digits, earlobes, nose) in patients with global (e.g., severe heart failure) or local (e.g., ischemic extremity, generalized peripheral vasoconstriction) poor perfusion. Pulse oximeters must track the pulse, so if the pulse indicated by the oximeter is discordant with the pulse you count or record on the ECG monitor, the SpO_2 indicated is not reliable and should be ignored. Pulse oximeters are accurate to ±2–3% over the usual range of clinical interest, and tend to be less reliable if the SaO_2 is <80%, but if the reading is that low, the details are not important, because you know your patient has a serious oxygenation problem. If working properly, pulse oximeter SpO_2 data is preferred over a PaO_2, because it is a better index of arterial oxygen content than a PaO_2, is easier to obtain and provides continuous real-time data that an ABG cannot.

Venous Blood Gases

Under most circumstances, there is good correlation between the pH, and PCO_2 values obtained by venous and arterial sampling.[17] In general, regardless of the absolute value, the $PvCO_2$ will always be about 5 mm Hg higher than the corresponding $PaCO_2$, and the venous pH only slightly lower. Obviously, the PvO_2 or SvO_2 cannot be used to assess the state of arterial oxygenation, and it is prudent to always check the source of the blood gas data, lest patients be unnecessarily intubated, for false hypoxemia, for example. Venous blood gases are easier to obtain and less traumatic for the patient, and the sample can be taken by anyone skilled at venipuncture.

End-Tidal CO_2

End-tidal CO_2 monitors are very useful for confirming correct position of the endotracheal tube and it is tempting to want to use them as a convenient, non-invasive means of estimating $PaCO_2$. However, although there is reasonable correlation of $PETCO_2$ and $PaCO_2$ ($PETCO_2 - PaCO_2 \sim 5$ mm Hg) in healthy individuals who have cardiovascular stability, critically ill patients are usually too unstable on several fronts to make $PETCO_2$ a reliable index of $PaCO_2$, in this setting.[18–22]

necessarily define the presence of dangerous gas exchange. Notwithstanding these observations, there are some important respiratory warning signs that should not be ignored. Although non-specific, a high respiratory rate is one of the most sensitive signs of respiratory failure. For example, in the setting of community-acquired pneumonia, a breathing rate above 30 per minute correlates with an increased

Table 11.1 – Clinical Signs and Symptoms of Respiratory Failure

General	Cardiovascular	Neurologic	
tachypnea	tachycardia	restlessness	asterixis
breathlessness	dysrhythmias	headache	seizures
diaphoresis	hypertension	confusion	drowsiness
central cyanosis (late)	hypotension	delirium	coma
		tremor	

risk of dying from the pneumonia.[23] Similarly, an increasing respiratory rate compared to baseline is of greater significance and urgency than an elevated but stable rate in a patient with COPD. Use of accessory breathing muscles, in particular use of the inspiratory parasternal and scalene muscles and abdominal muscles on expiration, indicates that the work of breathing is excessive and strongly suggests a serious underlying respiratory problem, which if not remedied, may progress to respiratory muscle fatigue and failure. In acute asthma or COPD, for example, use of inspiratory accessory muscles is usually a sign of worsening hyperinflation and use of abdominal muscles to assist exhalation signifies a high degree of airflow obstruction, even in the absence of audible wheezing. When breathing muscle fatigue occurs, the usual sequence of events is dyspnea, followed by tachypnea, then use of accessory breathing muscles, at which time the $PaCO_2$ may still be normal or even low. Only when diaphragm fatigue and failure supervene does $PaCO_2$ begin to rise as a relatively late manifestation. Thus, waiting for the $PaCO_2$ to rise to warning thresholds before intervening may delay the diagnosis and put patients at risk unnecessarily.

Patients in respiratory failure may present either in obvious respiratory distress or with a somewhat calm appearance, if the ventilatory drive is depressed. For example, the patient with primary central hypoventilatory failure usually presents with a depressed level of consciousness and a decreased respiratory rate. Not surprisingly, the most common cause of central hypoventilatory failure is sedative or narcotic overdose (either intentional or not) and, unfortunately, all too often the diagnosis is delayed, with the patient being found unresponsive in the middle of the night, having been presumed to be sleeping. Recognizing a patient with primary hypoxemic respiratory failure is usually more straightforward, particularly if the patient presents with a high respiratory rate, use of accessory muscles, intercostal indrawing and marked anxiety. However, the diagnosis can often be much more subtle. For example, older patients with a co-morbid illness such as COPD, may develop primary hypoxemic respiratory failure (e.g., pneumonia). However, due to weak respiratory muscles that quickly fatigue, they may paradoxically present with very few signs of overt breathing distress as they succumb to overwhelming fatigue. Clinically, they may seem merely to be very

drowsy, but blood gas analysis reveals a combination of hypoxemic and hypoventilatory failure. Similarly, the patient with Guillain-Barré syndrome may be in impending or even established respiratory failure, yet only present with a high respiratory rate, with few other signs, other than paralysis and a sense of air hunger, or dyspnea (be careful not to simply ascribe this to "anxiety"). Let's apply this discussion to our patient Mr. Puffer. Does he have respiratory failure?

As discussed earlier, labelling Mr. Puffer is not as important as recognizing that he is clearly in a precarious and potentially dangerous situation. Even without any blood gas data, it should be obvious that he is in danger of quickly progressing to cardiorespiratory collapse and could perish if not managed aggressively. He is tachycardic with new onset atrial fibrillation. Mr. Puffer is tachypneic and unable to speak without having to pause and catch his breath. Understandably, he is frightened, anxious, restless and drowsy. His work of breathing is high and he must use his accessory muscles of breathing. Clearly, he is manifesting signs of progressive air trapping and dynamic hyperinflation and is likely to progress to overt respiratory collapse without quick and aggressive intervention. The presence of dangerous blood gases is confirmed by the observation of an SaO_2 of only 85% despite the administration of supplemental oxygen, and venous blood gases indicate a significant acute respiratory acidosis. Action is required to save Mr. Puffer.

● Initial Management of Respiratory Failure: The Primary Assessment

When confronted with a patient with possible respiratory failure, the experienced clinician begins an instinctive, coordinated combination of assessment and concurrent initial management, based on basic principles and past experience. This is called the *primary assessment*, and involves a rapid initial evaluation for danger signs and the simultaneous institution of therapy, even before a firm diagnosis is reached. The conventional approach, which consists of a thorough history, followed by a complete physical examination, and then investigations and treatment is often inappropriate in critically ill patients, when things are moving quickly and time is limited. When you first walk into the room to assess your patient, you should quickly assess not only the patient, but also the overall situation including the resources available and any initial management that has already been started.

An example of a general approach to the primary assessment is to first scan the room and then scan the patient to answer several important questions. The scan of the room is to assess what is available and present in the immediate area. Is help—such as a nurse, respiratory therapist, physicians or family members—available or do you need to call for it? Has supplemental oxygen been started? Does the patient have an intravenous running? What monitors are available? Especially important is the use of an oximeter and an electrocardiogram. As you complete the scan of the room, your attention turns quickly to the patient and it is important to follow a logical approach to assessment. The ABC's again form the basis of assessing a patient in respiratory distress. First examine the patient for signs of upper airway obstruction. The ability to talk and the absence of inspiratory stridor, usually excludes upper airway pathology. The initial respiratory exam should be limited to a quick inspection, palpation and auscultation to quickly assess the respiratory system. The respiratory rate, use of accessory muscles of inspiration or expiration, midline trachea and asymmetrical movement of both hemithoraces (e.g., pneumothorax, large effusion) are important observations. Auscultation to identify asymmetry of breath sounds such as the absence of expiratory breath sounds (e.g., extreme hyperinflation, bilateral pneumothoraces) is critical to identify these life-threatening problems. Listening is also important to identify the presence of diffuse crackles (e.g., pulmonary edema, fibrosis), musical wheezes (e.g., asthma, COPD) or focal, monophonic wheezes (e.g., large airway obstruction). Finally, it is important to auscultate the expiratory sounds to identify air trapping, which is suggested by the air flow right up to the next inspiration.[24]

One should always assess the "vital pump" (the respiratory muscles, particularly the diaphragm) for signs of excess ventilatory loads that might foretell impending respiratory muscle failure.[25] Two of the signs that indicate excess loading of the respiratory muscles are *Hoover's sign* and *paradoxical abdominal breathing*. Hoover's sign is present when the lateral walls of the lower rib cage move inward instead of outward during inspiration and it caries a poor prognosis. This appears to be primarily related to the presence of very high airway resistance, which leads to exaggerated negative intrathoracic pressure during inspiration, and usually indicates severe airway obstruction (e.g., acute asthma, COPD and possibly upper airway obstruction). Paradoxical abdominal breathing is when the abdomen moves inward instead of outward with inspiration. This occurs when the inspiratory load becomes excessive due to advancing disease. Hyperinflation shortens the resting length of the diaphragm which then is no longer able to generate sufficient tension, and gets pulled up by the negative pressure created by the accessory inspiratory muscles. This results in a paradoxical inward displacement of the abdomen during inspiration. This is a sign of very high inspiratory loads and a weakened diaphragm in the patient with respiratory failure and usually indicates that ventilatory support will soon be needed.

Concurrent with this brief initial examination, ideally an oximeter should be placed for measurement of the oxygen saturation in all patients with respiratory distress. If an assistant is present, blood should also be drawn for initial biochemistry, hematology and venous blood gas assessment. Very few respiratory conditions necessitate immediate intervention at this stage, except possibly for an obvious tension pneumothorax. A tension pneumothorax is a rare occurrence unless a patient has had a procedure (e.g., line insertion, thoracentesis), or is a trauma victim. Even patients who are mechanically ventilated rarely develop a pneumothorax unless they are being ventilated with excessive volumes and pressures. If the clinical suspicion is high, or if the clinical examination leaves absolutely no doubt as to this diagnosis, immediately insert a needle into the second intercostal space followed by a chest tube. However, for patients at lower risk of developing a pneumothorax, there is often sufficient time to confirm the diagnosis with an x-ray.

● Empiric Oxygen Therapy

Usually, when respiratory failure is highly likely, the administration of empiric oxygen is the most prudent course. The methods of delivering initial oxygen therapy in respiratory failure are outlined below (Text Box 11.3). Regardless of the delivery method used,

Text Box 11.3 – Oxygen Therapy Options

Nasal Cannulae or Simple Face Masks

These devices deliver 100% oxygen from the oxygen source at flow rates that usually vary from 1 to 6 litres per minute (l/min). While the flow of oxygen is known, the exact concentration delivered to the patient is not known. The final concentration depends on the patient's inspiratory flow rates, as well as the oxygen flow rates. For example, imagine a patient who inhales at a modest flow rate of 18 l/min while receiving oxygen at a rate of 6 l/min. The mixture of 6 l/min of 100% oxygen with 12 l/min of room air (21% oxygen) determines the final concentration of oxygen, which in this instance will be 48%. Note that the concentration of oxygen varies throughout inspiration, with the highest concentrations observed at the end of a breath, when inspiratory flows are lowest. It follows that in critically ill patients, the use of either nasal prongs or simple masks is often inadequate in delivering a high and reliable oxygen concentration. If you have any doubt as to whether or not the delivery of oxygen is sufficient, simply measure the response using a pulse oximeter and adjust the oxygen concentration appropriately. With nasal cannulae, for every 1 l/min oxygen flow, the FiO_2 rises by 2–4 %. However, in somnolent patients with slow breathing rates, nasal O_2 at 4–6 l/min can provide an FiO_2 approximating 50%, if there is little entrainment of ambient air. Unless there is complete nasal occlusion, mouth breathing does not usually have a big impact on the FiO_2 delivered by nasal cannulae.

Fixed Performance Venturi Masks

These masks provide very reliable concentrations of oxygen from 24 to 50%. While these masks will not deliver more than the set oxygen concentration, they may deliver less if the patient entrains more air by hyperventilating. In addition, humidification of the oxygen source is not usually recommended with these masks, as condensation could change the inspiratory velocities and hence the resultant concentration of oxygen.

Non-rebreathing Masks

These masks are equipped with a plastic bag that fills with 100% oxygen and serves as a reservoir in the event that the inspiratory flow exceeds the delivered flow of oxygen. The inspiratory flow used with non-rebreathing masks varies from 10 to >15 l/min. Flows should be increased whenever the plastic bag is noted to deflate on inspiration. Even though non-rebreathing masks indicate that the patient is receiving 100% oxygen, entrainment of air around the masks usually limits them to delivering only 60–70% oxygen. Once again, it is more important to determine whether the oxygen being delivered is adequate by pulse oximetry, than to dwell on the theoretical FiO_2 being delivered. It is worth noting, however, that a non-rebreathing mask is the best we can do without resorting to either invasive or non-invasive positive pressure ventilation to improve the patient's oxygenation.

---

however, the most important principle is to assess the adequacy of the oxygen therapy often, and this is most conveniently done with a pulse oximeter.

Particularly in the setting of COPD, concern is frequently expressed that empiric administration of high concentrations of oxygen may result in a dangerous rise in $PaCO_2$, and CO_2 narcosis, secondary to elimination of the so-called hypoxic drive to breathe. As discussed earlier, this is probably an unwarranted fear, as the existence of CO_2 narcosis is controversial,[13] and more importantly, untreated hypoxia is much more dangerous than hypercapnia. It appears that when supplemental oxygen is administered to hypoxemic COPD patients, the subsequent rise in $PaCO_2$ is limited and the $PaCO_2$ eventually plateaus. In one study, even when 100% oxygen was given to hypoxemic COPD patients in respiratory failure, $PaCO_2$ rose on average 23 mm Hg over 15 minutes, but no change in level of consciousness was noted.[16] Studies in patients with COPD have shown that when $PaCO_2$ rises in response to oxygen therapy, the causes are multifactorial and certainly not solely due to suppression of the hypoxic drive to breathe.[16,26,27] The rise in $PaCO_2$ is also related to a release of CO_2 from the newly oxygenated hemoglobin (Haldane effect) and possibly also by an increase in V/Q mismatching and an increase in dead space ventilation.

In summary, although $PaCO_2$ may rise somewhat in hypoxic COPD in response to oxygen therapy, the magnitude of hypercarbia is small and not usually clinically relevant. Reduced minute ventilation in this setting is more commonly due to fatigue from the increased work of breathing due to the underlying pulmonary disease than to oxygen therapy.

In patients who are severely hypoxemic, it is probably best to start with an inspired oxygen concentration of as close to 100%, as possible, because the greatest danger is uncorrected hypoxemia. Rather than exposing the patient to a prolonged period of potentially dangerous hypoxemia, by starting therapy with low concentrations of oxygen, it is preferable to secure an adequate SpO_2 percentage using "enough" oxygen, and then to titrate down the oxygen concentration later. On the other hand, in patients with only modest hypoxemia, and in particular those with acute COPD, it is probably prudent to begin with low flow oxygen, or low FiO_2 Venturi masks, and to follow the SpO_2 response closely and often. The oxygen concentration need only be titrated to achieve a modest goal of arterial oxygenation, such as an SpO_2 percentage of 88–90% by pulse oximeter.

The response to oxygen therapy may provide important clues to the etiology of the respiratory failure. The hypoxemia of patients with central hypoventilatory failure, or with an exacerbation of COPD or asthma, for example, will usually easily correct with a relatively low concentration of oxygen. For example, a patient with a narcotic overdose and a $PaCO_2$ as high as 80 mm Hg could have an SaO_2 of 100% on an FiO_2 as low as 0.30 if the lungs were otherwise normal. On the other hand, failure to rapidly correct hypoxemia suggests diseases that produce a severe intrapulmonary shunt (i.e., alveoli that are perfused but not ventilated) such as a pneumonia, ARDS, or a right to left intracardiac shunt, as is occasionally seen in the patient with a patent foramen ovale and pulmonary hypertension (Chapter 10). Hypoxemia that is not corrected by a high inspired concentration of oxygen should be recognized early and should trigger the physician to consider alternative therapies, such as assisted ventilation (either invasive or non-invasive).

Non-invasive Ventilation by Bag and Mask

Patients with reduced breathing drive, or those with high drive but weak respiratory muscles may not be able to maintain safe blood gases without assisted ventilation. If there is time to work on reversible causes of respiratory failure (e.g., pulmonary edema, acute asthma, COPD, etc.), non-invasive ventilation may be preferable to intubation and mechanical ventilation (see below and Chapter 12).

Bag-mask ventilation is a short-term form of non-invasive ventilation that is most commonly used for patients with central respiratory failure and a depressed level of consciousness while waiting for more definitive intervention, such as the administration of naloxone, the establishment of non-invasive positive pressure ventilation (NPPV), or intubation and ventilation. A trial of bag-mask ventilation can also provide useful information about the patient and the nature of the breathing problem in a short period of time. For example: Is the patient easy to ventilate, or must you use a lot of force to generate shallow tidal breaths? High ventilating pressures indicate either obstruction to airflow (e.g., upper airway obstruction or diffuse bronchospasm), or low respiratory system compliance (e.g., pulmonary edema, high abdominal pressures). You may thus wish to bag-mask ventilate the patient yourself to get a "feel" for the patient's respiratory mechanics. Generally, it is prudent to delegate bag-mask ventilation to someone else who is qualified, as this frees your mind and hands. However, always take care to ensure that your assistant is performing the task well. One major concern with bag-mask ventilation is the possibility of insufflation of air into the stomach, which increases the risk of gastric aspiration. This is particularly likely to occur in patients who require high airway pressures for ventilation. Timing inspiration via the bag with the patient's own inspiratory effort often provides adequate ventilation using the lowest possible airway pressure and is also most comfortable for the patient.

Non-invasive Positive Pressure Ventilation

Non-invasive positive pressure ventilation (NPPV) provides both pressure support (PS) and positive end expiratory pressure (PEEP), also known as continuous positive airway pressure (CPAP). It is indicated as a temporizing measure in order to obviate the need for intubation and invasive ventilation. Implicit in choosing NPPV is the assumption that there is some reversible element of respiratory failure (e.g., pulmonary edema, bronchospasm, muscle fatigue) that can be corrected reasonably quickly (i.e., over a few hours at most). NPPV has been tried in numerous patient populations, and has been most successful in hypercapnic patients with COPD.

Aside from avoiding the many problems associated with tracheal intubation and invasive ventilation, a major advantage of NPPV is that it can be easily removed, even if only temporarily, facilitating assessment of the patient's response to therapy. Non-invasive ventilation is usually reserved for the patient with respiratory failure who is awake and co-operative. The patient must be able to tolerate a tight fitting facial mask, have a low risk of aspiration, and be able to easily clear airway secretions if present. Otherwise, tracheal intubation is usually indicated. Perhaps, Mr. Puffer would benefit from NPPV.

When last seen, our patient Mr. Puffer was not doing too well. He was clearly fatiguing and already had dangerous blood gas levels. While intubation and invasive ventilation was an option for him, he was relatively hemodynamically stable and was not showing signs of acute coronary ischemia. Therefore, it was decided to offer him a trial of NPPV in the hope that he could be rested and made more comfortable while bronchodilators, corticosteroids and antibiotics were given a chance to improve his lung function and reduce his work of breathing, so that intubation might not be necessary. Accordingly, he was given some fentanyl and lorazepam and started on NPPV with inspiratory and expiratory pressures of 10 and 5 cm H$_2$O respectively. Oxygen was titrated to achieve an SaO$_2$ of 88–92%.

● Intubation and Mechanical Ventilation

While non-invasive ventilation will prevent many intubations, as many as one third of patients with respiratory failure treated with non-invasive ventilation will end up requiring intubation. Intubation and mechanical ventilation are often life-saving procedures, however it is difficult to give clear recommendations on whether or not to intubate a given patient. The inability to adequately oxygenate or the inability to ensure adequate ventilation despite aggressive non-invasive therapy are the most common indications for intubation. Intubation is also often indicated for patients who are unable to clear airway secretions due to a weak cough, or who have a depressed level of consciousness and are unable to protect their airways. The patient in respiratory failure who shows signs of hemodynamic instability or who has ongoing cardiac ischemia is often best intubated early, in order to more quickly establish hemodynamic stability and myocardial protection. Intubation and mechanical ventilation can greatly reduce the metabolic demands that overactivity of the respiratory muscles places on the cardiovascular system. An experienced understanding of the specific disease process and the required investigations and therapy will also influence the decision of whether or not to electively intubate. For example, a patient in septic shock with multi-system organ failure who requires aggressive fluid resuscitation and whose oxygenation is deteriorating is often best intubated early, before florid respiratory failure develops. Similarly, patients are often electively intubated to ensure safe transport, or if numerous investigations such as CT scanning are being considered.

Although intubation and mechanical ventilation can save lives, it is important to continually reassess the patient once intubated, as this therapy is not without complications, which can jeopardize successful management of the patient. Once intubated, problems such as hypoxemia, hypercapnia, or hemodynamic instability are no longer only related to the patient's underlying disease, but may now also be related to problems associated with equipment such as the endotracheal tube and mechanical ventilator, or to discoordination between the patient and the ventilator (Table 11.2). For example, deterioration following intubation may be related to tube misplacement, such as a right main stem intubation, or an esophageal intubation, or to the sudden worsening of an existing pneumothorax coincident with the initiation of positive pressure ventilation. If not adequately sedated or given pain relief, the patient may become agitated and interfere with mechanical ventilation, or cause other problems such as biting down on the endotracheal tube, or even unplanned self-extubation.

Optimal ventilator management improves oxygenation and has even been shown to lower mortality in patients with ARDS.[28] Many measures can be undertaken to improve oxygenation during mechanical ventilation, including sedation to improve patient-ventilator synchrony, application of PEEP, alveolar recruitment manoeuvres, prone positioning, inhalation of nitric oxide, and other techniques.[29] Let's once again return to Mr. Puffer, who is still precariously unhappy despite attempts at NPPV.

Unfortunately, Mr. Puffer was not happy with attempts at NPPV, despite sedation and the ministrations of a skilled respiratory therapy staff. He became hypotensive and increasingly agitated, and the decision to intubate for invasive ventilation was made. Initially, following intubation, Mr. Puffer was stable and sleeping. His blood gases, BP and work of breathing all improved. However, a few hours later, at 3:00 AM, you are called by the nurse because Mr. Puffer is "fighting the ventilator." He is diaphoretic, agitated and turning blue. His respiratory rate is 35 bpm on SIMV mode (12 machine breaths and 23 spontaneous breaths). The ventilator is pressure-cycling and delivered tidal volumes of only 250 ml. Heart rate is 140 (atrial fibrillation), BP 90/50 mm Hg, SaO_2 80% with an FiO_2 0.60 and PEEP 10. What could be the problem? What should you do?

There are many possible reasons for Mr. Puffer's agitation and lack of synchronization with the ventilator (Table 11.2). As a first step to solving the problem, you disconnect Mr. Puffer from the ventilator and begin manual bag-mask ventilation. By timing your insufflation with his own rapid breathing efforts, you find that he is relatively easy to ventilate and that he calms down and his vital signs and SaO_2 begin to improve. This is gratifying, as it means that there is unlikely to be some unexpected catastrophe such as a pneumothorax, and that the solution is to give more sedation to Mr. Puffer, so that he will be more comfortable on the ventilator while his COPD exacerbation is being treated.

● Planning More Definitive Therapy

After the primary assessment and initial management, you should have a very good idea of whether or not intubation or the use of NPPV will be necessary. While preparations are being made, take the time to complete your assessment of the patient's hemodynamics (i.e., the *circulation* component of ABC's). If possible, this is also the time to delegate other tasks that need to be done in preparation for more definitive therapy (e.g., ordering medications, intravenous line insertion, preparing the equipment for intubation, etc.). This is

also often a good time to obtain additional history and to complete a more thorough physical examination prior to the institution of more definitive therapy.

Table 11.2 – Causes for Patient-Ventilator Asynchrony ("Fighting the Ventilator")

Ventilator Causes
  Inappropriate Settings
    - trigger sensitivity
    - inspiratory flow rate
    - pressure support level
    - inspiratory time
    - alarm settings
  Circuit Leak/Disconnect
  Device Malfunction
    - exhalation valve
    - humidifier
    - HME device

Endotracheal Tube (ETT) Causes
  Migration of ETT
    - right mainstem
    - larynx
  ETT cuff rupture or herniation
  ETT kinking or obstruction
  Tracheostomy tube problems

Patient Causes
  Airway Occlusion
    - bronchospasm, obstruction, secretions
  Lung Parenchyma
    - hyperinflation or atelectasis
    - pneumothorax
  Cardiovascular Pathology
    - myocardial infarction
    - heart failure
    - pulmonary embolus
  Altered Ventilatory Drive
    - pain, anxiety, fear, delirium, metabolic

Ventilator Set-Up
  Inappropriate tidal volume
  Inappropriate pressure target
  Inappropriate trigger sensitivity
  Inadequate FiO_2
  Inappropriate PEEP/CPAP level
  Inappropriate SIMV/rate

● Summary

Respiratory failure is a common problem in critically ill patients. Failure to rapidly correct hypoxemia associated with respiratory failure can have devastating consequences and thus management must be quick and to the point. Although it is usually easy to identify a patient with respiratory failure, a high degree of suspicion is required since respiratory failure sometimes presents in subtle ways. A patient presenting in respiratory failure should be rapidly evaluated and therapy instituted even before a firm diagnosis is reached. While the administration of oxygen remains the cornerstone of the management of hypoxemia, various manoeuvres and devices can be helpful in the management of respiratory failure, along with the institution of specific therapies directed at the underlying cause for respiratory failure.

Key Points

- Acute respiratory failure is any impairment of O_2 uptake and/or CO_2 elimination that is a threat to life.
- Respiratory failure can be divided into hypoxemic failure and hypercapnic failure.
- Primary assessment involves a rapid initial evaluation for danger signs and the simultaneous institution of therapy.
- A high respiratory rate is one of the most sensitive signs of respiratory failure.
- Blood gases should never be interpreted in isolation but always in the clinical context.
- Regardless of the mode of delivery, the most important principle is to assess the adequacy of the oxygen therapy often (e.g., with a pulse oximeter).
- Up to a third of patients treated with NPVV for respiratory failure will require intubation.

References

1. West J: Human limits for hypoxia: The physiological challenge of climbing Mt Everest. *Ann NY Acad Sci* 2000;899:15–27.

2. Basynat B, Murdoch D: High-altitude illness. *Lancet* 2003;361:1967–74.

3. British Thoracic Society Standards of Care Committee: Managing passengers with respiratory disease planning air travel: British Thoracic Society recommendations. *Thorax* 2002;57:289–304.

4. Schwartz J, Bencowitz H, Moser K: Air travel hypoxemia with chronic obstructive pulmonary disease. *Ann Int Med* 1984;100:473–7.

5. Jorgensen E, Holm S: The course of circulatory and cerebral recovery after circulatory arrest: Influence of pre-arrest, arrest, and post-arrest factors. *Resuscitation* 1999;42:173–82.

6. Balakrishnan I, Crook P, Morris R, et al: Early predictors of mortality in pneumococcal bacteremia. *J Infect* 2000;40:256–61.

7. Forsythe S, Schmidt G: Sodium bicarbonate for the treatment of lactic acidosis. *Chest* 2000;117:260–267.

8. Thorens J, Jolliet P, Ritz M, et al: Effects of rapid permissive hypercapnia on hemodynamics, gas exchange and oxygen transport and consumption during mechanical ventilation for the acute respiratory distress syndrome. *Crit Care Med* 1996;22:182–91.

9. Hickling K, Walsh J, Henderson S, et al: Low mortality rate in adult respiratory distress syndrome using low-volume, pressure-limited ventilation with permissive hypercapnia: A prospective study. *Crit Care Med* 1994; 22:1568–78.

10. Kiely D, Cargill R, Lipworth BJ: Effects of hypercapnia on hemodynamic, inotropic, lusitropic and electrophysiologic indices in humans. *Chest* 1996;109:1215–21.

11. Feihl F, Perret C: Permissive hypercapnia: How permissive should we be? *Am J Respir Crit Care Med* 1994; 150:1722–37.

12. Tuxen D, Williams T, Scheinkestel C, et al: Use of a measurement of pulmonary hyperinflation to control the level of mechanical ventilation in patients with acute severe asthma. *Am Rev Respir Dis* 1992;146:1136–42.

13. Caroll G, Rothenberg D: Carbon dioxide narcosis: Pathological or pathillogical? *Chest* 1992;102:986–8.
14. Meissner H, Franklin C: Extreme hypercapnia in a fully alert patient. *Chest* 1992;102:1298–9.
15. Laffey J, Kavanagh B: Carbon dioxide and the critically ill: Too little of a good thing? *Lancet* 1999;354:1283–6.
16. Aubier M, Murciano M, Milic-Emili J, et al: Effects of the administration of O_2 on ventilation and blood gases in patients with chronic obstructive pulmonary disease during acute respiratory failure. *Am Rev Respir Dis* 1980;122:747–54.
17. Laffey J, O'Croinin D, McLoughlin P, Kavanagh BP: Permissive hypercapnia: Role in protective lung ventilatory strategies. *Intens Care Med* 2004;30:347–56.
18. Rang L, Murray H, Wells G, et al: Can peripheral venous blood gases replace arterial blood gases in emergency department patients? *Can J Emerg Med* 2002;4:7–15.
19. Napolitano L: Capnography in critical care: Accurate assessment of ARDS therapy? *Crit Care Med* 1999;27:862–3.
20. Morley T, Giaimo J, Marozan E, et al: Use of capnography for assessment of the adequacy of alveolar ventilation during weaning from mechanical ventilation. *Am Rev Respir Dis* 1993;148:339–44.
21. Jardin F, Genevray B, Pazin M, et al: Inability to titrate PEEP in patients with acute respiratory failure using end-tidal carbon dioxide measurements. *Anesthesiology* 1985;62:530–3.
22. Soubani A: Non-invasive monitoring of oxygen and carbon dioxide. *Am J Emerg Med* 2001;19:141–6.
23. Boersma W: Assessment of severity of community-acquired pneumonia. *Semin Respir Infect* 1999;14:103–14.
24. Kress J, O'Connor M, Schmidt G: Clinical examination reliably detects intrinsic positive end-expiratory pressure in mechanically ventilated patients. *Am J Respir Crit Care Med* 1999;159:290–4.
25. Laghi F, Tobin M: Disorders of the respiratory muscles. *Am J Respir Crit Care Med* 2003;168:10–48.
26. Dunn W, Nelson S, Hubmayr R: Oxygen-induced hypercarbia in obstructive pulmonary disease. *Am Rev Respir Dis* 1991;144:526–30.
27. Sassoon C, Hassell K, Mahutte C: Hyperoxic-induced hypercapnia in stable chronic obstructive pulmonary disease. *Am Rev Respir Dis* 1987;135:907–11.
28. The Acute Respiratory Distress Syndrome Network: Ventilation with lower tidal volumes as compared with traditional tidal volumes for acute lung injury and the acute respiratory distress syndrome. *N Engl J Med* 2000;342:1301–8.
29. Tobin M: Advances in mechanical ventilation. *N Engl J Med* 2001;344:1986–96.

CHAPTER 12

INTRODUCTION TO MECHANICAL VENTILATION

LOIS CHAMPION,
PIERRE CARDINAL, AND
RICHARD HODDER

A 75-year-old woman presented with severe shortness of breath. She has been a heavy smoker for over 50 years and has been frequently admitted with COPD exacerbations. Despite resuscitation and initiation of bronchodilators, corticosteroids, antibiotics and oxygen, she continues to deteriorate. She was successfully intubated. You are asked what the initial settings for the ventilator should be. What do you say?

Clearly, the use of mechanical ventilators has saved the lives of countless patients. Mechanical ventilation is used in respiratory failure to oxygenate and ventilate the patient. Unfortunately, there are many different "modes" of ventilation, all with different names and initials, which can make it very confusing. In this chapter you will learn an approach to understanding mechanical ventilation, as well as some of the more commonly used modes of ventilation and the advantages and disadvantages of each. A discussion of positive end expiratory pressure (PEEP) is presented, including its role in managing hypoxemia and its relative contraindications. Intrinsic PEEP is discussed, along with its hemodynamic effects and those of positive pressure ventilation in general.

● Basics of Mechanical Ventilation

A *mode* is a particular pattern of spontaneous and mandatory breaths delivered by the ventilator. Common modes include pressure support, volume cycled and pressure controlled ventilation. In order to understand what a ventilator does, it is necessary to break down a breath into components, namely the different *phases of ventilation.* This will provide a way of organizing the concepts, and be useful in understanding some of the newer (and more complex) modes of ventilation.

A. Expiratory Phase

This is what happens during expiration. Positive end expiratory pressure (PEEP) is pressure applied throughout the ventilatory cycle, including during expiration. Continuous positive airway pressure (CPAP) is the same thing and is synonymous with PEEP. By convention, the term CPAP is used when patients are breathing spontaneously, and PEEP is used when expiratory pressure is applied in conjunction with positive pressure ventilation.

B. Ventilation Trigger

This describes the changeover from expiration to inspiration. A ventilator breath may be spontaneously initiated by the patient or be controlled—that is, initiated by the ventilator. A controlled trigger is based on a time window that is determined in part by the set respiratory rate. Typically, the ventilator is set to deliver a mandatory minimum number of breaths per minute and thus if the patient does not initiate a breath within a certain time frame, the ventilator automatically initiates a breath. A spontaneous triggered breath occurs if the patient initiates a breath by "triggering" the ventilator (i.e., the ventilator is able to sense the patient's inspiratory effort). There are two available mechanisms whereby the ventilator can detect that a patient is attempting to trigger a ventilator breath: pressure triggering and flow triggering.

Pressure triggering of the ventilator requires the patient to generate a small negative inspiratory pressure in the ventilatory circuit. Although the pressure sensitivity is adjustable, typically the patient must generate a negative pressure of 1–3 cm H_2O. The negative pressure is sensed by the ventilator and causes the machine to change over to inspiration and deliver the next breath.

Flow triggering requires the patient to generate a change that is detected by the ventilator. In flow triggering, a constant flow is provided in the patient circuit during expiration. The flow rate is measured both upstream and downstream of the patient. If the patient begins to take a breath, the downstream flow decreases relative to the upstream flow. The ventilator senses this difference in flow and a ventilator driven breath is delivered. Flow triggering is often set in the range of 1.5–3 l/min. Flow triggering may require less work for the patient when compared to pressure triggering.[1]

To demonstrate how important ventilation trigger is, a description of two modes of ventilation illustrates key differences in how the changeover from expiration to inspiration occurs. The *assist/control* (AC) mode refers to a combination of controlled (mandatory) breaths and breaths that the patient initiates by triggering the ventilator (assisted breaths). In the AC mode, the patient receives at least the number of breaths that are pre-set into the ventilator, but the patient can also trigger additional breaths. The additional breaths the patient triggers with AC have the same pre-set tidal volume or pressure that has been set for the mandatory breaths.

The *synchronized intermittent mandatory ventilation* (SIMV) mode is similar to the AC mode in that it also guarantees that the patient will receive a pre-set number of breaths per minute of a predetermined volume or a predetermined pressure. However, SIMV differs from AC when the patient's spontaneous respiratory rate exceeds the pre-set ventilatory rate. Whereas in the AC mode each breath above the pre-set rate has the same volume or pressure as mandatory breaths, the ventilator in a "pure" SIMV mode by contrast will not assist the extra breaths and the patient must perform all the inspiratory work. As discussed below, SIMV is often combined with pressure support (PS) to provide some support for the extra breaths above the pre-set rate. Thus, when both modes of ventilation are prescribed, the patient is guaranteed to receive a pre-set number of controlled SIMV breaths per minute, while PS assists only the extra breaths.

The *S* in *SIMV* stands for synchronized. When this ventilator mode was originally introduced, the extra breaths were delivered independently of the patient's innate breathing rate and effort (intermittent mandatory ventilation or IMV). For example, if the respiratory rate was set at 12 breaths per minute, the ventilator "fired" precisely every five seconds. Unfortunately, if the end of a spontaneous inspiration coincided with the onset of a ventilator breath, the patient ended up receiving two consecutive breaths with no time to exhale. This results in "breath stacking," which increases the risk of barotrauma and causes patient discomfort. In the SIMV mode, instead of delivering a fixed volume after a very precise time interval, the ventilator determines time periods that are either "assisted" or "spontaneous." During *assisted* periods, the ventilator delivers SIMV assisted breaths either in response to the patient's own inspiratory effort, or automatically if the patient does not attempt to initiate a breath. During the *spontaneous* period, the ventilator either lets the patient breathe on their own (SIMV alone), or delivers a pressure support breath (SIMV + PS). The manner in which the ventilator determines what are the assisted and spontaneous periods is more complicated than it may appear at first glance, and varies from one type of ventilator to the next. However, the principles of SIMV remain constant among different ventilators in that a minimum number of breaths is guaranteed per minute.

C. Inspiratory Phase

This is the phase of the ventilatory cycle that begins with the initiation of the breath and ends when the ventilator cycles into expiration.

D. Cycling

This is the parameter that ends inspiration and initiates the changeover from inspiration to expiration. Cycling defines how the ventilator recognizes that the inspiratory phase is over. Different modes of ventilation use different parameters to determine cycling. For example, pressure controlled ventilation is time cycled, whereas pressure support ventilation is flow cycled.

● Modes of Mechanical Ventilation

A wide variety of different modes are available, many of which are proprietary and ventilator specific. Examples include BiLevel®, BiPAP®, APRV (airway pressure release ventilation), PAV (proportional assist ventilation), VV+ (Volume Ventilation Plus™), ATC™ (Automatic Tube Compensation), Autoflow™, Volume Support and many more. The modes of ventilation that will be discussed in this chapter are pressure support ventilation, volume cycled ventilation and pressure controlled ventilation (Table 12.1). These modes are frequently used, and provide a framework for understanding some of the new options available. Note that the terms *AC* and *IMV* are often used to refer to volume cycled ventilation. In many centres, for example, if a patient is said to be on AC the implication is that they are being ventilated with volume cycled ventilation. The reason for this is that originally there was only one mode of controlled ventilation available on ventilators—volume cycled ventilation. Now there are other modes available; for example, pressure controlled ventilation can be used with AC or IMV, or one can combine IMV with pressure support for the spontaneous breaths.

A. Volume Cycled Ventilation

This is a controlled mode that also allows the patient to trigger additional breaths. The tidal volume is set,

Table 12.1 – Set Parameters and Ventilation Mode

Volume Cycled Ventilation	Pressure Support Ventilation	Pressure Controlled Ventilation
FiO$_2$	FiO$_2$	FiO$_2$
PEEP	PEEP	PEEP
respiratory rate	pressure support level (cm H$_2$O)	respiratory rate
trigger for spontaneous breaths	trigger for breaths	trigger for spontaneous breaths
- flow trigger	- flow trigger	- flow trigger
- pressure trigger	- pressure trigger	- pressure trigger
inspiratory flow rate	alarm settings	inspiratory time
inspiratory flow pattern	- rates (high or low)	inspiratory pressure limit (cm H$_2$O)
tidal volume	- tidal volume (high or low)	alarm settings
alarm settings		- tidal volume (high or low)
- peak pressure		- rates (high or low)
- rates (high or low)		

and the ventilator cycles into the exhalation phase once the tidal volume has been delivered, therefore this mode is volume cycled. Who benefits from assist/control volume cycled ventilation? Since there is a pre-set tidal volume and mandatory respiratory rate, this mode of ventilation is useful for patients with decreased ventilatory drive, patients who need hyperventilation, postoperative patients etc. This mode can provide virtually full ventilatory support, with little work of breathing if the respiratory rate, tidal volume and inspiratory flow are adjusted to meet the patient's needs. Usually, it is not useful for weaning patients. The phases of ventilation during volume cycled ventilation are described below (Figure 12.1).

a. trigger – The changeover from expiration to inspiration in volume cycled ventilation can be machine controlled or patient triggered. Volume cycled ventilation can be used with AC or SIMV modes. With the AC mode of ventilation, the ventilator rate is set (e.g., 12 breaths per minute). In addition, the AC mode allows the patient to initiate breaths in either a pressure or flow triggered manner. Each breath in the AC mode will have the same set

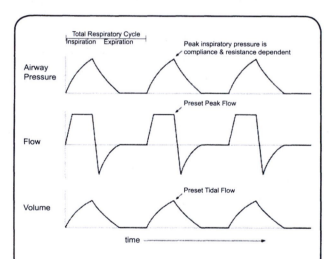

Figure 12.1 – Volume Controlled Ventilation

Figure 12.1 illustrates the tidal volume, flow and airway pressure curves in volume cycled ventilation. In this example the inspiratory flow is constant. Clinically inspiratory flow is often used with a decelerating pattern (a high initial flow rate early in inspiration with a decrease in flow rate over time), as this often seems to increase patient comfort and decrease airway pressures.

tidal volume that the controlled breaths have. When volume cycled ventilation is combined with SIMV, each additional breath the patient triggers above the set rate has a variable volume. The volume varies as it is dependent on the negative pressure the patient spontaneously generates and is supported in part by the machine with *pressure support* (see below).

b. inspiratory phase – For volume cycled ventilation, the tidal volume that the ventilator delivers is set (usually in the range of 6–8 ml/kg of predicted body weight). The inspiratory flow rate must also be set as this determines how fast the breath will be delivered by the ventilator. A very high inspiratory flow rate may lead to high airway pressures because the rapid flow generates more airway resistance. A low inspiratory flow rate, however, may lead to respiratory distress, since the patient may feel that the breath is coming too slowly, and may continue to exert an effort to breathe in during the inspiratory phase.[1] Typical inspiratory flow rates range from 50–80 l/min. The length of inspiration depends on the tidal volume and inspiratory flow rate that have been set.

c. cycling – The changeover from inspiration to expiration in this mode is typically volume cycled, since the ventilator switches to exhalation when the set tidal volume has been delivered.

d. expiratory phase – During this phase, pressure is often used for added benefit. This pressure is called *positive end expiratory pressure* (PEEP).

e. alarm settings – There is a high pressure alarm which is set at the peak airway pressure limit in volume cycled ventilation. The peak pressure that is generated during delivery of the tidal volume breath will vary with changes in resistance or compliance. If this pressure is exceeded, then the alarm will sound and the ventilator will default to a pressure cycled mode and not deliver the full tidal volume. This protects the patient from excessive airway pressures. There is also a high respiratory rate alarm.

B. Pressure Support Ventilation

This is a spontaneous mode of ventilation. The patient must initiate every breath. With each breath that the patient triggers, the ventilator provides a "push" of pressure with a high initial inspiratory flow of gas

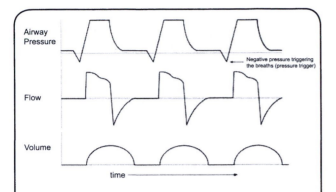

Figure 12.2 – Pressure Support Waveforms

Figure 12.2 shows pressure support waveforms: volume (VT), flow (shown as Q) and airway pressure. Note the high initial inspiratory flow rate to generate airway pressure; then the flow rate falls off and airway pressure is maintained constant throughout inspiration. On the airway pressure waveform you can see the negative pressure deflection the patient generated in order to trigger the ventilator.

to support the breath (Figure 12.2). When should you use pressure support ventilation? As this is a spontaneous mode of ventilation, the patient must be able to initiate every breath so they must have an adequate respiratory drive. Most patients find this to be a reasonably comfortable mode of ventilation. The patient is able to determine the respiratory rate, inspiratory flow rate, and inspiratory time. The tidal volume delivered depends on the amount of pressure support, the respiratory mechanics of the patient and the patient's effort. Pressure support is often used as a weaning mode.

a. trigger – The changeover from expiration to inspiration is solely patient triggered. The patient initiates each breath in pressure support ventilation using either pressure or flow triggering depending on the specific ventilator.

b. inspiratory phase – For pressure support ventilation a pressure is set. During inspiration, the ventilator delivers a high initial flow rate that declines in order to keep the set airway pressure constant throughout inspiration. The amount of pressure support can be set and adjusted so that the patient is able to generate adequate tidal volumes with a comfortable respiratory rate.

c. cycling – Pressure support is flow cycled. As the patient's inspiratory flow rate falls to a certain percentage of the peak flow rate, the ventilator cycles into the expiratory phase. Typically the ventilator will cycle into the expiratory phase as the patient's inspiratory flow rate falls below 10–25% of their peak inspiratory flow.

d. expiratory phase – Again PEEP can be combined with pressure support.

e. alarm settings – There is often a backup apnea rate that can be set.

C. Pressure Controlled Ventilation

This is a mode of ventilation in which the inspiratory airway pressure and inspiratory time are set (Figure 12.3). Who benefits from pressure control? Pressure control is sometimes used in patients with acute respiratory distress syndrome (ARDS). The advantage of this mode is that it allows for control of peak airway pressures, although tidal volume may vary from breath to breath. A longer inspiratory time may also allow for better alveolar recruitment and oxygenation.

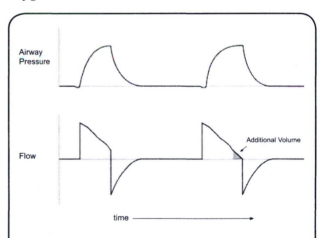

Figure 12.3 – Pressure Controlled Ventilation

Figure 12.3 illustrates the pressure-time and flow-time waveforms for pressure controlled ventilation. There is a high initial flow rate; then the flow rate decreases over time in order to maintain airway pressure constant. With a prolongation of the inspiratory time, the inspiratory flow may decrease to zero as seen for the second breath in the figure.

a. trigger – The changeover from expiration to inspiration is a combination of controlled and patient triggered breaths. The respiratory rate is set and a trigger is set to allow the patient to initiate additional breaths. Pressure controlled ventilation can be used with assist/control or SIMV.

b. inspiratory phase – In this mode, the ventilating pressure is set. This pressure is generated quickly and maintained constant throughout inspiration. The ventilator delivers a high initial flow rate in order to generate the set pressure. The flow rate then falls during inspiration as the amount of flow needed to maintain the set pressure decreases. With a prolonged inspiratory time, the inspiratory flow rate may fall to zero before the end of inspiration. The tidal volume delivered depends on the set pressure and inspiratory time, and on patient factors such as respiratory mechanics. Tidal volume may vary but the peak airway pressure is constant.

c. cycling – This mode is time cycled, which means that the ventilator cycles into expiration when the set inspiratory time is over. A longer inspiratory time will therefore increase the tidal volume delivered.

d. expiratory phase – Again PEEP can be combined with pressure support.

e. alarm settings – These include both high and low tidal volume limits as well as a high respiratory rate alarm.

● Positive End Expiratory Pressure (PEEP)

PEEP refers to a constant baseline pressure that is present throughout the ventilatory cycle (not just on expiration). PEEP is synonymous with continuous positive airway pressure (CPAP) but historically the term CPAP is used in the context of patients who are breathing spontaneously and the term PEEP is used when patients are ventilated with positive pressure ventilation.

A. Rationale

The rationale for using PEEP is that it can improve oxygenation by preventing end expiratory collapse of alveoli and by recruiting non-ventilated (shunt) or poorly ventilated (low V/Q) alveoli. PEEP may also help to prevent cyclic opening and closing of alveoli and distal bronchioles with each breath, which is thought to contribute to alveolar injury by depleting surfactant. PEEP does not decrease the amount of pulmonary edema in the lungs, but it does create hydrostatic forces that move fluid from the alveoli and airways into the interstitium where there is less effect on gas exchange. Although PEEP can recruit atelectatic alveoli and splint them open it may also create overinflation of alveoli; this can cause more lung injury and a worsening of ventilation due to an increase in dead space. Increased dead space ventilation with PEEP is more likely to occur with high levels of PEEP, in patients who are intravascularly volume depleted, and in patients with underlying lung diseases already associated with a high dead space such as COPD.

B. Hemodynamic effects

The effects of PEEP are essentially the same as the effects of positive pressure ventilation, except that PEEP is applied throughout the ventilatory cycle and not just during the inspiratory phase. The hemodynamic effects depend on the increase in intrathoracic pressure that occurs with positive pressure. Clinically, there is no way of knowing how much positive pressure is transmitted to the intrathoracic space unless there is a pleural or esophageal manometer inserted to actually measure the pleural pressure.

Positive pressure ventilation can cause a decrease in the venous return to the right ventricle. In dehydrated patients this can result in a precipitous fall in cardiac output and blood pressure. In addition, the use of narcotics and sedatives at the time of intubation decreases sympathetic drive, leading to vasodilation and more hypotension. When preload is adequate, the effect of an increased intrathoracic pressure on venous return is better tolerated.

If lung volume is recruited with PEEP, then pulmonary vascular resistance may decrease. However PEEP may cause overdistension of alveoli and an increase of pulmonary vascular resistance due to stretching of the perialveolar vessels. This can result in an increase in afterload to the right ventricle. PEEP may therefore contribute to worsening right heart failure and be associated with a shift of the interventricular septum to the left. This phenomenon is known as ventricular interdependence.

An increase in intrathoracic pressure will cause a decrease of left ventricular afterload, which is the wall tension the ventricle must generate to cause ejection. The positive pressure surrounding the left ventricle can assist systolic ejection. This means that patients with poor left ventricular function and adequate preload may actually benefit from the effects of positive pressure ventilation.

C. Relative contraindications

A relative contraindiction to the use of PEEP is when its adverse effects may outweigh the benefits. Although it is unlikely that low levels of PEEP are contraindicated, certainly higher levels may not be beneficial. PEEP is not always helpful in improving oxygenation. For example, an improvement in oxygen saturation may be outweighed by a decrease in cardiac output. Be aware that positive pressure ventilation and PEEP may cause profound hypotension in patients who are volume depleted or sensitive to changes in preload (e.g., those with cardiac tamponade) because of the decrease in venous return it causes. Thus, there are several different relative contraindications to the use of PEEP (Table 12.2).

Various cardiovascular conditions can worsen with the use of PEEP. A patient who is hypotensive, especially one who has low blood pressure due to volume depletion and dehydration, may not tolerate the application of PEEP. Likewise, a patient with right heart failure may experience worsening of right heart function due to PEEP because pulmonary vascular resistance and therefore right ventricular afterload may both be increased. This is in contrast to the patient with left heart failure who can benefit from PEEP. A patient with a right to left intracardiac shunt, such as an atrial septal defect, can experience a worsening of right to left shunting with the addition of PEEP.

Certain lung conditions tolerate the addition of PEEP poorly. Although a patient who is suffering from hyperinflation due to airflow obstruction and dynamic hyperinflation may benefit from some PEEP to overcome auto-PEEP (see below), PEEP levels above the auto-PEEP levels could affect expiration thereby worsening hyperinflation. Asymmetric or focal lung disease, such as severe unilateral pneumonia, can be adversely affected, since PEEP may end up hyperinflating the "good" lung without recruiting useful lung volume in the atelectatic lung. The hyperinflation would increase the pulmonary vascular resistance in the good lung and shift blood flow to the diseased lung, thus worsening oxygenation. A bronchopleural fistula may be adversely affected by high levels of PEEP, since it could increase the air leak and possibly prevent healing.

A final relative contraindication to PEEP is in patients with an increased intracranial pressure. If PEEP causes a rise in the central venous pressure, this may decrease cerebral venous drainage thereby further increasing the intracranial pressure. A PEEP of less than or equal to 12 cm H_2O will probably be well tolerated in these patients. Hypoxemia will certainly worsen brain injury, so that any risk of increased intracranial pressure must be weighed against an improvement in oxygenation with PEEP.

D. Dosing

How much PEEP should be used? Unfortunately, the answer is not known.[3-7] Most clinical trials in ARDS have used a protocol where PEEP was increased depending on the oxygen saturation and FiO_2. A recent study comparing a strategy of high PEEP with low FiO_2 versus low PEEP and high FiO_2 to maintain oxygenation showed no difference in clinical outcomes.[5,6] Clinically, many critical care units will use a standard baseline PEEP of 5 cm H_2O in virtually all patients to prevent end expiratory collapse of alveoli. As inspired oxygen is increased to 50% or more, PEEP is added, usually in increments of 2–3 cm H_2O. PEEP is titrated up slowly until oxygenation has improved, allowing a decrease in inspired oxygen concentration or until adverse hemodynamic effects are seen. Clinically the maximum PEEP that is used in most centres is in the range of 20 cm H_2O.

Table 12.2- Relative Contraindications to PEEP

1. Hypotensive Patients
2. Right Heart Failure
3. Right to Left Intracardiac Shunts
4. Increased Intracranial Pressure
5. Hyperinflation
6. Asymmetric or Focal Lung Disease
7. Bronchopleural Fistula

● Auto-PEEP

Auto-PEEP, also called intrinsic PEEP, describes the pressure that occurs when there is insufficient time for exhalation and the next ventilator breath "stacks" on the previous breath. As a result there is an increase in end expiratory pressure known as "auto-PEEP." Auto-PEEP cannot be detected just by looking at the pressure gauge of the ventilator since the airway pressure is set to the level of the external PEEP (the PEEP that is set) on exhalation.

A. Detection

There are several different ways to detect auto-PEEP. Clinically, patients at risk of developing auto-PEEP are patients with a high minute ventilation, high respiratory rate, short expiratory times and airway obstruction. Auto-PEEP can cause severe hyperinflation, and ventilator dysynchrony (also known as "fighting" the ventilator). On auscultation, if expiratory sounds are heard throughout the expiratory phase right up to the inspiratory phase

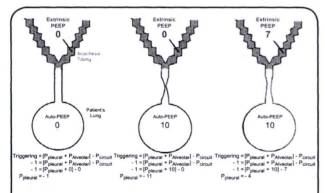

Figure 12.4 – PEEP and Patient Triggering Ventilator

Figure 12.4 illustrates how the addition of extrinsic PEEP can help the patient trigger the ventilator. To trigger the ventilator, the patient must generate a negative pressure of –1 cm H_2O in the circuit (the negative pressure a patient generates is measured as the P_{pleura} pressure). Thus, in the presence of an auto-PEEP of 10 cm H_2O and zero external PEEP, to trigger the ventilator, a patient must overcome both the auto-PEEP and the required triggering pressure of –1 cm H_2O, for a total of –11 cm H_2O. However, when an external PEEP of 7 cm H_2O is added, the patient only needs to generate –4 cm H_2O.

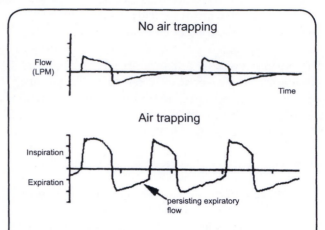

Figure 12.5 – Air Trapping on Flow versus Time Graph

Figure 12.5 illustrates the waveform for flow against time with the absence and presence of air trapping. Note that the flow is positive on inspiration with positive pressure ventilation and negative with exhalation. Inspiratory flow is above the time axis, and expiratory flow is below this axis. Expiratory flow does not reach zero before the next breath in the bottom diagram, demonstrating that there is an auto-PEEP effect from air trapping.

of the next breath, then suspect that auto-PEEP is present.[2] Remember that there will not be expiratory sounds or wheezing in the absence of airflow. Patients with high levels of auto-PEEP may fail to trigger the ventilator because auto-PEEP represents an inspiratory threshold load that the patient must first overcome before a ventilator breath can be triggered. In this situation, the patient will demonstrate inspiratory effort but the ventilator fails to sense the patient's effort (Figure 12.4).

Certain monitors, including the expiratory flow versus time curve graph on the ventilator, can be used to detect auto-PEEP (Figure 12.5). If expiratory flow does not return to zero before the next breath, then there may be a component of auto-PEEP (however one can not quantify the amount). Auto-PEEP cannot be detected or quantified using the expiratory airway pressure unless an expiratory hold or pause is performed. The expiratory circuit valves open to atmospheric pressure on expiration and therefore the expiratory airway pressure reflects the PEEP that has been applied by the operator, not the endogenous auto-PEEP. In order to quantify the amount of

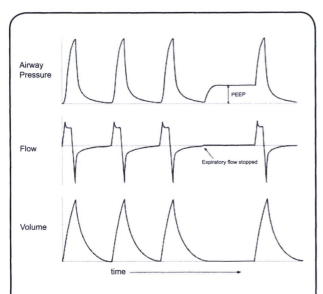

Figure 12.6 – Measurement of Auto-PEEP

Figure 12.6 shows an expiratory hold (or expiratory pause): Expiratory flow is stopped just prior to the next breath. This allows the pressure in the patient's lungs to equilibrate with the pressure in the ventilator circuit. In this example, the airway pressure increases to a plateau that represents the intrinsic or auto-PEEP (PI). If a patient is triggering the ventilator, an expiratory hold cannot be done because there will not be time for the equilibration of the airway pressure.

auto-PEEP, an expiratory hold is created (stop the expiratory phase with no flow just before the next inspiratory phase) and measure the pressure (Figure 12.6). The positive pressure measured by occluding the airway at the end of expiration may be related to hyperinflation (auto-PEEP) but may also be due to an increase in abdominal pressure produced by contraction of the abdominal muscles. It can be very difficult to quantify the amount of auto-PEEP even when using sophisticated techniques such as esophageal and gastric pressure measurements.

B. Clinical implications

Auto-PEEP causes an increase in intrathoracic pressure and therefore can cause all of the hemodynamic side effects discussed in the section on applied PEEP. In addition, auto-PEEP can increase the work of breathing required to trigger the ventilator. For

example if a negative pressure of 2 cm H_2O is set for a pressure trigger and there is an auto-PEEP of 10 cm H_2O, then the patient will need to generate negative 12 cm H_2O pressure before the ventilator will trigger the next breath. This additional imposed work of breathing can be very uncomfortable and fatiguing for the patient.

C. Management

Management of auto-PEEP is not always easy! One approach is to lengthen the time for exhalation (expiratory phase) by decreasing the respiratory rate or shortening the inspiratory time. However, a shorter inspiratory time may lead to an increase in airway pressure in volume cycled ventilation or lower tidal volumes in pressure controlled ventilation. Bronchodilators can be used to treat bronchospasm. Sedation is often required in patients who develop auto-PEEP to facilitate ventilation and improve patient ventilator synchrony. In some patients with COPD and expiratory air trapping external PEEP (5–8 cm H_2O) can be titrated to overcome auto-PEEP. However, excessive external PEEP may also be detrimental as it may limit expiratory flow and worsen hyperinflation and compromise blood pressure and cardiac output.

● Non-invasive Positive Pressure Ventilation

Non-invasive positive pressure ventilation (NPPV) is the delivery of positive pressure mechanical ventilation without the use of an endotracheal tube.[9,10] The use of NPPV has revolutionized the therapy of patients with respiratory failure. It offers the distinct advantages of being versatile in that it can be readily started and stopped. NPPV avoids the complications associated with intubation and can decrease morbidity and mortality in certain groups of patients with respiratory failure.[9–17] However, like most therapies, it has certain limitations and problems associated with its use. A rational approach to the use of NPPV, with a clear understanding of when to avoid or abandon the technique and institute intubation and invasive mechanical ventilation, is essential for the safe use of NPPV in acutely ill patients.

● Equipment

Non-invasive ventilation is defined as the delivery of mechanical ventilation without the use of an endotracheal airway. Non-invasive ventilation may be delivered using either negative or positive pressure. Negative pressure ventilators (e.g., "iron lung") were developed during the poliovirus epidemics. Although modern negative pressure ventilators exist, their use is strictly limited. Today, non-invasive ventilation is primarily delivered by positive pressure ventilation via a face mask.

Equipment needed for NPPV includes the mask (known as the "interface" between the patient and ventilator) and the ventilator. Masks used for NPPV include oronasal masks (partial or full face masks) and nasal masks held in place with head straps. Masks are available in different sizes, and proper fitting is essential in order to avoid excessive air leak and ensure patient comfort. Oronasal masks are designed to cover the patient's nose and mouth. Oronasal masks are used mainly in patients with acute respiratory failure. They tend to allow higher ventilation pressures without excessive leak, and allow for mouth breathing. The masks however can be uncomfortable; they are applied tightly to the face and can make patients feel claustrophobic. Cautious use of sedation may be required for patient comfort. Patients cannot eat or drink with the mask in place, and communication will be difficult. Nasal masks may be better tolerated and less claustrophobic than the oronasal masks and tend to be used in patients with chronic respiratory failure. Nasal masks however can result in air leak from the mouth, and less effective ventilation as a result. In acute respiratory failure a nasal mask could be tried for the patient who is unable to tolerate an oronasal or full-face mask because of claustrophobia.

The systems have various safety features incorporated into their design. Since the masks must be tightly occluded to the patient's face to ensure there is an air seal, it is necessary to have a "quick release" that allows the mask to be removed in one quick step (e.g., in case of vomiting). The masks also have a safety entrainment feature that allows the patient to breathe room air in case of ventilator failure or some disconnection from an oxygen source. Most of the devices have alarms that sound if there is excessive air leakage or if the patient becomes apneic. Some, but not all, devices can even begin to ventilate the patient with a backup mode of ventilation if they become apneic.

A NPPV ventilator can be the standard critical care ventilator or a ventilator designed specifically for NPPV (e.g., BiPAP® Vision® ventilator). Ventilators designed for NPPV have specially designed triggering capabilities and compensation for air leak. Standard critical care ventilators can deliver NPPV using a variety of ventilatory modes including continuous positive airway pressure (CPAP), pressure support, and volume cycled ventilation. Pressure support ventilation is often chosen as a ventilatory mode since the constant inspiratory pressure can compensate for air leaks. In pressure support ventilation, the patient initiates (triggers) every breath. Alternatively, a pressure control mode may be used with a set respiratory rate; the patient is also able to trigger additional breaths above the set ventilator rate.

The BiPAP® Vision® ventilator is an example of device specifically designed for non-invasive ventilation. This ventilator has a CPAP mode and a spontaneous/time (S/T) mode. The S/T mode delivers an inspiratory positive airway pressure (IPAP) at a set rate and when the patient triggers a breath. During exhalation the ventilator cycles to an expiratory positive airway pressure (EPAP). The BiPAP® Vision® differs from most other devices in that the IPAP value it displays is absolute (i.e., it includes the level of EPAP).[10] In contrast to this, most other devices in a pressure control ventilation or pressure support ventilation mode report an inspiratory pressure that does *not* include the constant underlying pressure (CPAP or PEEP). Thus, to calculate the peak inspiratory pressure that these devices are delivering, one must add the inspiratory pressure to the underlying PEEP. For example, a pressure support ventilation of 10 cm H_2O and PEEP of 5 cm H_2O would result in a peak inspiratory pressure of 15 cm H_2O; this would correspond to a setting of IPAP 15 cm H_2O and EPAP 5 cm H_2O using the BiPAP® Vision® ventilator.[10] Unfortunately, how ventilators report values has not yet been standardized and thus it is crucial that physicians become familiar with the devices found in their institutions.

Initial settings on the ventilator, whether using a conventional ventilator or one designed specifically for NPPV, should provide low levels of ventilating pressure (Table 12.3). This improves patient comfort and facilitates the transition to NPPV. Ventilating pressure (PS or IPAP) can be titrated up by 2–3 cm

Table 12.3 – Clinical Application of NPPV: Initial Settings

BiPAP® S/T	EPAP 4–5 cm H_2O IPAP 8–10 cm H_2O respiratory rate should be based on patient rate if using S/T mode
Pressure Support	PEEP 5 H_2O PS 5 H_2O
CPAP	5 cm H_2O
Hypoxemia	Increase FiO_2 to maintain O_2 saturation >88% Increase EPAP or PEEP by 2–3 cm H_2O Note: Clinically it is rare to exceed EPAP or PEEP of 10 cm H_2O with NPPV; if hypoxemia persists despite EPAP or PEEP of 10 cm H_2O then intubation and ventilation should be considered.
Hypercapnia	Increase IPAP or PS Note: Clinically peak airway pressures (IPAP or PS + PEEP) of >20 cm H_2O are rarely used, and a requirement for pressures in this range may be an indication that the patient requires intubation and ventilation.

n.b. These are guidelines only; individual patients will vary in their ventilatory requirements and ability to tolerate NPPV.

H_2O every few minutes using dyspnea, respiratory rate, and the use of accessory muscles to guide therapy. The goal is a decrease in respiratory rate and sense of dyspnea with reduced use of accessory muscles. In general ventilating pressures of over 20 cm H_2O will not be well tolerated by patients and may increase the risk of gastric distension. Patients requiring airway pressures of over 20 cm H_2O should be assessed for intubation.

● Indications

NPPV has been shown to decrease the need for intubation and decrease morbidity and mortality in patients with acute exacerbations of COPD. [10–12] NPPV has also been used in patients with cardiogenic pulmonary edema, acute respiratory failure with acute lung injury, and immunocompromised patients with respiratory failure.[1–3,5,7,9] NPPV initiated immediately after weaning and extubation of patients with COPD has been shown to decrease the risk of respiratory failure requiring reintubation.[14,16] Avoiding intubation avoids the complications of intubation itself, as well as allowing the patient to speak, and also to eat when NPPV is transiently discontinued. NPPV is also associated with a lower risk of ventilator-associated pneumonia.[19]

Table 12.4 – Relative Contraindications to the Use of NPPV

1. Hemodynamic instability or shock
2. Decreased level of consciousness and inability to protect airway
3. Inadequate respiratory drive
4. High risk of aspiration (e.g., upper gastrointestinal hemorrhage or bowel obstruction)
5. Facial trauma, burns or surgery interfering with application of mask
6. Upper airway obstruction
7. Agitated uncooperative patient
8. Inability to clear secretions or excessive airway secretions

Contraindications

NPPV should not be attempted on a patient who is unable to protect his or her airway (Table 12.4). The mask does not provide any protection against aspiration, and in fact may make it more difficult for a patient to avoid aspiration if actively vomiting. Patients who have upper GI bleeding, severe facial trauma or upper airway obstruction are likely not candidates for NPPV. Patients in respiratory failure who are unable to clear their secretions will probably not be helped by NPPV. Unstable patients (imminent respiratory arrest or hemodynamic instability) should not be tried on NPPV. In general, a patient should be awake and co-operative, but patients who are mildly obtunded due to hypercarbia may improve with NPPV.

Complications

Complications related to the mask include pressure necrosis of the skin, damage to the eyes such as corneal abrasions, and claustrophobia. A proper fit is essential. Patients are more likely to tolerate the mask if they have an explanation of how the mask works and what to expect. Gastric distension with air may occur. A nasogastric tube may be useful in these patients for decompression of the stomach, but is not needed routinely. A nasogastric tube may also make proper mask fitting more difficult and increase air leak. There is a risk of aspiration because the airway is not protected; this should be avoided by careful patient selection.

Monitoring and Identification of Patients Who Require Intubation

NPPV must be provided in a location able to monitor vital signs and continuous oxygen saturation (Table 12.5). NPPV is successful if a patient has improved oxygenation and a decrease in respiratory rate and is more comfortable with less dyspnea. This improvement is usually seen within a few hours.[20] Patients who have failed a trial of NPPV will have continued hypoxemia or hypercarbia, tachypnea and respiratory distress. These patients require intubation.

Table 12.5 – Documentation and Monitoring with NPPV

Clinical Information	Ventilator Data
- mask fit	- FiO_2
- level of consciousness	- mode (e.g., EPAP/IPAP)
- oxygen saturation	- ventilator pressures (PEEP/PS)
- patient comfort	- respiratory rate
- respiratory rate	- spontaneous
- use of accessory muscles	- controlled or timed if applicable
- ability to cough and clear secretions	- tidal volume
- degree of bronchospasm	- minute volume
- gastric distension	- air leak
- arterial blood gases for $Paco_2$ and pH	- alarms

Key Points

- The four phases of ventilation are trigger, cycling, expiratory phase and inspiratory phase.
- Different patients are more comfortable with different modes and trial and error is often required to find the best mode.

- PEEP recruits collapsed alveoli, which improves V/Q mismatch and lung compliance.
- PEEP can cause hemodynamic instability and hyperinflation.

- Auto-PEEP is likely if the patient has a high respiratory rate, bronchospasm, audible wheezing that lasts through to the next breath, or an expiratory flow wave form that does not reach zero before inspiration.
- Auto-PEEP can cause severe hemodynamic instability and increase the work of breathing.
- NPPV can decrease the need for intubation and reduce morbidity and mortality in patients with respiratory failure.

- It is important to become familiar with the NPPV devices since each is unique.
- NPPV should not be used in a patient with an unprotected airway.
- Patients on NPPV must be closely monitored to identify early those patients who are failing this form of ventilation.

References

1. Tobin M, Jubran A, Laghi F: Patient-ventilator interaction. *Am J Respir Care Med* 2001;163:1059–63.
2. Kress J, O'Connor M, Schmidt G: Clinical examination reliably detects intrinsic positive end-expiratory pressure in critically ill, mechanically ventilated patients. *Am J Resp Crit Care Med* 1999;159:290–4.
3. Levy M: Optimal PEEP in ARDS: Changing concepts and current controversies. *Crit Care Clin* 2002;18:15–33.
4. Rouby J, Lu Q, Goldstein I: Critical care perspective: Selecting the right level of positive end-expiratory pressure in patients with acute respiratory distress syndrome. *Am J Resp Crit Care Med* 2002;165:1182–6.
5. Dreyfuss D: Pressure-volume curves. *Am J Respir Crit Care Med* 2001;163:2–3.
6. National Heart, Lung, and Blood Institute ARDS Clinical Trials Network: Higher versus lower positive end-expiratory pressures in patients with ARDS. *N Engl J Med* 2004;351:327–36.
7. The Acute Respiratory Distress Syndrome Network: Ventilation with lower tidal volumes as compared with traditional tidal volumes for acute lung injury and the acute respiratory distress syndrome. *N Engl J Med* 2000;342:1301–8.
8. Tobin, M: Advances in mechanical ventilation. *N Engl J Med* 2001;433:1986–96.
9. Mehta S, Hill N: State of the art: Noninvasive ventilation. *Am J Respir Crit Care Med* 2001;163:540–77.
10. International Consensus Conferences in Intensive Care Medicine: Noninvasive positive pressure ventilation in acute respiratory failure. *Am J Respir Crit Care Med* 2001;163:283–91.
11. Stoller J K: Acute exacerbations of chronic obstructive pulmonary disease. *N Engl J Med* 2002;346:988–93.
12. McCrory D, Brown C, Gelfand B, Bach P: Management of acute exacerbations of COPD: A summary and appraisal of published evidence. *Chest* 2001;119:1190–1209.
13. Hilbert G, Gruson D, Vargas F, et al: Noninvasive ventilation is immunosuppressed patients with pulmonary infiltrates, fever, and acute respiratory failure. *N Engl J Med* 2001;344:481–7.
14. Nava S, Ambrosino N, Clini E, et al: Noninvasive mechanical ventilation in the weaning of patients with respiratory failure due to chronic obstructive pulmonary disease. *Ann Int Med* 1998;128:721–8.
15. Nava S, Carbone G, DiBattista N, et al: Noninvasive ventilation in cardiogenic pulmonary edema: A multicenter randomized trial. *Am J Respir Crit Care Med* 2003;168:1432–7.
16. Ferrer M, Esquinas A, Francisco A, et al: Noninvasive ventilation during persistent weaning failure. *Am J Respir Crit Care* Med 2003;168:70–6.
17. Antonelli M, Conti G, Rocco M, et al: A comparison of noninvasive positive-pressure ventilation and conventional mechanical ventilation in patients with acute respiratory failure. *N Engl J Med* 1998;339:429–35.
18. BiPAP® Vision® Ventilatory Support System clinical manual. Respironics Inc. 1997.
19. Tablan O, Anderson L, Bessr R, et al: Guidelines for preventing health-care associated pneumonia: 2003 recommendations of CDC and the Healthcare Infection Control Practices Advisory Committee. *MMWR Recomm Rep* 2004;53:1–36.

20. Celilek T, Sungur M, Ceyhan B, Karakurt S: Comparison of non-invasive positive pressure ventilation with standard therapy in hypercapnic acute respiratory failure. *Chest* 1998; 114: 1636–42.

Appendix 12.1 – Summary of Ventilator Modes

Variable	Volume-Cycled	Pressure Controlled	Pressure Support
Trigger	Set rate (AC or IMV) and flow or pressure trigger for patient trigger	Set rate (AC or IMV) and flow or pressure trigger for patient trigger	Spontaneous mode flow or pressure trigger for patient trigger
Limit*	Flow	Pressure	Pressure
Cycle	Volume	Time	Flow
Peak Pressure	Variable	Constant	Constant
Tidal Volume	Constant	Variable	Variable
Advantages	Guaranteed tidal volume	Limits airway pressure. May improve gas distribution with lengthened inspiratory time.	May be very comfortable for patients who can control their respiratory rate, inspiratory time, tidal volume.
Disadvantages	Inspiratory flow may not meet patient demand, causing inspiratory effort and work. Airway pressure is variable and depends on compliance and resistance of respiratory system.	Tidal volume varies with changes in compliance/ resistance or respiratory system and inspiratory effort of patient.	May increase work of breathing if level is too low for patient. Some patients, for example with high minute ventilation or very low compliance, will not be able to tolerate pressure support, even if the pressure support is increased. Tidal volume, minute ventilation and respiratory rate vary depending on changes in respiratory resistance and compliance, and patient effort. Respiratory drive required (this is a spontaneous mode).

*Limit refers to a variable that the ventilator maintains at a pre set value during inspiration, but which does not cause inspiration to end (or cycle). For example, in volume-cycled ventilation the peak inspiratory flow rate and flow rate pattern (constant flow, decelerating flow, ramped flow, etc.) are set.

Tidal Volume (VT) – The volume of a breath, either spontaneous or ventilated (normal VT is 6–10 ml/kg).

Minute Ventilation (VE) – The total ventilation in litres over one minute, also called minute volume. Normal minute ventilation for an adult is approximately 6–8 l/min. Minute ventilation depends on the respiratory rate (f) and tidal volume (**VT**).

VE = f × VT

Inspiratory Flow Rate (IFR) – The flow of gas measured in litres per minute. The IFR determines how fast a tidal volume is delivered. IFR is set in volume cycled ventilation.

a. High inspiratory flow rates will result in high peak airway pressures. This is not necessarily a concern, since the peak airway pressure does not represent the pressure to which the alveoli are exposed (there is a pressure gradient due to resistance along the airway through to the alveoli). Patients may find a high flow rate uncomfortable.

b. Low inspiratory flow rates will result in a longer inspiratory time and a lower peak airway pressure in volume cycled ventilation. A low IFR, however, may cause the patient to feel "air hungry" if the flow does not match this or her needs. This will result in the patient sustaining inspiratory effort throughout inspiration and will increase their work of breathing.

Inspiratory Time (TI) – The inspiratory interval of a breath, which depends on the tidal volume and inspiratory flow rate in volume cycled ventilation. In pressure controlled ventilation, the inspiratory time is set by the operator. Longer inspiratory times may improve oxygenation by allowing redistribution of gas to lung units that are slower to fill. A long inspiratory time, given a constant respiratory rate, however, decreases the time available for expiration and may result in auto-PEEP. Prolonged inspiratory times may not be comfortable for patients, who will feel as though the breath is continuing too long.

TI = VT / IFR (l/min)

Expiratory Time (TE) – The time in seconds for the expiratory phase.

I:E ratio – Ratio of inspiratory time to expiratory time (**TI:TE**). A typical I:E ratio is approximately 1:2. Much longer expiratory times are required in patients with bronchospasm, COPD or asthma, in order to avoid air trapping and auto-PEEP.

Inverse Ratio Ventilation (IRV) – A prolonged inspiratory time followed by a short expiratory time, so that the ratio of inspiratory time to expiratory time is less than 1.

CHAPTER 13

RESPIRATORY MECHANICS

Lois Champion,
Pierre Cardinal, and
Richard Hodder

You are asked to assess a patient who is on the ventilator because of acute respiratory failure due to an asthma exacerbation. The nurses are concerned because the high pressure alarms are sounding off as are the low volume alarms. A respiratory therapist is making adjustments but they are questioning why repeated changes are necessary.

Troubleshooting a mechanical ventilator requires an understanding of respiratory mechanics. The compliance of the lung, both static and dynamic, is a crucial element that influences respiratory mechanics. We will discuss this, along with other factors that contribute to resistance to air flow. Our goal is to illustrate how these components of the equation of motion for the respiratory system can influence patient care. Work is exerted with every breath, whether spontaneous or mechanical, to overcome elastic and resistive forces. An increased work of breathing will therefore occur with decreased compliance or distension of the respiratory system, or an increased resistance to airflow. Ultimately, the goal is to reduce the work of breathing for the patient thereby allowing the patient to be removed from the ventilator. This chapter will review the pertinent aspects of respiratory mechanics to allow physicians to better manage patients with altered pulmonary function.

● Compliance and Resistance

Compliance is the volume change per unit of pressure change (Table 13.1). Compliance is a measure of the stiffness of the respiratory system, and is inversely proportional to elastic recoil (i.e., elastance). Clinically, one cannot differentiate between lung and chest wall compliance (Figure 13.1). In order to achieve this distinction, it would be necessary to measure the pleural pressure. The insertion of an esophageal

Table 13.1 – Respiratory Mechanics Equations

Equation 13.1   compliance = change in volume / change in pressure

Equation 13.2 $\text{dynamic compliance} = \dfrac{\text{tidal volume}}{\text{PAWP} - \text{PEEP}_{total}}$

    n.b.   PAWP is peak airway pressure
            PEEP_{total} = applied PEEP + auto-PEEP

Equation 13.3 $\text{static compliance} = \dfrac{\text{tidal volume}}{\text{P}_{plateau} - \text{PEEP}_{total}}$

    n.b. $\text{P}_{plateau}$ is plateau airway pressure
            PEEP_{total} = applied PEEP + auto-PEEP

Equation 13.4   resistance = pressure / flow

Equation 13.5 $\text{resistance} = \dfrac{\text{PAWP} - \text{P}_{plateau}}{\text{inspiratory flow}}$

    n.b.   PAWP is peak airway pressure
            $\text{P}_{plateau}$ is plateau airway pressure

Equation 13.6   work = pressure × volume

Equation 13.7   Ventilation = Resistive + Elastic
                         Pressure   Pressure   Pressure

Equation 13.8   Time constant = compliance × resistance
                             ($\text{ml/cm H}_2\text{O}$)   ($\text{cm H}_2\text{O/ml sec} -1$)

manometer could estimate the pleural pressures, but this is invasive and can cause the patient discomfort and thus is not routinely performed. The consequence of this is that the airway pressures generated with mechanical ventilation depend not only on the stiffness of the lungs, but also upon the stiffness of the chest wall and abdomen. Compliance also depends on lung volume. Post pneumonectomy patients, for example, will have a lower measured compliance but an unchanged lung dispensability, or *specific compliance,* of the remaining lung. Specific compliance refers to compliance that has been corrected for actual lung volume.

Dynamic compliance is the tidal volume divided by the peak airway pressure minus the amount of positive end expiratory pressure (PEEP) in the system (Table 13.1). For example, a tidal volume of 600 ml with a PEEP of 5 cm H_2O that generates a peak airway pressure of 35 cm H_2O represents a dynamic compliance of 20 ml/cm H_2O (or .02 l/cm H_2O). The dynamic compliance is not considered to be a true measure of compliance since peak airway pressure reflects the pressure required to overcome not only the elastic forces of the lung but also the resistive forces to airflow. If the tidal volume of 600 ml was delivered with a high flow rate over a fraction of a second, the peak airway pressure would be much higher than if the same tidal volume was delivered over several seconds. The higher peak airway pressure reflects a change in resistance with the high flow rate, rather than a change in respiratory system compliance.

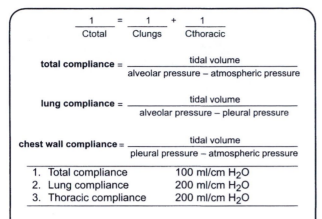

$$\frac{1}{C_{total}} = \frac{1}{C_{lungs}} + \frac{1}{C_{thoracic}}$$

$$\text{total compliance} = \frac{\text{tidal volume}}{\text{alveolar pressure} - \text{atmospheric pressure}}$$

$$\text{lung compliance} = \frac{\text{tidal volume}}{\text{alveolar pressure} - \text{pleural pressure}}$$

$$\text{chest wall compliance} = \frac{\text{tidal volume}}{\text{pleural pressure} - \text{atmospheric pressure}}$$

1. Total compliance   100 ml/cm H_2O
2. Lung compliance   200 ml/cm H_2O
3. Thoracic compliance   200 ml/cm H_2O

Figure 13.1 – Compliance Formulas and Normal Measurements

Figure 13.1 presents the formulas for the different types of compliance and the reported normal values.[1] Note that the lungs and chest wall are in series so that compliance of the lungs and chest wall add as reciprocals.

Static compliance is considered to be a better reflection of the compliance since the changes due to airflow resistance are no longer a confounder (Table 13.1). Thus, in order to measure the compliance without the confounding effect of airflow resistive forces, it is necessary to measure when airway pressure is static (i.e., no flow). A tidal volume is delivered and then "held" with a zero flow rate (known as an inspiratory hold). As shown in Figure 13.2, the airway pressure will decrease to a plateau pressure ($P_{plateau}$). The patient must not be attempting to trigger the ventilator in order to determine a plateau pressure. To achieve this lack of patient effort, the patient must be heavily sedated and sometimes even paralyzed. The concept of a plateau pressure is relevant for volume-cycled ventilation. With a pressure controlled or pressure support mode, pressure is maintained constant throughout inspiration. This means that the peak airway pressure and plateau pressure are the same. Prolonging inspiratory time will not result in a change in pressure, but will result in an increase in tidal volume. Total compliance can however change due to changes in the lung or other aspects of the system (Table 13.2).

Resistance to airflow depends both on frictional resistance (tissue resistance) and resistance to airflow (Table 13.1). Of these, resistance to airflow is the major determinant (>80%) of respiratory system resistance.

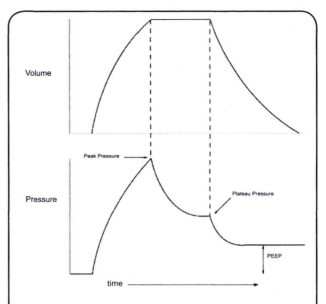

Figure 13.2 – Plateau Pressure and Inspiratory Pause

Figure 13.2 illustrates a waveform showing airway pressure versus time. Note the increase in airway pressure to peak airway pressure during inspiration. At the end of inspiration, the expiratory valve is closed creating a static or no flow state. The airway pressure then falls over about a second to a steady state plateau pressure. This is similar to the measurement of auto-PEEP, which requires an expiratory hold manoeuvre. The mean airway pressure is the area under the curve per change in time.

Clinically, resistance is not usually measured, but it can be quantified using a constant flow and an inspiratory hold manoeuvre in a fully relaxed patient.

● Airway Pressures with Mechanical Ventilation

Several different airway pressures can be measured during mechanical ventilation. Each has its own use in the management of patients (Figure 13.2).

A. Alveolar Distending Pressure

The actual alveolar distending pressure is the transmural alveolar pressure ($P_{alveolar} - P_{pleural}$).

Table 13.2 – Etiologies of Altered Compliance

Decreased Compliance		Increased Compliance
pneumonia	mainstem intubation	emphysema
atelectasis	kyphoscoliosis	open chest
obesity	congestive heart failure	flail chest
pulmonary fibrosis	generalized edema (anasarca)	
ARDS	abdominal distension	
pneumothorax	abdominal compartment syndrome	

Clinically, the pleural pressure is not routinely measured. However, it is known that pleural pressure will increase with PEEP and in patients with stiff chest walls. Experimentally, a static transpulmonary pressure of between 30 and 35 cm H_2O causes maximal alveolar inflation.[2]

B. Mean Airway Pressure

The mean airway pressure is the average pressure over the entire ventilatory cycle and therefore includes PEEP (although auto-PEEP does not contribute to the expiratory pressure). Mean airway pressure will correlate with the hemodynamic effects of positive pressure ventilation.

C. Peak Airway Pressure

The peak airway pressure (PAWP) is the highest pressure measured during inspiration. During volume-cycled ventilation, the PAWP depends on both the compliance of the respiratory system and the resistance to airflow. The PAWP does not always reflect the alveolar pressure because of the resistive component that contributes to PAWP. This results in a pressure gradient from the airway to the alveoli. In pressure controlled or pressure support ventilation, the PAWP will be equal to the set pressure plus the set PEEP.

D. Plateau Pressure

The plateau pressure ($P_{plateau}$) is measured after an inspiratory hold, or pause, with volume-cycled ventilation. The maximum pressure that the alveoli experience correlates is with the $P_{plateau}$, not the PAWP.

The reason for this is that there is additional pressure in the PAWP that overcomes the resistance to flow. When the $P_{plateau}$ is measured, there is no gas flow and thus there is no longer a pressure gradient between the site of measurement and the alveoli downstream. The $P_{plateau}$ is a more relevant parameter to monitor with respect to ventilator associated lung injury than PAWP. The ARDSNet trial for example used plateau pressure with volume cycled ventilation, with a goal of $P_{plateau} < 30$ cm H_2O.[2,4]

● Work of Breathing

The work of breathing represents the energy needed to ventilate the lungs. For the respiratory system, work is done when pressure changes the volume of the system (Table 13.1). Work is only done if movement takes place. The movement in the respiratory system is the air volume that changes the lung volume. Thus, no work is performed during isometric contraction (e.g., attempting to breath in against a closed glottis), despite the fact that effort is clearly expended.

The work that the respiratory muscles do is a combination of elastic work and resistive work. The elastic work opposes the elastic recoil of the lung and chest wall and the surface tension forces in the lung. Expiration during quiet breathing is usually passive, relying on the potential energy stored in the distended lungs and chest wall during inspiration. In many patients with respiratory failure, however, expiration also relies on the use of expiratory muscles (in particular abdominal muscles) to increase minute ventilation. The work of breathing is therefore greater.

The resistive work opposes the flow-resistive forces that develop as a result of gas flow through the airways, as well as the endotracheal tube and circuit of the mechanical ventilator. In addition, work is performed to overcome other forces, such as inertia and viscoelastic properties of the respiratory system (Table 13.3). Typically, the contribution of inertia and viscoelastic forces to the overall work of breathing is small.

At rest with quiet breathing, the respiratory muscles consume only a small proportion of our total oxygen consumption (in the order of 3%). With severe respiratory distress and shock there is both increased work of breathing and decreased oxygen delivery. In this situation the oxygen consumption of the respiratory muscles may be 25–30% of the total oxygen consumption (or higher).[1]

One of the indications for mechanical ventilation is to decrease the work of breathing in a patient with respiratory failure. Mechanical ventilation, however, may not decrease the work of breathing for a patient unless the ventilator rate and mode is carefully set and the patient monitored for signs of respiratory distress. There are many reasons why patients may have a high work of breathing, despite mechanical ventilation (Table 13.4). A low inspiratory flow rate, for example, in volume-cycled ventilation may cause persistent inspiratory effort as the patient continues

Table 13.3 – Work of Breathing

Elastic Forces – develop in the tissue of the lungs and chest wall when a volume change occurs

Flow-Resistive Forces – result from the flow of gas through airways

Viscoelastic forces – result from stress adaptation within the lung and chest wall

Plastoelastic Forces – a characteristic of stretchable materials. The plastoelastic forces of thoracic tissues help to explain the difference in the static elastic recoil of the respiratory system during inflation and deflation.

Inertial Forces –

Gas Compressibility – related to the compression and distension of intrathoracic gas

n.b. The respiratory muscles perform work against these forces.[1]

Table 13.4 – Causes of Increased Work of Breathing

1. Decreased compliance of the lungs or chest wall
2. Increased resistance to airflow
3. Active expiration
4. Ventilatory pattern
   a. compliance work is increased when breathing is slow and deep
   b. resistance work is increased with rapid shallow breathing (higher flow rates)
5. Added work is imposed by the ventilator or endotracheal tube

to try to breathe in from a limited available flow. Auto-PEEP can increase the work required to trigger a ventilator breath.[2,3] In this situation, the patient must first generate enough effort to overcome auto-PEEP (which may be 5–20 cm H_2O), before the ventilator can be triggered (Chapter 12). Patients may begin to try to breath out during inspiration, particularly if inspiratory time is prolonged.

● Equation of Motion

The pressure required to deliver a mechanical ventilator breath has two components (Table 13.1). The first is the pressure needed to cause flow through the airways and overcome the resistance to airflow. Resistive pressure is the product of resistance and flow. The second is the pressure required to overcome the elastic recoil of the lungs and chest wall. The required pressure to overcome the elastic recoil is the product of elastance (i.e., inverse of compliance) and volume. Ventilation pressures are therefore the sum of the negative intrathoracic pressure generated by the respiratory muscles during spontaneous ventilation and the positive airway pressure generated by the ventilator (Figure 13.3 and Figure 13.4).

The equation of motion has three important consequences.[1] First, one can calculate the compliance and resistance of the respiratory system if the ventilatory muscles are relaxed ($P_{mus} = 0$) and if flow, volume and pressure are measured. Second, when flow is zero (e.g., at end of inspiration) then ventilation pressure depends on volume and elastance (1/compliance). Finally, one cannot manipulate all of

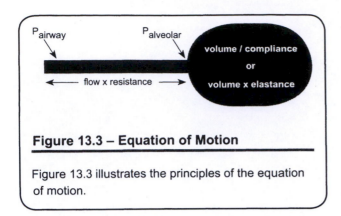

Figure 13.3 – Equation of Motion

Figure 13.3 illustrates the principles of the equation of motion.

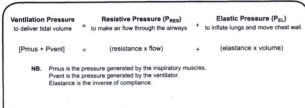

Figure 13.4 – Ventilation Pressure Formula

The pressures that the ventilator must overcome are the sum of both the resistive pressure to air flow and the pressure to overcome the elastic properties of the lung.

the variables involved in the equation of motion simultaneously. For example, if a ventilating pressure is set in a patient with a given elastance and resistance to flow, then a specific tidal volume will be delivered. If the tidal volume and inspiratory flow rate are set, the airway pressure that is generated depends on the elastance and resistance of the patient's respiratory system. One cannot simultaneously set both the tidal volume and the ventilating pressure.

● Pressure Volume Loops

Pressure volume loops plot pressure (on the x axis) versus volume (on the y axis) during inspiration and expiration. Pressure volume loops demonstrate a phenomenon called hysteresis. Hysteresis refers to how the pressure volume curve of inflation and deflation differ. The curve is larger on the deflation limb of the loop because the lung is more compliant once stretched. Clinically, the consequences of this is that once alveoli are opened (recruited), less pressure is required to keep these lung units open. A pressure

volume curve (as opposed to a loop) is generated only on inspiration, not on expiration.

Pressure volume loops can be generated under static (no flow) conditions or under dynamic conditions (with flow during a breath). Many newer generation ventilators have the capability of providing waveforms such as pressure-time, flow-time, pressure-volume, and others on a real-time (dynamic) basis. Some ventilators are also able to generate pressure volume loops under no flow (static) or low flow (quasi-static) conditions.

Static pressure volume loops allow assessment of the compliance of the respiratory system (both the lung and the chest wall). Since these loops are generated under static conditions, the effect of resistance on airway pressure is eliminated. Static pressure volume loops have been suggested as a method for assessing the severity of lung injury and optimizing PEEP.

Several methods have been described for producing a static pressure volume loop but they all require the patient to be sedated and paralyzed since spontaneous inspiratory efforts will interfere with measurements (Table 13.5).[5] The *super syringe* method requires that the patient be preoxygenated with 100% oxygen and then disconnected from the ventilator so that the lungs empty to functional residual capacity. A large syringe is used to inflate the lungs using 50–100 ml increments up to a volume up to 1.5–3 litres. Airway pressures are measured with each volume increment. The same manoeuvre is performed on deflation withdrawing 50–100 ml of volume with each step. The entire procedure takes about a minute. The *inspiratory occlusion* technique consists of the measurement of plateau pressures that correspond to different tidal volumes using volume-cycled ventilation. The pressure volume inspiratory curve is developed using the plateau pressure corresponding to the administered tidal volumes and this procedure takes up to 15 minutes. Finally, the *quasi-static* method creates the inspiratory pressure volume curve by using continuous inflation at a constant inspiratory flow. The flow is very low, thus minimizing (although

Table 13.5 – Techniques to Measure Static Pressure Volume Loop

1. Super Syringe Method
2. Inspiratory Occlusion Technique
3. Quasi-static Method

not eliminating) the contribution of airway resistance to the airway pressures generated.

When interpreting static pressure volume loops, there are several aspects that must be considered (Figure 13.5). With positive pressure ventilation the loop is generated in a counter-clockwise direction. With spontaneous ventilation a loop would be plotted in a clockwise direction. The expiratory limb does not return to zero, which is likely due to oxygen consumption that occurs during the measurement (this accounts for the volume change). The slope of the curve represents compliance (pressure/volume). An important spot is the *lower inflection point* where compliance increases. The lower inflection point has been considered to represent a point where alveoli have been recruited and the lung becomes more compliant (i.e., less stiff because the lung volume has increased with the opening of these alveoli). There is also an upper inflection point where compliance decreases which is thought to represent over-distension of alveoli.

It has been suggested that the ideal amount of PEEP should be titrated to 2–3 cm H_2O above the lower inflection point and that ventilation should take place within the linear compliance area (between the lower and upper inflection points). There are however problems with using a static pressure volume curve clinically (quite apart from the difficulties in trying to obtain a curve).[5-7] The compliance and therefore the pressure volume curve are affected by chest wall compliance, not just lung compliance. There is also no consensus on how best to obtain these curves

safely and accurately in a clinical environment, thus limiting their value. Pressure volume curves are also affected by the tidal volumes and PEEP before the curve is done. Further, often the curve does not have an easily discernable inflection point and interobserver variation in identifying an inflection point limits their value. The value of PEEP to prevent derecruitment of alveoli may be more important on the deflation limb of a pressure volume loop, rather than the inflation limb. Finally, recruitment of alveoli is not an all or nothing phenomenon that occurs at a specific pressure. Alveolar recruitment occurs throughout inspiration, co-existant with distension of other alveoli. For these reasons, static pressure volume loops have not gained widespread acceptance for determination of optimal PEEP values.

Other forms of pressure volume loops can be generated. *Dynamic pressure volume loops* that are generated during mechanical ventilation do not reflect the true compliance of the respiratory system because the gas flow generates a pressure gradient due to the resistive components of the system. The loops obtained will depend on the mode of ventilation as well as changes in flow rates (Figure 13.6). The pressure volume loops obtained in pressure controlled ventilation differ (Figure 13.7). In pressure controlled ventilation, the inspiratory pressure is preset and the inspiratory flow decreases throughout inspiration (decelerating flow pattern).

● Time Constant (t)

Exponential functions are characterized by time constants, which describe the rate of variation of a function over time. A system with a long time constant will react slowly to a stimulus. For the respiratory system the time constant depends on the compliance and resistance of the system (Table 13.1). The time constant for a normal respiratory system is approximately 0.79 seconds. Since time constants describe an exponential function, an event is approximately 95% complete after 3 time constants (Figure 13.8). In lung disease there is increased non-homogeneity of lung units. Thus, with the use of a short inspiratory time, gas may be preferentially delivered to stiff alveoli (short time constant). There is some suggestion experimentally that lengthening inspiratory time may improve distribution of ventilation to alveoli that are more compliant or have high resistance ("slow alveoli") (Figure 13.9).

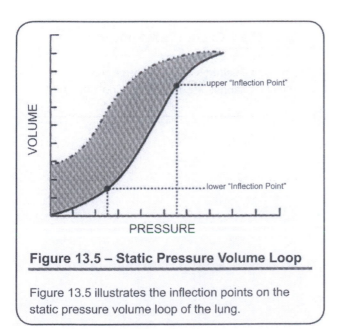

Figure 13.5 – Static Pressure Volume Loop

Figure 13.5 illustrates the inflection points on the static pressure volume loop of the lung.

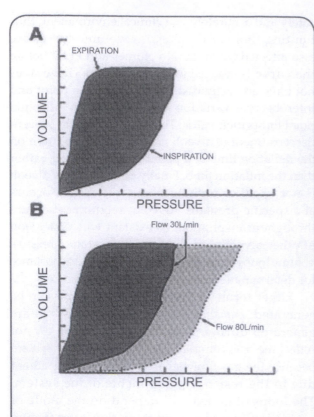

Figure 13.6 – P-V Loops in Volume-Cycled Ventilation

Figure 13.6a shows a typical loop generated with constant flow and volume ventilation. During inspiration the lung is inflated with a set tidal volume and the airway pressure increases throughout inspiration. This pressure will depend on the compliance of the respiratory system, the resistive properties and the inspiratory flow rate. With exhalation the ventilator opens the exhalation valve and the pressure decreases to the set level of PEEP.

Figure 13.6b illustrates loops obtained with a change in the inspiratory flow rate using a constant inspiratory flow. Note that with an increase in flow rate the inspiratory airway pressure is higher. Different loops would be obtained with different inspiratory flow patterns (for example, a decelerating pattern).

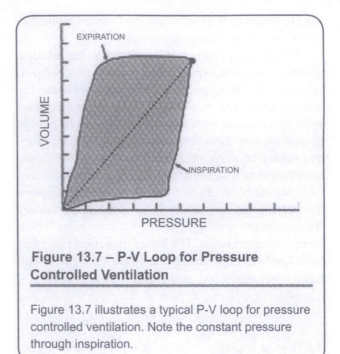

Figure 13.7 – P-V Loop for Pressure Controlled Ventilation

Figure 13.7 illustrates a typical P-V loop for pressure controlled ventilation. Note the constant pressure through inspiration.

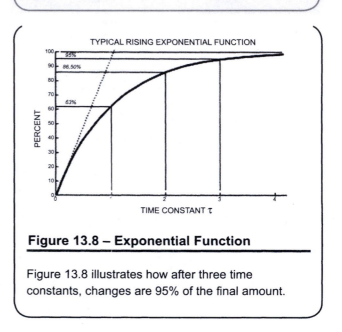

Figure 13.8 – Exponential Function

Figure 13.8 illustrates how after three time constants, changes are 95% of the final amount.

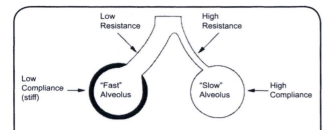

Figure 13.9 – Slow and Fast Filling Alveoli

Figure 13.9 demonstrates alveoli that can be thought of as "fast" and "slow." The low resistance, low compliance alveoli will fill quickly, and gas flow will be preferentially directed to these alveoli. The "slow" alveoli will have longer time constants and therefore require a longer inspiratory time for filling. A prolongation of inspiratory time may improve distribution of ventilation and gas exchange.

Key Points

- The work of breathing includes work done to oppose the elastic forces of the respiratory system and the resistance to airflow.
- Mechanical ventilation does not necessarily decrease work of breathing—you just need to observe a tachypneic distressed patient with patient-ventilator dysynchrony to recognize this.

- Peak airway pressure is not the same as alveolar pressure; with volume-cycled ventilation the plateau pressure more closely reflects alveolar pressure.
- The equation of motion incorporates the concepts of elastance (the inverse of compliance) and resistance into one equation.

References

1. Tobin M: *Principles and practices of mechanical ventilation.* McGraw Hill, New York, 1994.
2. Tobin M: Advances in mechanical ventilation. *N Engl J Med* 2001;344:1986–96.
3. Tobin M, Jubran A, Laghi F: Patient-ventilator interaction. *Am J Respir Crit Care Med* 2001;163:1059–63.
4. The Acute Respiratory Distress Syndrome Network: Ventilation with lower tidal volumes as compared with traditional tidal volumes for acute lung injury and the acute respiratory distress syndrome. *N Engl J Med* 2000;342:1301–8.
5. Lu Q, Rouby JJ: Measurement of pressure-volume curves in patients on mechanical ventilation: Methods and significance. *Crit Care* 2000;4:91–100.
6. Crottic S, Mascheroni D, Caironi P, et al: Recruitment and derecruitment during acute respiratory distress syndrome. *Am J Respir Crit Care Med* 2001;164:131–40.
7. Dreyfuss D: Pressure volume curves: Searching for the grail or laying patients with adult respiratory distress syndrome on Procrustes' bed? *Am J Respir Crit Care Med* 2001;163:2–3.

CHAPTER 14

PRACTICAL APPROACH TO MECHANICAL VENTILATION

**LOIS CHAMPION,
PIERRE CARDINAL, AND
RICHARD HODDER**

You are asked to reassess a patient you placed on a mechanical ventilator earlier that evening. She is a 63-year-old female who was intubated and ventilated because of respiratory failure due to a community acquired pneumonia. She has a significant history of chronic obstructive pulmonary disease (COPD). Her arterial blood gas reveals a pH of 7.06 with a $PaCO_2$ of 68 mm Hg and a PaO_2 of only 55 mm Hg. When you arrive, she is tachypneic and agitated. Alarms on the ventilator are sounding off repeatedly.

Mechanical ventilation is used to help provide oxygenation and ventilation for patients with respiratory failure. Unfortunately, mechanical ventilation can cause lung injury, hemodynamic instability and patient distress if not applied carefully and appropriately. The goal of this chapter is to discuss ventilator-induced lung injury and present strategies to prevent it. We will cover mechanical ventilation strategies for various lung diseases such as acute respiratory distress syndrome, COPD and asthma. Finally, we will discuss an approach to management of patient-ventilator dysynchrony, including identification of any contributing factors.

● Concepts in Mechanical Ventilation

A. Ventilator-Induced Lung Injury

Traditional recommendations have been to use a tidal volume of 10–15 ml/kg during mechanical ventilation. These large volumes were recommended despite the fact that normal tidal volumes during spontaneous ventilation is only 4–6 ml/kg. The use of a relatively large tidal volume, however, seemed to improve oxygenation in patients during anesthesia and was thought to compensate for the decrease in functional residual capacity that occurs with the supine position and anesthesia. It was apparent, however, that mechanical ventilation with such large tidal volumes was associated with complications such as pneumothorax, pneumomediastinum and interstitial emphysema of the lung. These complications, collectively known as *barotrauma*, tended to occur in patients with severe lung injury and those who had high pressures during ventilation. Over the past decade it has become increasingly clear that mechanical ventilation can contribute not only to air leaks but also to other forms of lung injury (Table 14.1). This concept is known as ventilator-induced lung injury (VILI) or ventilator-associated lung injury.

Animal studies demonstrate that ventilation with large tidal volumes damages the alveolar epithelium and capillary endothelium with increased microvascular permeability and pulmonary edema. Morphologically, these changes are the same as those seen in acute respiratory distress syndrome. Release of inflammatory mediators have been demonstrated in human and animal studies where mechanical ventilation using high volumes was used.

Animal studies demonstrate that VILI is primarily related to increases in lung volume with alveolar distension rather than increases in airway pressure in the absence of volume change. Large increases in lung volume are associated with lung injury, even if airway pressures do not increase or rise only minimally. Lung injury can be caused by negative pressure ventilation with large tidal volumes or in animals with the chest wall removed allowing high volume ventilation with minimal airway pressures. Similarly, high airway pressures, in the absence of large lung volume changes, do not result in lung injury. Animals that were ventilated with high airway pressures but whose abdomens and chest walls were splinted to prevent large increases in lung volumes, did not develop VILI. The term *volutrauma* therefore more accurately reflects the mechanism of lung injury in VILI—as opposed to *barotrauma*.

Cyclic opening and closing of lung units with ventilator breaths also causes a form of lung injury sometimes called *atelectactic trauma*. The underlying mechanism is that the cyclic changes create large shearing forces in the walls of the terminal bronchioles. In addition, the architecture of the lung means that alveoli and small bronchioles are interdependent. Thus, forces affecting one lung unit are transmitted to other units, and over-distension or collapse results in tractional forces that affect adjacent lung units to cause further lung damage.

The different categories of lung injury appear to release cytokines that not only potentiate lung injury but also contribute to a systemic inflammatory response. Thus, injury to the lung from mechanical ventilation can impair the function of other organs. The concept of *biotrauma* has thus been used to describe the underlying detrimental effects of mechanical ventilation.

Table 14.1 – Proposed Mechanisms of Ventilator-Induced Lung Injury[1,2]

1. Alveolar overdistension with damage to alveolar epithelium and capillary endothelium ("volutrauma")
2. Shear stress due to cyclic opening and closing of airways with each breath ("atelectactic trauma")
3. Interdependence of alveoli and bronchioles, so that the forces acting on one lung unit are transmitted to adjacent areas. Alveolar collapse, for example, causes tractional forces on adjacent alveoli
4. Release of inflammatory mediators including cytokines from lung tissue with alveolar overdistension ("biotrauma")
5. Translocation of bacteria from injured lung into the circulation

B. Lung Protective Ventilation

Lung protective ventilation strategies are designed to try to decrease lung injury due to mechanical ventilation. There are still many unanswered questions about how best to ventilate patients and thus it is unclear as to what is the best tidal volume, mode of ventilation, ventilating pressure or PEEP to use for a given patient.[3-6] Evidence however supports the premise that alveolar distending pressures of 30–35 cm H_2O will maximally distend normal alveoli. It is clear that large tidal volumes are associated with VILI and alveolar and epithelial damage. There have been several clinical trials of mechanical ventilation in humans. The largest study, the ARDSNetwork trial,[7] compared patients randomized to a control arm (tidal volume of 12 ml/kg predicted body weight and plateau pressure < 50 cm H_2O) versus patients randomized to a protective lung ventilation strategy (tidal volume of 6 ml/kg and plateau pressure of < 30 cm H_2O). There was a decrease in mortality in patients with the lower tidal volume ventilation (31.0% vs. 39.8% p = 0.007). Although this trial is not the "final answer" in the lung protective ventilation story, it certainly added considerable evidence towards the prevention of VILI. Regardless, there is ongoing debate in the literature and significant variation clinically in the approach to mechanical ventilation in patients with lung injury (Tables 14.2 and 14.3).[5-24] The good news is that there are further trials in progress that will help to answer our questions. Lung protective ventilation strategies that incorporate the use of PEEP to splint alveoli open to prevent shearing forces and improve oxygenation are in progress.

C. Permissive Hypercapnia

Carbon dioxide levels depend on carbon dioxide production and alveolar ventilation. Alveolar ventilation depends on minute ventilation and the proportion of dead space ventilation. Patients with severe lung injury have increased alveolar dead space and require higher minute ventilation. Thus, to maintain a "normal" $PaCO_2$ and pH, an increase in either the tidal volume or respiratory rate, or both, will be required.

Permissive hypercapnia is a ventilatory strategy that gives priority to lung protective ventilation (limiting tidal volumes and/or airway pressures) rather than to maintaining a normal pH and $PaCO_2$. Hypercapnia and acidosis are usually well tolerated, and the risk-benefit balance favours allowing mild to moderate hypercapnic acidosis (pH > 7.20) rather than attempting to increase tidal volume or respiratory rate excessively in patients with lung injury.[4] Presently, it is unknown what the lower level is for a "safe" pH. Many clinicians will begin to correct hypercapnic acidosis using bicarbonate once the pH falls below 7.20–7.25. An increase in $PaCO_2$ and respiratory acidosis is relatively contraindicated in patients with cerebral edema because the increase in $PaCO_2$ is associated with cerebral vasodilatation that could worsen edema.

$$PaCO_2 \propto \frac{\text{carbon dioxide production}}{\text{alveolar ventilation}}$$

Table 14.2 – Lung Protective Ventilation — What We Know (or Think We Know)

1. Tidal volumes that are very large (e.g., >12 ml/kg) can cause alveolar overdistension and are bad for lungs.
2. Ventilation with tidal volumes of 8–12 ml/kg appears to be safe, even for prolonged periods, with normal lungs.
3. With lung injury, for example ARDS, some of the lung is collapsed or filled with debris, and is not ventilated. This means that the tidal volume is distributed to only a portion of the lung; a tidal volume of 10 ml/kg in this situation may be ventilating only a fraction of the lung and causing overdistension of the ventilated alveoli.
4. Ventilation at low lung volumes is bad: This causes cyclic collapse and opening of lung units, which may be prevented by PEEP
5. PEEP can help to prevent end expiratory collapse of alveoli and improve oxygenation and ventilation.
6. Too much PEEP can cause overdistension of compliant alveoli.
7. Alveoli are recruited throughout inspiration; there is no one level of PEEP that works for all the alveoli (no surprise).
8. With severe lung injury there are areas of the lung that will not be recruited/opened up/ventilated no matter what pressures we use.
9. Transplumonary pressures (alveolar pressure minus intrathoracic pressure) > 30–35 cm H_2O will cause overdistension of alveoli and lung damage.
10. Peak airway pressure is not the same as alveolar pressure. There is a pressure gradient from the airway to the alveoli due to resistance and gas flow.
11. With volume-cycled ventilation, plateau pressure more closely reflects alveolar pressure.
12. Alveolar pressure is not the same as transpulmonary pressure. A patient with severe chest wall edema and a distended abdomen will have a high intrathoracic pressure; a higher ventilating pressure in these patients may be safe.

Table 14.3 – Lung Protective Ventilation — What We're Not Sure About

1. Should we use volume-cycled ventilation with a constant tidal volume or pressure controlled ventilation for patients with severe lung injury? Or should we be using another form of ventilation such as high frequency oscillation?

2. How much PEEP should we use in a patient? And how do we decide?

3. Should we measure auto-PEEP and try to avoid it? Or is it somehow a beneficial side effect of high respiratory rates? (The ARDSNetwork study didn't measure auto-PEEP)

4. Is a tidal volume of 6 ml/kg predicted body weight a reasonable goal, or is 7–8 ml/kg safe?

5. Are recruitment manoeuvres a helpful adjunct to mechanical ventilation?

6. Should we tolerate mild to moderate acidosis due to permissive hypercapnia, or should we treat with bicarbonate?

7. If we have patients with a noncompliant thorax can we safely allow higher ventilating pressures? If so, how high, and how do we decide?

8. Many, many more questions…

● Acute Respiratory Distress Syndrome

Acute respiratory distress syndrome (ARDS) is a syndrome characterized by an acute onset, hypoxemia ($PaO_2/FiO_2 < 200$), bilateral infiltrates on chest x-ray and no evidence clinically or using invasive monitoring that the cause is left atrial hypertension (cardiogenic pulmonary edema). Acute lung injury (ALI) is present if the PaO_2/FiO_2 is < 300.[6] There are many different causes of ARDS, but they can be divided into primary pulmonary causes (for example aspiration, pneumonia, inhalation injury, near drowning, lung contusion) and extrapulmonary causes (e.g., sepsis, trauma, pancreatitis, drug overdose, etc.).

Pathologically, ARDS is characterized by an initial inflammatory or exudative phase. Computed tomography of lungs in patients with ARDS in this stage show that the lung involvement is not nearly as homogeneous as suggested by simple chest x-rays.

A model of the ARDS lung that divides the lung into three zones has been suggested based on CT images.[7,8] The first zone is made up of areas of normal lung with normal compliance and is usually located in the non-dependent regions. The second zone is made up of areas of lung that are collapsed but can be recruited and ventilated with the use of PEEP. The third zone is made up of areas of lung (usually dependant), that are consolidated, and either represent collapse of alveoli or alveoli that are filled with debris. These areas are not recruitable and do not contribute to gas exchange but do cause shunting and therefore contribute to hypoxemia. The exudative phase of ARDS evolves to a second phase, called the fibroproliferative phase, over a week to 10 days. This phase involves fibrosis of the lung and has been associated with an increase in dead space and development of bullae and lung cysts.

The underlying consequences of the pathology in ARDS is that ventilation gets distributed to only a small portion of the lung. A tidal volume that would not cause injury in a normal lung may be associated with VILI in ARDS because it is distributed to a small fraction of the lung volume, resulting in over-distention of those alveoli. There is general agreement that a lung protective strategy should be used to ventilate patients with ARDS. One approach is to use the strategy of the ARDSNetwork study (Tables 14.4 to 14.6). Hypoxemia can be a major problem in patients with ARDS due to intrapulmonary shunting and ventilation-perfusion mismatch. A reasonable approach is to accept an oxygen saturation of 88–93%, with the recognition that a saturation in this range will provide a safe oxygen content in arterial blood.

In the hypoxemic ARDS patient, start with an FiO_2 of 1.0 and titrate the oxygen down to maintain a saturation greater than approximately 88%. Positive end expiratory pressure can be used to try to recruit alveoli and improve oxygenation. One approach is to use a PEEP nomogram such as that studied in the ARDSNetwork trial (Table 14.5). It is important to remember that PEEP has adverse effects and may not improve oxygenation in some patients (e.g., using PEEP to improve oxygenation in a patient with a pneumothorax would not work!).

In severe ARDS, hypoxemia may persist despite 100% oxygen and attempts to optimize PEEP. For these patients, other options to improve oxygenation can be used (Table 14.7). The use of lung recruitment

Table 14.4 – Ventilator Management Protocol Used in the ARDSNetwork Study

1. Ventilator mode: assist/control volume cycled ventilation
2. Tidal volume: 6 ml/kg predicted body weight (Table 14.6)
3. Goals:
    - plateau pressure ($P_{plateau}$) < 30 cm H_2O
    - tidal volume to as low as 4 ml/kg to limit $P_{plateau}$ as needed
    - oxygen saturation 88–95%
    - PEEP titrated as per algorithm (Table 14.5)
    - pH 7.30–7.45
    - increase in ventilator rate to maximum 35 bpm for pH < 7.30
        - for continued acidosis and ventilator rate 35, or PCO_2 < 25 mm Hg, then bicarbonate infusion suggested (clinician discretion)
        - if pH < 7.15 a bicarbonate infusion is required
        - if ongoing acidosis with pH < 7.15 despite bicarbonate, then tidal volumes increased by 1 ml/kg until pH > 7.15

source: The Acute Respiratory Distress Syndrome Network.[7]

Table 14.6 – Calculation of Predicted Body Weight (PBW) Based on Height

Male: PBW = 50 + 0.91 [height (cm) – 152.4]
Female: PBW = 45.5 + 0.91 [height (cm) – 152.4]

source: The Acute Respiratory Distress Syndrome Network.[7]

Table 14.7 – Strategies for Refractory Hypoxemia in ARDS

1. Lung Recruitment Manoeuvres
2. Decreasing Oxygen Consumption
3. Prone Positioning
4. Extracorporeal Membrane Oxygenation
5. Inhaled Nitric Oxide
6. Ensure Adequate Oxygen Delivery
    a. Cardiac Output
    b. Hemoglobin
7. Rule Out Intracardiac Right to Left Shunts

manoeuvres to open up collapsed alveoli may help but presently there is no evidence from clinical trials that these manoeuvres are beneficial. Prone positioning has been shown to improve oxygenation but clinical trials have not shown improved survival. Extracorporeal membrane oxygenation has also been used as a "rescue" therapy. Clinical trials have not shown improved outcome. Inhaled nitric oxide has also been shown to temporarily improve oxygenation by increasing ventilation-perfusion matching but once again clinical trials have not shown improved survival with its use. Since shunting in the lung contributes to hypoxemia in ARDS, increasing the mixed venous oxygen saturation by improving oxygen delivery can be beneficial. Oxygen delivery is improved by ensuring an adequate cardiac output and hemoglobin. The mixed venous saturation levels are also improved by reducing oxygen consumption. Decreasing oxygen consumption with the use of sedation and/or muscle paralysis with neuromuscular relaxants and treating fever to maintain normothermia thus may also improve refractory hypoxemia in ARDS patients. Finally, refractory hypoxemia may

Table Table 14.5 – Algorithm for Management of PEEP Used in the ARDSNetwork Study

FiO$_2$	0.3	0.4	0.4	0.5	0.5	0.6	0.7	0.7	0.8	0.9	0.9	0.9	1.0
PEEP	5	5	8	8	10	10	10	12	14	14	16	18	20–24

source: The Acute Respiratory Distress Syndrome Network.[7]

be due to the presence of an intracardiac right to left shunt. ARDS patients with right heart failure and high right sided filling pressures may open up a foramen ovale and shunt blood from the right atrium to the left atrium. The diagnosis can be made with a bubble study during echocardiography. Right to left intracardiac shunting has been described in patients with ARDS and pulmonary embolism. If this is the cause of the hypoxemia, PEEP may make oxygenation worse by increasing pulmonary vascular resistance and right-sided intracardiac pressures.

Chronic Obstructive Pulmonary Disease (COPD)

Mechanical ventilation of a patient with severe COPD and expiratory airflow obstruction can be a challenge. Management should focus on treating bronchospasm and avoiding patient ventilator dysynchrony and auto-PEEP. Following intubation, be very careful to avoid "bagging" the patient too aggressively. Aggressive insufflation can cause hyperinflation with auto-PEEP, leading to barotrauma (such as pneumothorax) or cardiovascular collapse due to high intrathoracic pressures. Additionally, many patients with severe COPD who require ventilation have a degree of chronic hypercapnia with a compensatory metabolic alkalosis. Inadvertently ventilating these patients to a $PaCO_2$ of 40 l/min would cause a severe alkalosis. Remember that ventilation is guided by pH, not $PaCO_2$.

Initial ventilator settings should include a tidal volume of 7–8 ml/kg, but this may need to be decreased if airway pressures exceed 35–40 cm H_2O. The respiratory rate should be low enough to allow a prolonged expiratory time with complete emptying of the preceding breath. Alternatively, pressure support ventilation could be used, however, this may not be well tolerated if the patient is fatigued and the work of breathing is high. Remember that pressure support ventilation can also be associated with air trapping and auto-PEEP (Chapter 12). Flow-time waveforms can be helpful in these patients; documenting expiratory flow that does not reach zero before the next breath implies a degree of air-trapping or auto-PEEP.

The long expiratory time, and therefore low respiratory rate, that is required to avoid hyperinflation may result in hypercapnia. Clinically this is usually not a concern, and many clinicians would find a pH > 7.20–7.30 acceptable. A lower pH can be managed with bicarbonate. Any degree of acidosis however is a powerful stimulus for ventilation, and usually requires sedation to prevent tachypnea and patient-ventilator dysynchrony. Neuromuscular relaxants should be avoided if at all possible because of the association with myopathy and neuropathy, particularly with concomitant use of parenteral steroids.

Asthma

Patients with severe asthma or status asthmaticus, requiring intubation and ventilation, are also at risk for hyperinflation, barotrauma and hemodynamic collapse due to increased intrathoracic pressures. Many of these patients are volume depleted at the time of intubation, and hypotension due to decreased venous return with positive pressure ventilation should be anticipated.

The principles of mechanical ventilation in these patients are similar to those for patients with severe COPD. The respiratory rate should be low in order to allow a prolonged expiratory time and to minimize auto-PEEP. Plateau pressures of < 30 cm H_2O are recommended.[25,26] The low respiratory rate and focus on preventing high airway pressures will almost undoubtedly result in hypercapnia. Sedation will likely be required to prevent respiratory distress, and tachypnea with attempts at triggering the ventilator. As with COPD, neuromuscular relaxants should be avoided if possible.

Obesity

The obese patient typically has decreased lung volumes due to their large abdomens and increased airway resistance.[27] The compliance of the respiratory system is decreased, in large degree because of a decrease in chest wall compliance. The tidal volumes that are used should be based on ideal body weight or predicted body weight as opposed to actual body weight. Positioning the patient head up or in a reverse Trendelenberg position may improve compliance and airway pressures.

Patient-Ventilator Dysynchrony

Numerous different problems can cause patient-ventilator dysynchrony. This problem, sometimes referred to as the patient "fighting the ventilator," is a common problem for a patient on a ventilator. Although sedation is often required to help to settle the patient, it is also important to identify and manage the causes, rather than just heavily sedate or paralyze the patient without thinking the problem through.

The most important principle is to rule out hypoxemia or acidosis as a cause for agitation and/or tachypnea. Check the oxygen saturation, and also look at the patient's spontaneous breathing rate and pattern. A patient who is tachypneic and gasping may be acidotic. Ensure that agitation and tachypnea associated with mechanical ventilation is not due to pain, myocardial ischemia, urinary retention, shock or delirium, for example.

Is the patient tachypneic and triggering or trying to trigger extra breaths on an assist/control mode? If the AC rate is set so low that the patient is triggering the majority of the breaths, simply increasing the ventilator rate to match the patient's demand may make the patient more comfortable. Look at the patient's chest: Is it moving symmetrically? Are breath sounds equal bilaterally? It is important to rule out mucous plugging, pulmonary edema, pneumothorax, bronchospasm and mainstem intubation since these are treatable causes of respiratory distress.

It is often helpful to take the patient off the ventilator and ventilate manually with a self-inflating bag. This will allow you to get a "feel" for whether the problem is with the ventilator settings or with the patient or endotracheal tube. If the patient settles with bagging, then modifying the ventilator settings or changing the mode of ventilation may help. If high airway pressures are generated with bagging, make sure the endotracheal tube is patent and not kinked or blocked. The easiest way to ensure that the tube is patent is to insert a suction catheter down it. Also ensure that the expiratory time is adequate and that there is no component of auto-PEEP contributing to the patient's distress.

Help — the Oxygen Saturation Is Falling!

Although it is easier said than done, try not to panic. Place the patient on 100% oxygen as the first step and reassess the ABC's. It is often helpful to take the patient off the ventilator and to temporarily ventilate manually. An exception to this approach is a patient on high levels of PEEP since manual ventilation will not be able to continue to provide PEEP and thus will further worsen the hypoxemia. As always, it is important to ensure that the patient is monitored and frequently reassessed.

Never hesitate to call for help! Recheck the vital signs including the heart rate, blood pressure and respiratory rate. Closely monitor the heart rate, oxygen saturation and the blood pressure. Ideally, an arterial line is in place. Failing this, the blood pressure should be monitored by a cuff in the STAT mode on an automatic non-invasive machine. Reassess the airway to ensure that the endotracheal or tracheostomy tube is patent and in place. If there is a lot of resistance to bagging, a kinked or plugged tube may be the problem. A suction catheter should pass through the tube easily. If you are unable to pass a catheter through the tube then you need to consider reintubation.

Reassess the patient's breathing. Is the trachea midline? Is the chest moving up and down symmetrically? Are breath sounds present bilaterally? Are breath sounds normal? Is there subcutaneous emphysema? Is abdominal distension contributing to high airway pressures and difficulty with ventilation? Clinically, it is important to rule out a mainstem bronchus intubation, mucous plugging with lung collapse, a pneumothorax, pulmonary edema, bronchospasm, aspiration, pulmonary hemorrhage and numerous other causes of lung pathology. More difficult to clinically diagnose are causes of hypoxemia and desaturation such as microatelectasis, worsening of an underlying disease process such as pneumonia or ARDS or a pulmonary embolism. A chest x-ray may help diagnose some of these problems. Call for a STAT chest x-ray unless the desaturation was transient and resolved completely.

Therapy can include sedation for a patient who is hypoxemic and agitated or tachypneic until the underlying problem can be identified and corrected. Consider increasing PEEP if saturation does not improve with an increase in Fio_2 especially if hypoxemia is due to pulmonary edema or ARDS. Be aware of the limitations and relative contraindications to the use of PEEP.

● Lung Recruitment Manoeuvre

A lung recruitment manoeuvre (LRM) is a sustained lung inflation designed to recruit alveoli. The idea is that very high pressures may be required to open up lung units so that they can be ventilated, and once opened they can be maintained open with the use of PEEP (it takes more pressure to open up lung units than to keep them open).[28] There are several different approaches to applying an LRM. These include "sigh" breaths several times a minute, or the use of temporary increases in PEEP or tidal volume, or a sustained inflation pressure as described below.[28] A trial studying the use of recruitment manoeuvres and high PEEP using pressure control ventilation as compared to the ventilatory protocol used in the ARDSNetwork study is currently in progress.[29]

A recruitment manoeuvre can be done using a sustained inflation of 40 cm H_2O for 40 seconds, with an Fio_2 of 1.0. There are several different contraindications to an LRM.[29] An LRM may decrease the blood pressure and thus should be avoided in hypotensive patients. The increase in intrathoracic pressures with an LRM can worsen an air leak or emphysema. Thus, LRMs should be avoided in patients who have a persistent air leak through a thoracostomy tube or have spontaneous subcutaneous emphysema (i.e., not related to trauma, procedures, etc.) or pericardial or mediastinal emphysema. Finally, the presence of underlying pneumatoceles is a relative contraindication to the use of an LRM.

An LRM may need to be stopped early if a patient does not tolerate the sustained high airway pressure. Reasons for stopping an LRM include oxygen saturation < 85%, heart rate < 60 or > 140, onset of a new arrhythmia, hypotension or the development of a new air leak through a chest tube.

Key Points

- Consider lung-protective ventilatory strategies for patients with ARDS, including limitation of tidal volumes and ventilating pressures and permissive hypercapnia.
- For bronchospastic patients such as those with COPD and asthma to avoid auto-PEEP they require prolonged expiratory times, a low respiratory rate and tidal volumes low enough to prevent high airway pressures.
- Severe hypercapnia with acidosis can be managed with bicarbonate.
- Ventilated patients may become agitated and tachypneic and thus may require sedation, but it is important to rule out treatable causes of patient-ventilator dysynchrony.

References

1. Whitehead T, Slutsky A: The pulmonary physician in critical care: Ventilator induced lung injury. *Thorax* 2002;57:635–42.
2. Adams A, Simonson D, Dries D: Ventilator-induced lung injury. *Respir Care Clin N Am* 2003;9:343–62.
3. Brower RG, Rubenfeld GD: Lung-protective ventilation strategies in acute lung injury. *Crit Care Med* 2003;31(4 suppl):S312–6.
4. Hickling KG: Permissive hypercapnia. *Resp Care Clinics N Am* 2002;8:155–69.
5. Brower RG: Mechanical ventilation in acute lung injury and ARDS: Tidal volume reduction. *Crit Care Clin* 2002;18:1–13.
6. Ware LB, Matthay MA: The acute respiratory distress syndrome. *N Engl J Med* 2000;342:1334–49.
7. The Acute Respiratory Distress Syndrome Network: Ventilation with lower tidal volumes as compared with traditional tidal volumes for acute lung injury and the acute respiratory distress syndrome. *N Engl J Med* 2000;342:1301–8.
8. Gattinoni L, Caironi P, Pelosi P, Goodman LR: What has computed tomography taught us about the acute respiratory distress syndrome? *Am J Respir Crit Care Med* 2001;164:1701–11.
9. Rouby JJ, Puybasset L, Nieszkowska A, Lu Q: Acute respiratory distress syndrome: Lessons

from computed tomography of the whole lung. *Crit Care Med* 2003;31(4suppl):S285–95.

10. Amato MB, Barbas CS, Medeiros DM, et al: Effect of a protective-ventilation strategy on mortality in the acute respiratory distress syndrome. *N Engl J Med* 1998;338:347–54.

11. Stewart TE, Meade MO, Cook DJ, et al: Evaluation of a ventilation strategy to prevent barotrauma in patients at high risk for acute respiratory distress syndrome. *N Engl J Med* 1998;338:355–61.

12. Critical Care Medicine, National Institutes of Health: Meta-analysis of acute lung injury and acute respiratory distress syndrome trials testing low tidal volumes. *Crit Care Perspective* 2002;166:1510–4.

13. Steinbrook R: How best to ventilate? Trial design and patient safety in studies of the acute respiratory distress syndrome. *N Engl J Med* 2003;348:1395–1401.

14. Tobin MJ: The role of a journal in a scientific controversy. *Am J Respir Crit Care Med* 2003;168:511–5.

15. Lenfant C: Clinical research to clinical practice: Lost in translation? *N Engl J Med* 2003;349:868–74.

16. Drazen JM: Controlling research trials. *N Engl J Med* 2003;348:1377–80.

17. Miller FG, Rosenstein DL: The therapeutic orientation to clinical trials. *N Engl J Med* 2003;348:1383–6.

18. Miller F, Silverman H: The ethical relevance of the standard of care in the design of clinical trials. *Am J Respir Crit Care Med* 2004;169:562–4.

19. Steinbrook R: Trial design and patient safety: The debate continues. *N Engl J Med* 2003;349:629–30.

20. Grunberg SM, Cefalu WT: The integral role of clinical research in clinical care. *N Engl J Med* 2003;348:1386–8.

21. Ricard JD: Are we really reducing tidal volume—and should we? *Am J Respir Crit Care Med* 2003;167:1297–8.

22. Rouby JJ, Lu Q, Goldstein I: Selecting the right level of positive end-expiratory pressure in patients with acute respiratory distress syndrome. *Am J Respir Crit Care Med* 2002;165:1182–6.

23. Hubmayr RD: Perspective on lung injury and recruitment: A skeptical look at the opening and collapse story. *Am J Respir Crit Care Med* 2002;165:1647–53.

24. Levy MM: Optimal PEEP in ARDS: Changing concepts and current controversies. *Crit Care Clin* 2002;18:15–33.

25. Rodrigo GJ, Rodrigo C, Hall JB: Acute asthma in adults: A review. *Chest* 2004;125:1081–102.

26. McFadden ER: Acute severe asthma. *Am J Respir Crit Care Med* 2003;168:740–59.

27. El-Solh A: Clinical approach to the critically ill, morbidly obese patient. *Am J Respir Crit Care Med* 2004;169:557–61.

28. Halter JM, Steinberg JM, Schiler HJ, et al: Positive end-expiratory pressure after a recruitment maneuver prevents both alveolar collapse and recruitment/derecruitment. *Am J Respir Crit Care Med* 2003;167:1620–6.

29. Lung Open Ventilation Study. Study in progress.

SECTION IV

CIRCULATION

Objectives

1. Recognize and manage the patient with shock.
2. Learn the important principles of fluid resuscitation.
3. Review the indications for, and problems with, blood and blood product transfusions.
4. Develop a working knowledge of the available vasoactive medications.
5. Understand the limitations and advantages of hemodynamic monitors.
6. Develop an approach to the rational use of central venous monitoring.

CHAPTER 15

MANAGEMENT OF SHOCK

DAVE NEILIPOVITZ,
PIERRE CARDINAL, AND
PETER BRINDLEY

A 42-year-old woman has presented to your hospital with a severe subarachnoid hemorrhage. She is intubated and unconscious. Her blood pressure is 164/92 with a heart rate of 62. She has a very poor urine output, is peripherally mottled and has poor peripheral perfusion. What would you do?

The patient above is clearly not doing well. Aside from her significant neurologic problems, she appears to have impaired circulation. Is she in shock? John Collins Warren described shock as "... a momentary pause in the act of death."[1] Although this pragmatic definition aptly describes a potential outcome despite therapy, it fails to assist the physician. Indeed, despite the common use of the term shock, it is often poorly understood. Since shock has a high associated morbidity and mortality, it is essential that it be promptly recognized and aggressively treated. The goal of this review is to aid rapid diagnosis and treatment primarily by understanding the physiology of shock.

● Overview of Shock

The definition of shock is controversial. Once synonymous with hypotension, it is now clear that this definition is overly simplistic. In addition, in those in whom hypotension is present correction of the blood pressure does not always reverse shock. Further, while some hypotensive patients may not be in shock, others may be hypertensive, yet be in shock.[2] Shock exists whenever oxygen delivery is inadequate to meet tissue oxygen requirements. This is not to say that other physiologic parameters are not important. Blood pressure is important insofar as pressure differences are the forces that drive blood through the vessels. Severe hypoxemia or anemia may also cause tissue ischemia regardless of pressure or blood flow.[3] Failure to promptly correct any of these parameters can result in organ dysfunction and possibly death.[4-7]

The commonly accepted classification of shock is from Hinshaw and Cox,[8] who in 1972 subdivided shock into four major categories (Table 15.1). Their classification, a modification of what Blalock proposed in the 1930s,[9] is sensible, but in practice has limitations especially early when diagnoses are not yet confirmed. Often it is difficult to classify a patient in a specific category and multiple categories of shock coexist. For example, a septic patient may have an element of myocardial impairment[10-12] and relative hypovolemia, as well as a distributive problem. Early management is often not guided by the different categories of shock. Thus, although it is important to identify the type of shock as it helps us to refine our therapy, it should not delay the initiation of therapy. An alternative to the categorical approach to shock is to use a physiologic approach to simplify early management. Essentially, the approach is to optimize blood flow, blood pressure and oxygen content to ultimately improve tissue oxygen delivery.

● Basic Physiology

A. Blood Flow

Blood flow is tightly regulated to meet the metabolic needs of each tissue and organ.[13] This occurs through local vasodilatation or vasoconstriction in response to increased or decreased local needs. Whenever the metabolic needs of a specific organ increase, blood flow increases through local vasodilatation; whenever metabolic needs decrease, blood flow decreases through local vasoconstriction. This tight regulation of local blood flow is mediated by the local release of various cellular metabolic by-products and other vasoactive agents produced by the endothelium.

B. Blood Pressure Regulation

Just as blood flow is precisely regulated to meet the metabolic needs of the various tissues, cardiac output is in large part regulated by the sum of all local tissue flows. When local vasodilatation increases tissue perfusion, this immediately increases venous return, which the heart in turn is able to eject. However, the nervous response also assists the heart and circulation to make changes in blood pressure that are independent of blood flow and to better respond to changing metabolic needs especially in times of stress. For example, a small reduction in blood pressure activates the sympathetic nervous system, which increases heart rate and contractility and causes vasoconstriction of arterioles and, more importantly, venoconstriction. The increased sympathetic discharge thus restores blood pressure and flow but also redirects blood flow to more vital organs.

● Management

The therapy of shock, however crude, attempts to mimic the finely tuned physiological response of the heart and circulation to meet the body's metabolic needs. The goals of therapy are therefore twofold: first, to restore the balance between metabolic supply and demand; and second, to avoid hypotension. Restoring the balance between metabolic supply and demand is achieved by optimizing blood flow and oxygen content and reducing oxygen consumption. Since the blood pressure is the product of blood flow times the systemic vascular resistance, restoring

Table 15.1 – Classification of Shock

Hypovolemic	Cardiogenic	Distributive	Obstructive
Hemorrhagic	Infarction	Septic	Cardiac Tamponade
Dehydration	Rhythm Disturbances	Anaphylactic	Pulmonary Embolus
		Neurogenic	Tension Pneumothorax
		Adrenal Insufficiency	
		Liver Failure	

blood flow would ideally also restore blood pressure. However, in diseased states, it may become impossible to increase blood pressure solely through increases in blood flow. Thus, blood pressure must be raised by the induction of arteriolar vasoconstriction. The potential reduction in perfusion of non-vital organs is the price that must sometimes be paid in order to preserve blood flow to the heart and brain.

A. Restoring the Balance between Supply and Demand

1. Improving Oxygen Supply

a. heart rate – The cardiac output is the product of the heart rate and stroke volume (Table 15.2). Increases in the heart rate initially raise the cardiac output but once the rate has increased above 120 bpm, further increase produces minimal benefit.[14] At rates above 150 bpm, the cardiac output may actually begin to fall due to inadequate filling of the heart. The disadvantages of a higher heart rate are the increased myocardial oxygen consumption and the reduced myocardial oxygen supply both of which increase the risk of myocardial ischemia.[15] Therefore, increasing the heart rate is rarely the preferred manner of increasing the cardiac output unless the rate is inordinately low. Thus, to increase cardiac output, the focus should be on raising the stroke volume, which is primarily influenced by preload, contractility and afterload.

Table 15.2 – Common Formulas

$$CO = HR \times SV$$
$$BP = CO \times SVR$$
$$CaO_2 = (SaO_2 \times 0.134 \times Hgb) + (PaO_2 \times 0.0031)$$
$$DO_2 = (CO / BSA) \times CaO_2$$

CO = cardiac output
HR = heart rate
SVR = systemic vascular resistance
BP = blood pressure
SV = stroke volume
CaO_2 = arterial oxygen content
SaO_2 = oxygen saturation
Hgb = hemoglobin (g/L)
PaO_2 = arterial oxygen pressure
DO_2 = delivery of oxygen
BSA = body surface area

b. preload – Preload refers to the amount of stretch exerted on cardiac myofibrils at end diastole by a volume of blood.[16,17] It is influenced by both blood volume status and ventricular compliance (stiffness) — with a stiffer ventricle being less distended at a given pressure than a more compliant ventricle. Traditional teaching is that greater filling of the ventricle increases the cross-linkage of the muscle fibres,[18] which in turn increases the force and velocity of each contraction (recent evidence suggest it is more related to calcium regulation).[19] Either giving fluids, decreasing the venous capacitance or decreasing the resistance to venous return to improve venous return will therefore increase preload. The major advantage of augmenting the preload is that it increases the cardiac output with little increase in myocardial oxygen consumption (i.e., it improves the efficiency of the heart).[20] Unfortunately, increasing preload carries the risk of an increase in pulmonary capillary pressure to a level at which pulmonary edema may occur. This is especially likely in those with poor left ventricular function or those with increased pulmonary capillary permeability. In addition, solely increasing preload often fails to fully correct shock in patients with a cardiogenic or a septic component.

c. contractility – Contractility refers to the intrinsic ability of the heart to generate the force and velocity for contraction. Although many variables influence it, the primary mechanism is an alteration in intracellular calcium. A rise in free intracellular calcium will increase the magnitude of cardiac contraction. Inotropic drugs such as beta agonists and phosphodiesterase inhibitors raise intracellular calcium levels to increase cardiac contractility and thus increase the stroke volume. Unfortunately, improved contractility is often accompanied by an increase in myocardial oxygen consumption. Furthermore, increasing contractility offers little benefit when the heart has a relatively normal systolic function or is under filled.[21,22]

d. afterload – Afterload refers primarily to the forces that oppose cardiac emptying during systole.[17,23] Strictly speaking it refers to the wall stress of the ventricle. Although many variables influence afterload, an important component is the systemic vascular resistance (SVR). It is easier for the ventricles to empty when the resistance vessels (i.e., arterioles) are relaxed than when they are contracted. Thus, reducing the SVR will increase the stroke volume and the cardiac output. The beneficial effects of increasing blood flow are, however, tempered by the reduction in blood pressure that often accompanies a fall in SVR. Note that medications that vasodilate arterioles, usually considered as strict afterload reducing agents, also increase venous return by decreasing the resistance to venous return and thus may also increase preload. The effect of these agents on the right atrial pressure will depend on the relative contribution of increasing venous return (which increases right atrial pressure) versus the improved performance of the heart, which empties more easily when afterload is reduced (which in turn lowers right atrial pressure). Other important variables that significantly affect the afterload include blood viscosity and, especially, myocardial wall tension.[17,24] Thus, these variables can alter the cardiac output independent of changes in the SVR.

e. optimizing oxygen content – The delivery of oxygen to the tissues is the product of cardiac output and the oxygen content of the blood. The oxygen content is the summation of bound and dissolved oxygen. Since the amount of dissolved oxygen is negligible, oxygen content is primarily that bound to hemoglobin. Hemoglobin levels and oxygen saturation levels are thus the major determinants of the oxygen content of blood. The goal is to aim for saturations equal to or just above 90%, since efforts to further increase the oxygen saturation will have limited benefit in increasing oxygen delivery and may subject the patient to harm. The optimal hemoglobin value is unknown. Although transfusion practice must be individualized, present recommendations suggest that transfusions are usually beneficial if hemoglobin levels are below 70 g/L but unlikely to be helpful if levels are above 90 g/L.[25] An increase in the hemoglobin from 70 to 90 g/L will increase oxygen by over 20%. The benefits of transfusion must always be weighed against the risks. Most physicians would set a lower transfusion threshold in patients who are actively bleeding or are at risk of cardiac ischemia.

2. Reducing Oxygen Demands

Although the focus of therapy is primarily directed at increasing the delivery of oxygen, the oxygen demand component should always be considered. Oxygen demand can be greatly reduced by removing the work of breathing through intubation and the institution of mechanical ventilation.[26–28] The treatment of pain and agitation with analgesia and sedation will also reduce the oxygen requirements. Treating fever and even pharmacological paralysis are other measures that can further reduce oxygen consumption.

B. Blood Pressure

Blood pressure is required to perfuse organs and tissue beds. Increasing blood pressure disproportionately increases blood flow, because it not only increases the driving pressure but also distends blood vessels thus lowering resistance. Formula 2 in Table 15.2 states that blood pressure is the product of the cardiac output and the systemic vascular resistance (SVR) and thus can be raised by increasing either the cardiac output or the SVR. As discussed above, increasing preload and contractility augment both blood flow and blood pressure. While vasodilators also increase blood flow, they often cause a fall in pressure due to the fall in SVR. Conversely, arterial vasoconstriction usually increases pressure but sometimes at the expense of a fall in blood flow. However, because the vascular response to vasoconstrictors differs amongst various organs, arteriolar vasoconstriction can preserve blood flow to the brain and heart—at the expense of reducing flow to the skin, gut, and kidneys. Unfortunately, this offers only a temporary reprieve since persistent ischemia to the gut and kidneys would ultimately cause death. Administration of pure vasoconstrictors, however, might also increase blood flow since vasoconstrictors not only exert their effects on arterioles but also on veins and venules. If the predominant activity is to decrease venous capacitance, the resulting effect will be an increase and not a decrease in cardiac output.

● Recognition of Shock

Despite medical advances, the morbidity and mortality with all forms of shock remains high.[4–7] Evidence now suggests that duration of shock is a major determinant of morbidity and mortality.[5,6,29] Early intervention should therefore be the primary management goal. The principle of "time is tissue" stresses the fact that shock must be quickly identified and corrective therapy rapidly instituted for it to be most effective.

The patient in a profound state of shock is usually easy to identify. The presence of multi-organ failure along with grossly abnormal vital signs makes the diagnosis obvious. The challenge is to identify the patient who is in the early stages of shock when symptoms are less severe yet the situation is more readily reversible. While there is no doubt that prompt recognition of shock is essential, it is difficult to offer guidance on how to recognize early shock. There has not been any study evaluating the sensitivity and specificity of the different clinical symptoms, signs and tests in shock. There is also no gold standard test available to diagnose shock. Furthermore, shock is a syndrome with multiple etiologies each of which may lead to different manifestations. For example, shock may present with low, normal or high blood pressure.

The clinical setting and a high index of suspicion are key factors that will allow for an early diagnosis. For example, a patient involved in a trauma or presenting with obvious external bleeding should be considered in shock until proven otherwise. Similarly, subtle changes in vital signs will be interpreted as much more clinically significant in one setting versus another. Abnormalities in the vital signs of a febrile immunocompromised patient carry much more weight than the same abnormalities in a patient who is otherwise well. It is therefore important to actively search for clues that may indicate an early shock state (Table 15.3). Since a patient can actually look good, it can be easy to miss the diagnosis unless the subtle signs and symptoms are actively looked for. The principle of reassessment is invaluable in identifying the patient with an early, albeit milder, form of shock. The changes or trends in the vital signs or end organ function provide more information than can a single reading at one point in time and thus can help one to identify this problem. A progression, even subtle in nature, can suggest a worsening of the situation. Further, it is often the global clinical picture that facilitates the diagnosis. For example, a slightly confused patient with a low-grade temperature and poor urine output may be in early shock, whereas each of these problems alone is unlikely to signify shock.

● Early Treatment of Shock

The approach to the patient suspected of being in shock should start with an evaluation of the ABC's. Once the primary survey of airway and breathing is completed, a rapid assessment of the circulation follows and focuses on vital signs, assessment of peripheral perfusion and a brief auscultation of the heart. The goal of this rapid assessment is to identify acute life-threatening problems that require immediate therapy (e.g., tension pneumothorax). Before moving on to a more detailed history and physical examination, it is important to immediately institute therapy, especially if gross abnormalities are identified.

All patients believed to be in shock should have a large-bore intravenous catheter inserted. Most patients will require the rapid infusion of a fluid bolus (see below). Exceptions to this may be the patient who is in cardiogenic shock and pulmonary edema and is obviously already fluid overloaded. Even such patients may benefit from careful fluid administration once intubated and mechanically ventilated.[17] It is also important to correct hypotension immediately. The administration of vasoconstrictors in this situation may be life-saving. In the early treatment of shock, the primary goals of therapy are to restore the perfusion to the brain and heart. Given the relative paucity of alpha receptors in the cerebral and coronary circulation, the administration of alpha agonist redirects blood flow from non-vital organs to the brain and heart. In addition, venoconstriction may also improve venous return and therefore restore cardiac output. However, the administration of vasoconstrictors alone should be perceived as a bridge and not as a long-term solution. Therapy will need to be reassessed once the blood pressure has been restored and a more definitive diagnosis established.

A. Airway and Breathing

Immediate intubation of the airway is only required if there is a life-threatening airway obstruction.

Table 15.3 – Impaired End Organ Function

1. Central Nervous System – agitation, altered LOC
2. Peripheral Perfusion – colour, temperature
3. Cardiovascular System – HR, BP, ischemia
4. Renal System – urine output, creatinine
5. Gastrointestinal System – ileus, feed tolerance

More commonly, the primary survey of airway and breathing will include therapies such as an airway, bag-mask ventilation and oxygen. Early intubation is commonly indicated in shock but only once the assessment of circulation has been completed, including IV access and treatment of hypotension. Mechanical ventilation can reduce the work of breathing allowing blood to travel to vital organs rather than the respiratory muscles. In respiratory failure, which often accompanies shock, the respiratory muscles may receive as much as 30% of the cardiac output.[26-28] Intubation also allows for adequate sedation without the risk of aspiration and for more aggressive fluid resuscitation since positive pressure decreases the risk of developing pulmonary edema. Finally, positive pressure ventilation also assists the failing left ventricle by reducing afterload.[17,30] Thus, it is often preferable to consider intubation and ventilation earlier rather than later in the treatment of patients in shock.

B. Fluid Management

The administration of fluids is a mainstay for the management of shock. Although controversy exists over what type of fluid to use, it is important to infuse a sufficient volume at a rapid rate to quickly correct any deficits. With very few exceptions, it is *much better to give too much than too little fluid.* Two notable exceptions are the patient with penetrating trauma who could get to an operating room within 30 minutes[31] and the patient in florid pulmonary edema.

The administration of fluids has several advantages over the use of inotropes to improve cardiac output. While the heart performs more work (greater stroke volume), it does so with little or no increase in myocardial oxygen consumption (i.e., improved efficiency or free output).[20] Inotropes raise myocardial oxygen consumption, increase the likelihood of tachycardia and may induce arrhythmias. Fluid administration is also advantageous since it increases the cardiac output without decreasing the blood pressure (many inotropes also reduce afterload, which can drop the pressure). The primary disadvantage of fluid administration is the possibility of worsening gas exchange. In general, gas exchange problems are more easily managed than refractory shock and thus fluid administration should not be

restricted except in exceptional circumstances (which do not include the initial stages of shock).

The best type of fluid to use is very controversial. The long-standing debate over the use of crystalloids versus colloids continues and is unlikely to be solved in the near future. Presently, there is no firm evidence to suggest a difference in morbidity or mortality with the use of colloids versus crystalloids.[32-35] In general, both fluid types are used to treat patients in shock. The initial fluid however, is an isotonic crystalloid solution such as lactated Ringer's solution or normal saline. Hypotonic solutions including D5W or 2/3rds 1/3rds are inappropriate since these solutions have minimal effects on the circulating blood volume. As illustrated in Figure 15.1, crystalloid solutions rapidly redistribute into the different body compartments. The half-life for this redistribution is influenced by several variables, but is usually around 10–15 minutes. Thus, after an hour the fluid has redistributed. In addition, the increase in venous return that immediately follows the infusion of a fluid bolus is transient and thus it is important to reassess the volume status regularly.

Fluid therapy for shock typically begins with a bolus of 500–1000 mL of an isotonic crystalloid solution. The bolus should be given as quickly as possible (i.e., within a couple of minutes), which

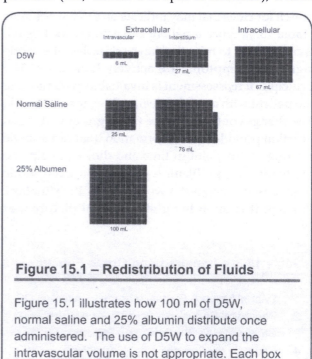

Figure 15.1 – Redistribution of Fluids

Figure 15.1 illustrates how 100 ml of D5W, normal saline and 25% albumin distribute once administered. The use of D5W to expand the intravascular volume is not appropriate. Each box represents 1 mL of fluid.

precludes the use of a volumetric pump. Volume deficits must be rapidly corrected. Simply increasing an intravenous rate is inadequate and may jeopardize the patient. The bolus should be repeated if the blood pressure or heart rate improve or if beneficial changes are only transient. The volume status of the patient should be re-evaluated after each bolus.

Assessment of volume status is initially done by a clinical examination of the patient. The blood pressure and heart rate are indirect measures of blood volume. The jugular venous pressure can be used to help estimate the central circulating volume. Signs of dehydration such as poor tissue turgor and peripheral perfusion can be supportive but are not specific. Invasive monitors such as an arterial line and central lines provide continuous monitoring of the systemic and central venous pressures but do not replace the need for repeated examinations. Clear lungs and low inspired oxygen requirements indicate that fluid can be safely administered with minimal risk of causing an immediate and life-threatening deterioration in gas exchange. While the presence of crackles or significant hypoxemia does not preclude the administration of fluid, it does render frequent reassessments even more important. Often, assessing the patient's response to a fluid bolus is the only way of determining whether or not fluid was indeed needed. While such a retrospective assessment is not perfect, it is always preferable to err on the side of fluid administration. Withholding fluid in a hypovolemic patient is far more injurious than giving fluid to a patient who is euvolemic or even somewhat hypervolemic. The adverse consequences of excessive fluid administration, namely worsening gas exchange and edema, are much less serious and easier to treat than the consequences of protracted shock, namely multi-system organ failure and death.

C. Vasoactive Medications

Patients who fail to respond to fluid therapy alone will usually require the initiation of a vasoactive drug in order to improve the delivery of oxygen to peripheral tissues (Figure 15.2). Although there is no perfect strategy for determining which vasoactive medication to use, several principles should guide their administration. Always ensure optimal volume status. The use of vasoactive drugs does not replace the need for adequate volume resuscitation. Vasoactive drugs should be titrated to some desired effect (e.g.,

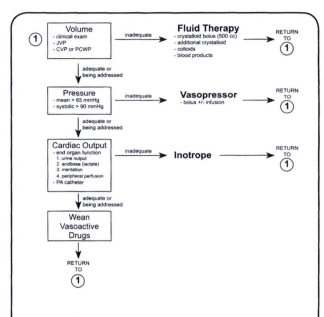

Figure 15.2 – Approach to Shock Management

Figure 15.2 presents a simple approach to the management of shock. The emphasis is on always optimizing the volume resuscitation and continuously re-evaluating the patient's need for fluid and vasoactive medications.

vasopressors for a target mean arterial pressure). As the condition improves, attempts to wean off the medication should be pursued with vigour.

Although several factors can influence which vasoactive drug to use, the decision is often guided by the therapeutic goals (Chapter 18). A simple approach is to divide vasoactive drugs into one of three categories: drugs aimed to increase blood pressure (phenylephrine and norepinephrine), drugs aimed to increase cardiac output (dobutamine and milrinone), or drugs with combined effects (dopamine and epinephrine). Drugs aimed at increasing blood pressure always elevate the blood pressure but may either increase or decrease cardiac output (i.e., blood flow). The typical vasopressor is an alpha agonist, which vasoconstricts the peripheral vasculature. Phenylephrine (pure alpha agonist) and norepinephrine (alpha and beta 1 agonist) are examples of vasopressors that can be titrated to improve the blood pressure. These medications are often used early in the treatment of shock even before a diagnosis is established. Blood pressure usually increases in response to these drugs unless the volume status is so poor that additional vasoconstriction is ineffective. These drugs may increase cardiac output by decreasing the venous capacitance thereby improving venous return. However, they preferentially vasoconstrict arterioles feeding the skin, gut and kidneys. Therefore, the improvement in cerebral and cardiac perfusion usually comes at the expense of hypoperfusion of other organs. While this is an acceptable short-term solution, it may ultimately be quite detrimental. Thus, if a vasopressor has "normalized" the blood pressure, it does not mean that the shock state has been corrected.

Drugs aimed at increasing blood flow almost always increase cardiac output but may also cause hypotension. Dobutamine and milrinone are two drugs commonly used to increase flow. Their effects are usually titrated to optimize the cardiac output or some marker of it (e.g., end organ function). The mixed group of vasoactive drugs are those medications that can increase either pressure or flow but in a dose dependent manner. Dopamine and epinephrine are vasoactive drugs with mixed effects that are commonly used. The advantage of these drugs is that they usually improve both the blood pressure and the cardiac output. The disadvantages are that they increase myocardial oxygen consumption, are more arrhythmogenic and may have a less predictable effect on either blood pressure or cardiac output.

D. Definitive Therapy

Acute resuscitation involves addressing the ABC's and giving fluids and vasoactive medications in an attempt to quickly stabilize the patient thereby minimizing end organ damage. However, once stabilized, it is important to diagnose the specific etiology of shock and institute definitive therapy. Septic shock requires drainage of infectious collections and antibiotics. Cardiogenic shock may require thrombolytics or an interventional cardiac procedure. Hemorrhagic shock requires that bleeding be stopped.

● Summary

As with all critically ill patients, an approach stressing concurrent management, reassessment, and re-evaluation along with the ABC's approach is invaluable in the treatment of shock patients. The goals of treatment are to restore both blood flow and pressure. Fluid boluses are infused rapidly over minutes and the patient's response immediately re-evaluated. Repeated fluid boluses are the rule rather than the exception. Drugs aimed at increasing the pressure, such as phenylephrine or norepinephrine, are often administered early in the resuscitation of hypotensive patients. While these drugs may protect the heart and brain, they may also produce hypoperfusion of other organs. Therefore, it is important to refine the therapy once a diagnosis has been reached and to reassess frequently.

Key Points

- Shock is when oxygen delivery is inadequate to meet tissue requirements.
- The goals in the treatment of shock are to restore the supply-demand balance and avoid hypotension.
- Cardiac output is a product of heart rate and stroke volume.
- Blood pressure is required for perfusion.
- A high index of suspicion must be had at all times to identify shock in the early stages.
- It is better to err on the side of giving too much fluid rather than too little fluid.
- Normalization of blood pressure does *not* ensure that the shock state has been corrected.

References

1. Warren JC: *Surgical pathology and therapeutics*. WB Saunders, Philadelphia, 1895.

2. Cheatham ML, Block EFJ, Nelson LD: Chapter 177. Shock: An overview. In Irwin RS, Cerra FB,

Rippe JM: *Intensive Care Medicine.* 4th ed. Vol. II. Lippincott-Raven, Philadelphia, 1999.

3. Schumacker PT, Samsel RW: Oxygen delivery and uptake by peripheral tissues: Physiology and pathophysiology. *Crit Care Clin* 1989;5:255–69.

4. Vincent JL, Dufaye D, Berre J, et al: Serial lactate determinations during circulatory shock. *Crit Care Med* 1983;11:449–51.

5. Crowl AC, Young JS, Kahler DM, et al: Occult hypoperfusion is associated with increased morbidity in patients undergoing early femur fracture fixation. *J Trauma* 2000;48:260–7.

6. Blow O, Magliore L, Claridge JA, et al: The golden hour and the silver day: Detection and correction of occult hypoperfusion within 24 hours improves outcome from major trauma. *J Trauma* 1999;47:964–9.

7. Shoemaker WC, Appel PL, Kram HB: Role of oxygen debt in the development of organ failure, sepsis, and death in high-risk surgical patients. *Chest* 1992;102:208–15.

8. Hinshaw LB, Cox BG: *The fundamental mechanisms of shock.* Plenum Press, New York, 1972.

9. Blalock A: Shock: Further studies with particular reference to the effects of haemorrhage. *Arch Surg* 1937;29:837.

10. Parker MM, Shelhamer JH, Bacharach SL, et al: Profound but reversible myocardial depression in patients with septic shock. *Ann Intern Med* 1984;100:483–90.

11. Parrillo JE, Burch C, Shelhamer J, et al: A circulating myocardial depressant substance in humans with septic shock: Septic shock patients with a reduced ejection fraction have a circulating factor that depresses in vitro myocardial cell performance. *J Clin Invest* 1985;76:1539–53.

12. Carmona RH, Tsao T, Dae M, Trunkey DD: Myocardial dysfunction in septic shock. *Arch Surg* 1985;120:30–35.

13. Johnson PC: Autoregulation of blood flow. *Circ Res* 1986;59:483–95.

14. Canty JM Jr, Giglia J, Kandath D: Effect of tachycardia on regional function and transmural myocardial perfusion during graded coronary pressure reduction in conscious dogs. *Circ Res* 1990;82:1815–25.

15. Hjalmarson A: Significance of reduction in heart rate in cardiovascular disease. *Clin Cardiol* 1998;21(suppl 2):II3–7.

16. Sarnoff SJ, Berglund E: Ventricular function: I. Starling's law of the heart studied by means of simultaneous right and left ventricular function curves in the dog. *Circulation* 1954;9:706–18.

17. Kumar A, Parrillo JE: Chapter 20. Shock: Classification, pathophysiology, and approach to management. p. 371–420. In Parrillo JE, Bone RC (eds): *Critical care medicine: Principles of diagnosis and management.* Mosby, Toronto, 1995.

18. Gordon AM, Huxley AF, Julian FJ: The variation in isometric tension with sarcomere length in vertebrate muscle fibres. *J Physiol* 1966;184:170–92.

19. Lakatta EG: Starling's law of the heart is explained by an intimate interaction of muscle length and myofilament calcium activation. *J Am Coll Cardiol* 1987;10:1157–64.

20. Suga H, Goto Y, Futaki S, et al: Systolic pressure-volume area (PVA) as the energy of contraction in Starling's law of the heart. *Heart Vessels* 1991;6:65–70.

21. Appleton C, Olajos M, Morkin E, Goldman S: Alpha-1 adrenergic control of the venous circulation in intact dogs. *J Pharmacol Exp Ther* 1985;233:729–34.

22. Schuster DP, Lefrak SS: Chapter 74. Shock. p. 891–908. In Civetta JM, Taylor RW, Kirby RR: *Critical care.* JB Lippincott, New York, 1988.

23. Sonnenblick EH: Force-velocity relations in mammalian heart muscle. *Am J Physiol* 1962;202:931–9.

24. Pouleur H, Covell JW, Ross J Jr: Effects of alterations in aortic input impedance on the force-velocity-length relationship in the intact canine heart. *Circ Res* 1979;45:126–36.

25. Expert Working Group: Guidelines for red blood cell and plasma transfusion for adults and children. *CMAJ* 1997;156(11 suppl):S1–S24.

26. Aubier M, Trippenbach T, Roussos C: Respiratory muscle fatigue during cardiogenic shock. *J Appl Physiol* 1981;51:499–508.

27. Hussain SN, Graham R, Rutledge F, et al: Respiratory muscle energetics during endotoxic shock in dogs. *J Appl Physiol* 1986;60:486–93.

28. Walley KR, Wood LDH: Chapter 20. Shock. p. 277–301. In Hall JB, Schmidt GA, Wood LDH (eds): *Principles of critical care.* 2nd ed. McGraw-Hill, New York, 1998.

29. Rivers E, Nguyen B, Haustab MA, et al: Early goal-directed therapy in treatment of severe sepsis and septic shock. *N Engl J Med* 2001;343:1368–77.

30. Calvin JE, Driedger AA, Sibbald WJ: Positive end expiratory pressure does not depress left ventricular function in patients with pulmonary edema. *Am Rev Respir Dis* 1981;124:121–8.

31. Bickell WH, Wall MJ, Pepe PE, et al: Immediate versus delayed fluid resuscitation for hypotensive patients with penetrating torso injuries. *N Engl J Med* 1994;331:1105–9.

32. Schierhout G, Roberts I: Fluid resuscitation with colloid or crystalloid in critically ill patients: A systematic review of randomised trials. *BMJ* 1998;316:961–4.

33. Cochrane Injuries Group Albumin Reviewers: Human albumin administration in critically ill patients: Systematic review of randomized controlled trials. *BMJ* 1998;317:235–40.

34. Choi PT, Yip G, Quinonez LG, Cook DJ: Crystalloids vs. colloids in fluid resuscitation: A systematic review. *Crit Care Med* 1999;27:200–10.

35. Wilkes MM, Navickis RJ: Patient survival after human albumin administration: A meta-analysis of randomized, controlled trials. *Ann Intern Med* 2001;135:149–64.

CHAPTER 16

FLUID RESUSCITATION: THEORY AND PRACTICE

PETER BRINDLEY

You are managing a 64-year-old male who you believe has septic shock due to urosepsis. You have administered 2 litres of normal saline but his blood pressure is still only 75/42 and his heart rate is 124 in sinus tachycardia. One nurse asks you if you should give some albumin, but another is concerned about giving any more fluid because the patient has a "cardiac" history. What would you do?

The overall purpose of fluid resuscitation in the critically ill is simple: namely, to prevent premature death. However, there are numerous controversies surrounding the putative benefits and detriments of various fluid types. The absence of a "one-treatment-fits-all" approach or universal algorithms could lead to delays at a time when rapid intervention may be the difference between success and failure. The physician must be able to aggressively and immediately treat despite the lack of a definitive therapy and often without a clear etiology. The purpose of this chapter is to outline essential physiology and some common mistakes, but more specifically to provide recommendations as to what fluids to give, how to administer them, and when enough has been given. In short, it is to attempt to provide life-saving strategies. While practitioners must be wary of the complex issues surrounding resuscitation, this should not induce inaction. Rather this mandates an appreciation of the controversies and hence the need for frequent reassessment. This combination of knowledge, practical application and the willingness to intervene makes resuscitation one of the most interesting areas of medicine and potentially one of its most rewarding.

● Physiology of Fluid Resuscitation

Fluids are given to unstable patients in order to preserve intravascular volume and organ perfusion.

Unfortunately, the clinical criteria that confirm this goal has been achieved are poorly defined. Direct measurement of blood volume such as by indicator dilution is not feasible in critically ill patients. Therefore surrogates are used, and these include systolic, diastolic and mean arterial blood pressure (SBP, DBP, MAP), the central venous pressure (CVP), urine output (U/O) and sometimes pulmonary artery catheter (PAC) – derived numbers such as pulmonary capillary wedge pressure (PCWP) and cardiac output (CO). Many physicians wish to obtain as many numeric values as possible prior to administering therapy. However, the acuity of illness may preclude this luxury and the physiologic changes of critical illness complicate the interpretation of these values. For example, we routinely measure indices that use a pressure (e.g., CVP) in order to make inferences as to the volume status of a patient. Alterations in vascular tone and cardiac compliance mean that the usual relationship between pressure and volume is altered.[1] Typically, the decreased compliance means that pressure measurements underestimate the volume status in a sick patient as compared to a healthy person.[2,3] If physicians fail to appreciate this, then an elevated CVP may purvey a false assurance that the patient is adequately fluid loaded. The end result of this is that physicians should err towards over- rather than under-fluid resuscitating (i.e., better to give too much than too little).

Physicians must also be cognizant that grossly excessive fluid volumes can cause complications and can impair subsequent recovery.[4] This is because altered vascular permeability means fluid distribution in an acutely ill patient is different than in the healthy individual. Increased extravascular volume with associated tissue edema despite the presence of an inadequate intravascular volume is typical. For example, endothelial leakiness is central to acute respiratory distress syndrome[5] and in that case fluid may expand the extravascular/interstitial space more than the intravascular. This is why aggressive fluid resuscitation must be tempered with frequent reassessment. The physician must be wary that life-saving fluids can lead to poor oxygenation, impaired wound healing, impaired gut mobility and increased intracranial pressure. This "capillary leakiness" may also diminish the utility of daily weights and daily fluid totals.

The errors associated with monitoring devices are beyond the scope of this review but do mandate further caution. In addition, the effects of critical illness are frequently heterogeneous between organ systems and even within a single tissue bed. Systemic blood pressure does not indicate the exact perfusion to each organ and a serum lactate does not separately quantify the oxygen debt of each organ system. Therefore, single parameters cannot be the sole determinant of how much fluid to give. Instead, multiple pieces of the puzzle such as oxygen requirement, coagulation status, vasoactive medication requirements and urine output provide a more powerful amalgam of information. For example if we treat a single number rather than the patient, then simply seeing an increase in CVP may suggest that the fluid status has improved—and perhaps it has. However, CVP also increases in the patient who requires increased mechanical ventilatory pressures or develops worsening myocardial contractility. Such information would suggest that this patient is in a more—rather than less—perilous state. In short, the goal of fluid resuscitation is to save the patient not just the heart or just the lungs. This all means that we must assess the whole patient and not simply normalize one or two aberrant hemodynamic numbers. The complexity of treatment should be clear by now, but the patient must be treated nonetheless. In short, basing fluid therapy on numeric values is only as good as the numbers are accurate and clinically meaningful and is only useful providing there are treatments that will reverse the pathology. It is also important to understand the basic science of fluid distribution in order to understand the next stage—namely, which fluid should be used.

● Resuscitation Fluid Selection

Total body water (TBW) is roughly 60% of body weight, though this varies by age, sex and body habitus. TBW is divided into intracellular fluid (⅔) and extracellular fluid (⅓) (Figure 16.1). Extracellular fluid is further divided into three-quarters interstitial and one quarter intravascular. The partitioning of fluid between compartments is determined by the Starling equation and lymphatic flow (Figure 16.2). In short, fluid is more likely to leave the intravascular space if there is high capillary permeability or a high hydrostatic pressure gradient between the intravascular space and the interstitum. Furthermore, fluid is less likely to leave if the oncotic pressure

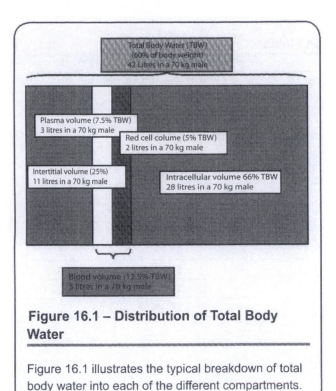

Figure 16.1 – Distribution of Total Body Water

Figure 16.1 illustrates the typical breakdown of total body water into each of the different compartments.

$$J_V = K_F \, [P_{MV} - P_T] - R \, (O_{PMV} - O_{PT})$$

J_V = TRANSCAPILLARY FLUID FILTRATION RATE

K_F = ULTRAFILTRATION COEFFICIENT (DETERMINED BY CAPILLARY PERMEABILITY AND SURFACE AREA)

P_{MV} = MICROVASCULAR HYDROSTATIC PRESSURE

P_T = TISSUE HYDROSTATIC PRESSURE

R = REFLECTION COEFFICIENT (REPRESENTING ABILITY OF MEMBRANE TO EXCLUDE MOLECULES)

O_{PMV} = MICROVASCULAR ONCOTIC PRESSURE

O_{PT} = INTERSTITIAL ONCOTIC PRESSURE

Figure 16.2 – The Starling Equation for Fluid Movement Across a Semi-permeable Membrane[39]

gradient (generated by plasma proteins) favours the intravascular space. As an example, if 1 litre of D5W is given, it will distribute throughout all body compartments. As a result only 1/12 (1/4 × 1/3) or roughly 83 cc will be in the intravascular space. D5W is therefore a very poor resuscitative fluid. Within the family of crystalloid fluids, saline has the greatest propensity to reside solely in the extracellular space. However this still means that three-quarters will go to the interstitum and only one quarter or 250 cc of 1 litre will remain in the intravascular space. This means that 4 litres of normal saline is required to restore 1 litre of intravascular volume. Notably, this is also prior to fluid loss from the vascular space, which can occur in acute illness due to increased capillary permeability and in chronic illness due to low albumin, the major determinant of vascular oncotic pressure.

If crystalloids result in interstitial edema rather than intravascular expansion, then frankly, they have not achieved their primary task, namely that of augmenting organ perfusion. For this reason many physicians administer various colloid solutions, which include albumin or one of the ethylated starches such as hetastarch (Hespan®) or pentastarch (Pentaspan®). Five percent albumin has a plasma oncotic pressure similar to that of a healthy adult and should therefore increase plasma volume at least equal to the volume infused, whereas 25% albumin could increase plasma volume by five times that (Table 16.1). Pentastarch gives an effective circulating volume of one to two times the volume infused and has a half-life of roughly 2.5 hours. Hetastarch has a lower oncotic pressure and increases plasma volume by the amount infused, but has a half-life of at least 24 hours (as compared to 16 hours for albumin).[8] Colloids contain large molecules that ought not to diffuse rapidly through cell membranes, and should in theory stay intravascular longer. Furthermore if colloids have a higher oncotic pressure than the vascular space, then osmosis should further expand vascular space as water is drawn from the interstitum. As such, colloids can increase effective circulating volume by more than their actual volume at the same time as decreasing interstitial edema. The effect may be further amplified because many chronically ill patients have subnormal oncotic pressure. These are the physiologic justifications for colloids in the critically ill. However it is at this point that contradictory clinical studies complicate the discussion regarding the optimal fluid to use.

● Colloid Solutions

Albumin has been used for over 50 years, and was previously believed to be extremely safe

Table 16.1 – Characteristics of Common Resuscitation Fluids[40]

Category	Solution	[Na+] mEq/L	Osmolality mOsm/l	Oncotic Pressure	Price (CA$)	Expansion/ 500cc
Plasma	reference	130–145	300	20–30	N/A	500
Colloids	5% albumin	130–160	300	20–30	$80 for 500cc	500
	25% albumin	130–160	1500	100	$100 for 500cc	1700
	pentastarch	154	326	40	$40 for 500cc	600–800
	hetastarch	154	310	30	$40 for 500cc	500–700
Crystalloids	D5W	0		–	$1 for 1 litre	38
	0.9% NaCl	154	308	–	$1 for 1 litre	125
	Ringer's lactate	130	272	–	$2 for 1 litre	125
Hypertonic	3% NaCl	513	1026	–	$1 for 250cc	750–1000
	7.5% NaCl	856	2560	–	$1 for 250cc	1500–2000
PRBC					$200–300 for 1U	500

Expansion/500 cc refers to plasma volume expansion after 500 cc of product. Estimated costs (in Canadian dollars) are from the University of Alberta Hospital Pharmacy, 2004.

and beneficial.[6,7] However, albumin is prepared from fractionated heated blood and as such can cause reactions similar to transfusion reactions such as chills, urticaria and fever. It has also been associated with a possible decrease in myocardial contractility and renal function.[8] Potential issues with the starches include allergic reactions (0.85–1.0%), a dilutional coagulopathy and alterations in coagulation parameters such as PT, PTT, platelet adhesiveness and factor VIII activity. For this reason, most physicians limit starch administration to 20 ml/kg or 2000 cc per 24h. However, this is despite very few reports of actual bleeding, even in excess of 3500 cc.[9] There is the theoretical concern that if capillary permeability is markedly increased by disease such that colloids enter the interstitum, then they can paradoxically exert the opposite oncotic force to that required.[8,10] Colloids are also expensive and, for a similar initial volume expansion, cost up to 50 times that of crystalloids (Table 16.1). However it was a 1998 meta-analysis by the Cochrane Injuries Group that really ignited concerns against colloids. The authors found mortality higher in albumin recipients as compared to those receiving fluids with no albumin.[11] Many physicians began resuscitating with only crystalloids or demanding that in excess of 3 litres of crystalloid be given before any colloid. However this excess albumin mortality has not been duplicated

in other studies. Numerous counter arguments include concerns regarding the omission of relevant trials, heterogeneity of those trials included in the analysis, inadequate assessment of trial quality, and the absence of a clear etiology for harm. A subsequent meta-analysis included all of the trials in the Cochrane meta-analysis plus relevant others and found no overall difference in mortality with albumin except among trials of higher methodological quality where albumin actually lowered mortality.[12] This debate has become a favourite in critical care. However, at this time the choice of resuscitative fluid remains largely empiric, providing enough is given, providing the physician remains open to the possible need to change fluids and providing the patient is frequently reassessed.

● Hypertonic Saline

Hypertonic (7.5%) saline is not widely used but has strong potential particularly in military and disaster resuscitations. It may be considered to have colloid-like effects, although the principal component is sodium chloride. Studies show that hypertonic saline: increases plasma volume far more than its administered volume; decreases fluid requirements including blood transfusions; normalizes pH, base excess and lactate; and decreases whole body edema. Seven and half percent saline (usually combined with 6% dextran 70) can expand plasma volume 8–10 times more than a similar normal/isotonic (0.9%) saline.[13] Again, this is because water is osmotically shifted from the extravascular to the intravascular space. Potential adverse effects include hyperosmolarity, hypernatremia, central pontine myelinolysis and perhaps bleeding. However, studies involving more than 1500 patients have failed to show any of these side effects conclusively.[13–17]

In hemorrhagic shock, hypertonic saline can normalize blood pressure for hours, but should cause no significant blood pressure change with normovolemic patients. It augments cardiac output by increasing venous return, but also through direct chronotropic and inotropic effects. Afterload is also decreased, presumably by vasodilatation of the systemic and pulmonary circulations. The combination of increased cardiac output and capillary dilatation should increase microperfusion to struggling organs. A renewed interest has occurred with hypertonic saline when the focus changed from hemodynamics to immunomodulation. Inhibition of neutrophil margination may reduce the excessive systemic inflammatory response syndrome (SIRS) response, which may subsequently reduce the progression to irreversible organ dysfunction. In addition, enhanced lymphocyte and macrophage function may decrease late immunosuppression and sepsis. Studies have also suggested less lung morbidity, a decreased need for mechanical ventilation and shorter ICU stays.[13–17] Hypertonic saline has the potential to be widely used if larger studies show a benefit. In the meantime we will focus on more commonly used fluids.

● Isotonic Crystalloids

Normal saline contains 154 mEq/L of sodium and 154 mEq/L of chloride. This high sodium concentration means the solution has a greater chance of remaining extracellular when compared to lower sodium solutions. It is therefore used widely in resuscitation but is not without its own concerns: For example, in the critically ill, acidosis is multifactorial, but is in large part from inadequate tissue oxygen, which results in lactic acidosis. Generations of physicians have been taught to divide metabolic acidosis into those cases with an anion-gap due to the presence of a new anion/acid versus non-anion gap acidosis

caused by inadequate bicarbonate. This approach is still helpful to guide resuscitation. In fact, in the "heat of battle," physicians have commonly assumed that continued acidosis must mean continued tissue dysoxia (or ketoacidosis) and have therefore given yet more saline. Instead, physicians must be cognizant that a large volume of saline (or colloids) can actually cause a further acidosis but of a hyperchloremic non-anion gap type. These sorts of fixation errors are extremely common in Critical Care[18] and require vigilance. Confirming if lactate levels are still the sole cause of acidosis or whether the acidosis is still purely of an anion-gap type can be a useful clue as to whether saline should now be substituted. While discussion of the strong ion theory[19–20] is beyond the scope of this review, it is important to realize that while the traditional anion gap/non-anion gap dichotomy serves our purposes, it may be a gross oversimplification. Use of fluids with lower chloride concentrations may cause less perturbation to the acid-base status of the patient and less acid load upon the respiratory and renal systems.

Ringer's lactate (RL) has a higher pH (6.5 vs. 5.5) than saline, contains less sodium (130 mEq/L) and has considerable less chloride (109 mEq/L). It does not cause a hyperchloremic acidosis. RL also contains potassium (4 mEq/L), calcium (1.4 mEq/L) and sodium lactate (metabolized to bicarbonate) in concentrations similar to plasma. The calcium could also bind to citrate used to anticoagulate blood products and thus should not be used. It is contraindicated as a diluent for packed red cell transfusions. Overall very few adverse effects have been reported, and RL, like saline, is a very safe crystalloid option.

The physician should now appreciate that to increase vascular volume with crystalloids will take at least four times more fluid volume than if colloids were used. This means that resuscitation might take longer and the beneficial effects may be shorter lived. It again mandates that whatever fluid is chosen it be aggressively administered and frequently re-evaluated. The discussion therefore now shifts to general principles to employ during attempted fluid resuscitation.

● Approach to Fluid Resuscitation

Systemic inflammatory response syndrome (SIRS) is a non-specific response to illness secondary to the release of pro-inflammatory mediators. It is usually defined by tachycardia (HR > 90 bpm), tachypnea (RR > 20 or $Paco_2$ < 32 mm Hg), leukocytosis (WBC > 12) or leukopenia (WBC < 4) or bandemia (> 10% immature white cells).[21] SIRS can be self-limiting or if untreated can progress to septic shock, multi-system organ failure and death. If the physician intervenes early, then that progression may be halted and the patient "rescued" while tissue is still recoverable. In short, "time is tissue." Treatment must begin as soon as the patient arrives, and the patient must be maintained in an area where this aggressive intervention can continue. The urban emergency room is not just a holding area until a critical care bed becomes available. This means treatment should be proactive not just reactive and means having the confidence to request help—often before obvious deterioration. This may mean a shift in mindset: With the resource pressures of medicine, it is frequently easier to justify intervention only when obvious deterioration has occurred. However, studies suggest the need to modernize our mindset. Expressed another way, resuscitation delayed may be resuscitation denied.

In a study of "early goal directed therapy" in the emergency room, Rivers et al. aimed for a goal CVP of 8–12, a MAP > 65 mm Hg and a urine output of > 0.5 ml/kg/hr in all patients.[22] In the treatment arm, Rivers also aimed for a $ScvO_2$ = 70%.[22] $ScvO_2$ may provide an early warning of tissue hypoxia and may obviate the need for a PAC, which in turn has its own potential risks.[23] This study achieved one life saved for every six treated—and this with only six hours of therapy. It is likely that the later one waits, the more invasive the required therapy will be and the lower the quality of recovery. It may be appropriate to regard early aggressive therapy as akin to preventative therapy, with early fluid boluses preventing controversial and expensive therapies such as the PAC, large volume "rescue" colloids or blood products.

In a study of penetrating torso trauma with rapid transport times to a trauma centre, a survival benefit was actually found for patients who received delayed as opposed to immediate fluid resuscitation.[24] This study created a lot of controversy as its conclusion was contrary to the central tenant of this review, namely the need to give fluids early and aggressively. It is unclear whether the survival benefit with resuscitation delayed until the operating room resulted from a decrease in bleeding or hydraulic disruption of immature clot, was due to study design

or statistical aberrance or simply emphasized the effectiveness of resuscitating in the operating room. There is also no evidence that this study can be generalized to far more common etiologies of shock such as septic shock or even non-penetrating trauma. Regardless, numerous experts have appealed to physicians to continue to resuscitate as they have before and continue to emphasize that to under-resuscitate is probably a bigger sin than to over-resuscitate.[25]

Resuscitative zeal should be tempered by the fact that there has not been a conclusive benefit found from studies where patients were resuscitated to supernormal levels. It appears that once circulating volume is restored, there is no clear survival benefit from additional oxygen delivery—and there may, in fact, be detriments. Therefore this review will now focus on resuscitative strategies and how to determine when adequate oxygen delivery and fluid resuscitation have probably occurred.[26–29]

● Assessing Adequacy of Fluid Resuscitation

Clinical goals must always be individualized. As such there are no universally appropriate hemodynamic numbers to achieve. However with the complexity of critical illness, minimal prescriptive goals might help. As per the work of Rivers et al.,[22] this review recommends a minimum MAP of > 65 mm Hg, a minimum CVP of 8, a U/O of 0.5 ml/kg/hr, an oxygen saturation of > 90%, and a pH of = 7.2 (Figure 16.3).

Fluid should be given rapidly and therefore requires large bore intravenous lines. Ideally whether a fluid has helped is determined immediately after the fluid has been given and before it has redistributed from the vascular space. Redistribution half-life varies depending on the presence and absence of pathophysiology, but is usually around 10 minutes. This means when a litre of crystalloid or 500 cc of colloid is given, it should be infused as quickly as possible and not over more than a half hour. To achieve a target CVP may take over a dozen litres of crystalloid or it may take just one or two. As such, there is not a specific amount of fluid to give but rather minimum goals to achieve.

Shoemaker developed resuscitative algorithms[39] based on the premise that hypovolemia causes most of the mortality in acute shock, and these have been incorporated into the recommendations of this review (Figure 16.4). He suggested that one litre of RL is given without delay if the MAP is < 60 or SBP < 90 mm Hg. The next decision is the choice of fluid. For those younger than 45 and with no cardiac history, the assumption is that they can tolerate increased salt and water and therefore Shoemaker suggested an additional litre of RL. Alternatively 500 ml colloid (either starch or albumin) should be given. The next decision point is what to do as the CVP increases; Shoemaker chose a value of > 15 whereby fluid administration is slowed to compensate just for ongoing losses. The next decision point is when the hematocrit (HCT) is < 25% (corresponds to a Hgb of < 75), and if so then 2 units of packed red cells would be given. The MAP response to therapy determines whether to repeat or whether one can proceed to the next step.[30] In short, hypotension is the criterion for starting fluid; age, cardiac history and HCT determine the type of fluid given; and a CVP of over 15 determines when to re-evaluate the need for further fluid boluses. This algorithm can be viewed as analogous to a journey with the MAP being the car's accelerator, and the CVP and MAP response as the brake. There is unlikely to be a significant downside to aiming for a CVP of 15 rather than 8–12, but as always resuscitation must be individualized. This requires vigilance as well as a rudimentary knowledge of how best to clinically assess the patient.

In terms of physical exam, the jugular venous pressure (JVP) in the critically ill is probably accurate as a gross assessment of hypovolemia. By inference,

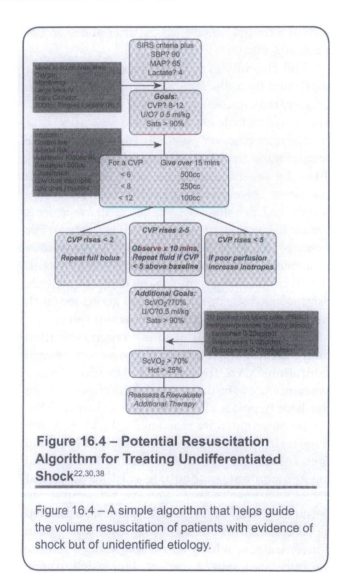

Figure 16.4 – Potential Resuscitation Algorithm for Treating Undifferentiated Shock[22,30,38]

Figure 16.4 – A simple algorithm that helps guide the volume resuscitation of patients with evidence of shock but of unidentified etiology.

fluid therapy based upon JVP is reasonable.[31] However, regardless of experience levels there is considerable inaccuracy. Observers are able to determine with accuracy when a JVP is low but not the exact number or even when patients are volume overloaded. The effect of positive pressure ventilation further decreases the utility of JVP interpretation. The presence of dry mucous membranes, dry tongue, dry axilla, urine specific gravity and postural hypotension are unfortunately even less useful. Postural blood pressure changes are infrequently used in the critical care setting simply because the tenuous state of the patient precludes raising the patient in bed. Blood pressure cuffs are also notoriously poor when blood pressures are low. As such the low utility of physical findings means they may need to be supplemented with early insertion of invasive pressure monitors such as a central venous line, an arterial line and/or a urinary catheter.

The difficulty in volume assessment is further confirmed by a discrepancy between echocardio-graphic, radionucleotide and PAC derived values.[32] In terms of bedside hemodynamic values there may even be inter-observer variability from nurse to nurse or from nurse to physician. For example a CVP may differ by several mmHg between well-qualified examiners. This does not necessarily mean one person is right and the others wrong but rather represents routine fluctuations or just stages of respiration. While a change in CVP of 1–2 mm Hg may be statistically significant, it is less often clinically significant. However, following trends, particularly of multiple parameters, decreases the chance of giving too much credence to a single potentially aberrant value.

Measuring central venous oxygen saturation from a central line (ScvO$_2$ or mixed venous oxygen saturations MVo$_2$ from a PAC) also adds a crude assessment of tissue oxygen extraction and the resultant hypoxia. The factors that influence ScVo$_2$ can be determined by rearranging Fick's equation (Figure 16.4). If venous saturation is suboptimal then it is likely because of inadequate arterial oxygen content, inadequate cardiac output or excessive oxygen consumption (Vo$_2$). Therapies can be attempted to redress this imbalance. Packed red blood cell transfusions should increase hemoglobin concentration, which could markedly increase the calculated oxygen content. Increasing oxygen saturation from 90% to perhaps 100% will increase oxygen content in blood but to a much lesser degree than packed red blood cell transfusions. Administering antipyretics, initiating mechanical ventilation, sedation and paralysis—as well as disease specific therapies—might lower the oxygen demand. Unfortunately, each strategy is less straightforward than this equation suggests. However, using Fick's principle does provide a theoretical basis for both treatment and reassessment. It is generally recommended to aim for a ScvO$_2$ of 70% or greater and an MvO$_2$ of 65% or greater.

The physician has other bedside "low-tech" assessments that can be used to ensure minimum fluid resuscitation. For example, pulsus paradoxus is seen with hypovolemia. This respiratory systolic pressure variation is typically defined as the decrease in SBP of more than 10 mm Hg with inspiration as compared with expiration. In addition to the "respiratory swing," hypovolemia may be associated with a lowering of the dicrotic notch and narrowing of the arterial pressure tracing.[33] This is an exaggeration of the normal inspiratory decrease in left ventricular stroke volume. It is seen with hypovolemia as well as respiratory distress and pericardial disease and therefore lacks specificity. However, if rapid fluid resuscitation continues until such signs are extinguished then the clinician has another crude assessment that the vascular volume status may be improving.[34,35]

The comparatively simple combination of an upper extremity central venous line and a Foley catheter ("the poor man's Swan-Ganz catheter") may replace the need for a PAC in many cases. The central line provides an assessment of filling pressure from the CVP.[36] In addition, the shape of wave tracings provides a clue as to volume status, right heart compliance and the relationship between pericardium and myocardium. A central line also permits the measuring of central venous oxygen saturation (ScvO$_2$). While admittedly even cruder, the urine output does suggest the heart's ability to pump sufficient blood to generate urinary output. The PAC remains a controversial device and its discussion is beyond the realm of this review. Suffice it to say that the PAC should be used sparingly in the acute stages of resuscitation in part because surrogates are available, but more so because its insertion may cause time delays and distract from continuous evaluation of the patient.

If the cardiac chambers are thought of as fluid filled balloons, then they will reach a point at which any additional volume will cause a large increase in pressure for a minimal increase in volume. In other words, if other variables are constant then cardiac compliance will decrease when the chambers become full. This has been summarized as the 5/2 strategy for CVP. What this means is that fluid boluses are deemed necessary if the CVP increases by less than 2 and not if the CVP increases by more than 5. If the CVP rises between 2 and 5 then the patient is observed for at least 10 minutes to allow for fluid redistribution (Figure 16.3). Following that time period if the CVP is not 2 or more above baseline then fluid is rebolused. There is a comparable 3/7 strategy for the PCWP. Of course, changes in perfusion—rather than merely changes in pressure—are the goal. Therefore once the target CVP is reached the patient may be assumed to have been minimally fluid resuscitated. At this time concomitant inotropes, vasopressors and assessments of organ perfusion (cardiac index, urine output, level of consciousness) become the next focus[26,37–39] and will be discussed in subsequent chapters.

● Conclusions

Whilst willingness to treat aggressively and re-evaluate frequently are the hallmarks of successful resuscitation, some rudimentary background knowledge is needed. The practitioner must appreciate the differences in physiology between healthy and unhealthy subjects, and how this can influence the hemodynamic parameters derived and the therapy that the numbers provoke. The implication is that the whole patient must be treated rather than just normalizing hemodynamic numbers. The dynamic nature of critical illness mandates frequent reassessment as well as the willingness to re-examine both hypothesis and treatment. This is how lives can be saved.

The basic physiology of fluid distribution must also be appreciated. There are suggestions that large volume colloid resuscitation might be associated with increase complications, but this remains an area of fertile debate. At this time, this review cannot dictate the type of fluid to use. Rather the practitioner should realize that it is most important to avoid under-resuscitating the patient. It is also far better to treat in the early potentially reversible stages of SIRS than to try to salvage the patient in the late potentially irreversible stages of multi-organ system failure. There are, however, downsides to vastly over-resuscitating the patient such as impaired oxygenation, poor wound healing and inability to close surgical wounds. The leakiness of capillaries associated with critical illness can make this balancing act difficult, which again emphasizes the need for frequent reassessment. This is facilitated by the rapid initiation of hemodynamic monitors such as an arterial line, a central venous catheter and a urinary catheter. The physician should also appreciate how much information can be obtained without a PAC.

The goals of resuscitation must always be based on overall patient progress and as such there are no universal hemodynamic numbers to achieve. However attaining a CVP of at least 8, a U/O of 0.5 ml/kg/hr, a MAP of > 65 mm Hg, a saturation of > 90% and a $ScvO_2$ of > 70% will avoid under-resuscitation to a large degree. Successful resuscitation requires the willingness to intervene, the foresight to treat before deterioration, the humility to ask for help, the insight to re-evaluate, the tenacity to react to change and the personality to direct a team towards a single goal. It is one of the most challenging areas of medicine and one of the most rewarding.

Key Points

- Physicians should err towards giving slightly more fluid rather than potentially under dosing.
- Crystalloids and colloids are important for volume resuscitation but it is unclear if one is preferable to the other.

- Hypertonic saline may have a role in volume resuscitation, but its present role is unknown.
- Assessing the adequacy of volume resuscitation is essential but this assessment must be individualized to each patient.

References

1. Packman MI, Rackow EC: Optimal left heart filling during fluid resuscitation of patients with hypovolemic and septic shock. *Crit Care Med* 1993;11:165–9.

2. Shippy CR, Appel Pl, Shoemaker WC: Reliability of clinical monitoring to assess blood volume in critically ill patients. *Crit Care Med* 1984;12:107–12.

3. Wo CC, Shoemaker WC, Appel Pl, et al: Unreliability of blood pressure and heart rate to evaluate cardiac output in emergency resuscitation and critical illness. *Crit Care Med* 1983;21:218–23.

4. Twigley AJ, Hillman KM: The end of crystalloid era? A new approach to peri-operative fluid administration. *Anaesthesia* 1985;40:860–71.

5. Ware LB, Matthay MA: Medical progress: The acute respiratory distress syndrome. *N Engl J Med* 2000;342:1334–49.

6. Wilkes MM, Navickis RJ: Does albumin infusion affect survival? Review of meta-analytic findings. p. 454–63. In JL Vincent (ed): *Yearbook of intensive care and emergency medicine.* Springer Press, Berlin, 2002.

7. Sort P, Navasa M, Arroyo V: Effect of intravenous albumin on renal impairment and mortality in patients with cirrhosis and spontaneous bacterial peritonitis. *N Engl J Med* 1999;341:403–9.

8. Roberts JS, Bratton SL: Colloid volume expanders: Problems, pitfalls and possibilities. *Drugs* 1998;55:621–30.

9. Nearman HS, Herman ML: Toxic effects of colloids in the intensive care unit. p. 713–33. In Carlson RW, Gehgeb MA, Blumer JL, Bond GR (eds): *Critical care clinics.* Saunders, Philadelphia, 1991.

10. Rackow EC, Mecher C, Astiz ME, et al: Effects of pentaspan and albumin infusion on cardiorespiratory function and coagulation in patients with severe sepsis and systemic hypoperfusion. *Crit Care Med* 1989;17:394–8.

11. Cochrane Injuries Group Albumin Reviewers: Human albumin administration in critically ill patients: Systematic review of randomized controlled trials. *Br Med J* 1998;317:235–40.

12. Wilkes MM, Navickis RJ: Patient survival after human albumin administration: A meta-analysis of randomized, controlled trials. *Ann Intern Med* 2001;135:149–64.

13. Vasser MJ, Fischer RP, O'Brien PE, et al: A multicenter trial for resuscitation of injured patients with 7.5% sodium chloride: The effect of adding dextran 70. The Multicenter Group for the Study of Hypertonic Saline in Trauma Patients. *Arch Surg* 1993;128:1003–11; discussion 1011–3.

14. Vasser MJ, Perry CA, Holcroft JW: Analysis of potential risks associated with 7.5% sodium chloride resuscitation of traumatic shock. *Arch Surg* 1990;125:1309–15.

15. Mattox KL, Maningas PA, Moore EE, et al: Prehospital hypertonic saline/dextran infusion for post-traumatic resuscitation. The USA Multicenter Trial. *Ann Surg* 1991; 213:482–91.

16. Younges RN, Aun F, Accioly CQ, et al: Hypertonic solutions in the treatment of hypovolemic shock: A prospective randomized study in patients admitted to the emergency room. *Surgery* 1992;111:380–5.

17. Younges RN, Aun F, Ching CT, et al: Prognostic factors to predict outcome following the administration of hypertonic/hyperoncotic solution in hypovolemic shock. *Shock* 1997;7:79–83.

18. Gaba DM, Fish KJ, Howard SK: *Crisis management in anesthesia.* Churchill Livingstone, New York, 1994.

19. Stewart PA: How to understand acid-base. p. 1–286. In Stewart PA (ed): *A quantitative acid-base primer for biology and medicine.* Elsevier, New York, 1981.

20. Stewart PA: Modern quantitative acid-base chemistry. *Can J Physiol Pharmacol* 1983;61:1444–61.

21. Levy MM, Fink MP, Marshall JC, et al: 2001 SCCM/ESICM/ACCP/ATS/SIS International Sepsis Definitions Conference. *Crit Care Med* 2003;31:1250–6.

22. Rivers E, Nguyen B, Haustab MA, et al: Early goal-directed therapy in treatment of severe sepsis and septic shock. *N Engl J Med* 2001;343:1368–77.

23. Reinhart K, Rudolph T, Bredle DL, et al: Comparison of central venous to mixed venous saturations during changes in oxygen supply/demand. *Chest* 1989;95:1216–21.

24. Bickell WH, Wall MJ, Pepe PE, et al: Immediate versus delayed fluid resuscitation for hypotensive patients with penetrating torso injuries. *N Engl J Med* 1994;331:1105–9.

25. Siegal JH, Veech RL, Lessard MR, et al: Immediate versus delayed fluid resuscitation in patients with trauma. *N Engl J Med* 1995;332:681–3.

26. Shoemaker WC, Appel PL, Waxman K, et al: Clinical trial of survivors cardiorespiratory patterns as therapeutic goals in critically ill postoperative patients. *Crit Care Med* 1982;10;398–403.

27. Shoemaker WC, Appel PL, Kram HB, et al: Prospective trial of supranormal values of survivors as therapeutic goals in critically ill postoperative patients. *Chest* 1988;94:1176–86.

28. Hayes MA, Timmins AC, Yau EH, et al: Evaluation of systemic oxygen delivery in the treatment of critically-ill patients. *N Engl J Med* 1994;330:1717–22.

29. Gattinoni L, Brazzi L, Pelosi M, et al: A trial of goal-orientated hemodynamic therapy in critically-ill patients. *N Engl J Med* 1995;333:1025–32.

30. Shoemaker WC: Resuscitations algorithms in acute emergency situations. p. 47–59. In Shoemaker WC (ed): *Textbook of critical care*. WB Saunders, Philadelphia, 2000.

31. Cook DJ: Clinical assessment of central venous pressure in the critically ill. *Am J Med Sci* 1990;299:175–8.

32. Thys DM, Hillel Z, Goldman ME, et al: A comparison of hemodynamic indices derived by invasive monitoring and two-dimensional echocardiography. *Anaesthesiology* 1987;67:630–4.

33. Dolesnska S: Principles of measurement of flow in gases and liquids. p. 105–127. In Dolesnska S (ed): *Anesthetic data interpretation*. Greenwich Medical Media, London, 2000.

34. Lazrove S, Waxman K, Shippy C, Shoemaker WC: Hemodynamic, blood volume, and oxygen transport responses to albumin and hydroxyethyl starch infusions in critically ill postoperative patients. *Crit Care Med* 1980;8:302–6.

35. Tavernier B, Makhotine O, Lebuffe G, et al: Systolic pressure variation as a guide to fluid therapy in patients with sepsis induced hypotension. *Anesthesiology* 1998;36:496–9.

36. Dolesnska S: Intravascular pressure waveforms and the ECG waveform. p. 105–27. In Dolesnska S (ed): *Anesthetic data interpretation*. Greenwich Medical Media, London, 2000.

37. Bland R, Shoemaker WC, Shabot MM: Physiologic monitoring goals for the critically ill patient. *Surg Gyn Obstet* 1978;147:833–41.

38. Weil MH, Shubin H: The VIP approach to the bedside management of shock. *JAMA* 1969;207:337–40.

39. Darby JM, Nelson PB: Fluid, electrolyte & acid-base balance. p. 133–57. In Andrews BT (ed): *Neurosurgical intensive care*. McGraw-Hill, New York, 1993.

40. Bongard FS: Shock and resuscitation. p. 242–67. In Bongard FS, Sue DY (eds): *Current critical care diagnosis and treatment*. McGraw-Hill/Lange, New York, 2002.

CHAPTER 17

BLOOD PRODUCTS IN CRITICALLY ILL PATIENTS

PETER BRINDLEY AND
SUSAN N. NAHIRNIAK

A man presents to the hospital with a massive upper gastrointestinal bleed. The man is well known since he has cirrhosis and has experienced multiple bleeds in the past, which have required repeated transfusions. Blood is ordered but the blood bank informs you that the patient has multiple antibodies and they are having difficulties finding blood that is safe for the patient. They are also questioning whether other products will be required as they only have a couple of units of platelets. What do you do?

Amongst all of the recent advances in the care of the critically ill, the field of transfusion medicine has experienced some of the most dramatic. The tendency to liberally transfuse in an effort to normalize hemoglobin, platelets or coagulation indices is simply no longer appropriate, necessarily safe, or even justified by science.

The physician must aggressively resuscitate the hemorrhaging patient. Frequently, the most appropriate and expeditious way to do this is with blood products. However, the physician must also manage a scarce and expensive resource and be cognizant of the potential risks from indiscriminate transfusion. Studies have shown that some previous assumptions regarding transfusion were specious—that is, initially plausible but ultimately untrue. As a result, the purpose of this chapter is to guide when to transfuse and what to use. The art of transfusion is that of preserving life and organ function while minimizing the risks. This demands a review of the literature, as well as basic physiology, hematology, immunology and biochemistry. It is simple to order blood products, it is tougher to know when this is the optimal strategy.

● Physiologic Basis for Transfusion

Blood loss in the critically ill is common and often multifactorial. It can result from surgical or traumatic loss, gastrointestinal loss, hemolytic conditions, marrow suppression and abnormal coagulation. Transfusion is not given to provide primary volume expansion or simply normalize aberrant laboratory values. Rather, red blood cell transfusions are intended to reverse or prevent tissue dysoxia and therefore minimize subsequent organ failure.

To maintain oxygen delivery in the setting of low hemoglobin, tissues are able to augment blood flow through compensatory mechanisms such as increasing cardiac output, increasing the extraction ratio or decreasing oxygen consumption. When compensatory limits are reached, however, end organ dysfunction can result.[1] If untreated, then dysfunction can magnify into multi-system organ failure and ultimately death. Therefore, at first glance, the rationale to transfuse freely seems compelling— whether it is to augment oxygen delivery using packed red blood cells (PRBCs) or prevent loss of hemoglobin using platelets or plasma. However, while PRBCs do increase global oxygen delivery, there is no guarantee that this increases regional oxygen delivery or the ability of tissues to extract that oxygen and use it.

Transfused blood, whether allogeneic or autologous, is simply not the same as that already in circulation. Firstly, stored blood can be as much as 42 days old. Biochemical changes occur during this time that can be collectively referred to as the "storage lesion."[1] For example, stored blood typically has low 2,3-diphosphoglycerate. This can shift the oxygen dissociation curve leftward and impair unloading of oxygen from hemoglobin.[2] Stored blood can also have a suboptimal rheology (due to decreased deformability) and this impairs its ability to reach the microcirculation.[2] For the most part, these anomalies reverse following transfusion with the resumption of normal metabolism. In the setting of massive transfusion, however, which is typically defined as one whole blood volume in less than 24 hours,[3] or in those with no reserve, exposure to this suboptimal product can exacerbate an already perilous situation. There is also a theory that "older units" have a higher concentration of cytokines, which may cause immunosuppression. This immunosuppression theoretically increases the risk of infections or even the recurrence of neoplasia.[4] Regardless, transfusion is not innocuous and might paradoxically worsen cellular oxygen utilization at the very time that a physician is desperate to improve it. As with any

treatment for the critically ill, this mandates a well thought out rationale for giving blood products.

Many considerations affect the perceived need to transfuse. For example, transfusion is more justified after an acute drop in hemoglobin as compared to a slower and therefore better-compensated anemia. Blood transfusion is more acceptable in the setting of coronary and cerebral vascular disease, where the patient is presumably less able to tolerate decreases in oxygen delivery.[5,6] Evidence suggests that transfusion might benefit the patient who has difficulty weaning from a mechanical ventilator.[7] However, the single most common reason that blood is ordered is for a low hemoglobin value rather than for obvious bleeding or organ dysfunction.[6,8] Alternative strategies could be to use a physiologic rather than numeric indication of the need for transfusion, such as when the patient becomes acidotic or has an oxygen extraction greater than 50%.[9] A physiologic approach appears to be more reasonable and would encourage a more comprehensive patient evaluation. However, this is still complicated by factors that affect oxygen extraction independent of hemoglobin and the many other causes of acidosis. The heterogeneity of illness demands a thorough assessment and individualization of therapy, rather than just a cursory review of blood work. Despite this, the complexity of critical illness means that laboratory values will probably always substantially impact when transfusions are given. As such, it is important to understand the evidence that guides just what hemoglobin levels are recommended as a *trigger* for transfusion.

● Hemoglobin Transfusion Triggers

Historically, though based upon limited data, a threshold hemoglobin of less than 100 g/L (hematocrit <30) was used to trigger a transfusion of PRBCs.[10,11] It is possible that some peri-operative patients benefit from a hemoglobin of this level.[12] In addition, chronically ill or elderly patients with less adept compensatory mechanisms might not be able to tolerate anemia. However, overall there is little evidence to support maintaining the hemoglobin at greater than or equal to 100 g/L.

Present evidence supports the use of a considerably lower transfusion trigger. Typically, cardiac output in previously healthy individuals does not increase dramatically until the hemoglobin falls below 70 g/L or a > 15% blood loss is experienced.[1,7]

Literature suggests that for many patients, a hemoglobin below 50 g/L is the threshold at which organ dysfunction begins to increase.[13] Anecdotally, Jehovah's Witness patients have tolerated hemoglobin levels below 50 g/L without experiencing systemic acidosis. The landmark study regarding PRBC transfusion triggers is the Transfusion Requirements in Critical Care (TRICC) trial of Hebert et al.[6] This randomized controlled trial compared a restrictive strategy (hemoglobin goal of 70–90 g/L, with a trigger of 70 g/L) with a liberal strategy (hemoglobin goal of 100–120 g/L with a trigger of 100 g/L). One hundred percent of the liberal transfusion group required blood. The ubiquity of transfusion in the Intensive Care Unit becomes apparent given that two-thirds of those in the restrictive group also required blood. This landmark study found a non-significant decrease in 30-day mortality in favour of using a transfusion trigger of 70 g/L. In terms of secondary end points, there were also significantly fewer acute myocardial infarctions and less pulmonary edema in the restrictive transfusion group. Furthermore, in those less than 55 years old as well as those who had a lower severity of illness score (APACHE II score < 20), the restrictive transfusion strategy was associated with a statistically significant lower mortality. The conclusion of the TRICC trial is that a transfusion trigger of 70 g/L is at least as good as and potentially better than a trigger of 100 g/L. With the following caveats, this is the recommendation of this review. It is important, however, to note that patients with active bleeding, acute coronary syndromes and those undergoing cardiac surgery were excluded from the study. As such, it is crucial to remember that this study does not dictate that a hemoglobin of 70 g/L is universally applicable nor ideal for all patients. Instead, 70 g/L may serve as the preferable trigger for PRBC transfusion. The physician must still individualize the trigger for patients. For example, in patients who are actively bleeding, few would criticize for transfusing at a higher hemoglobin level in order to stay ahead of ongoing losses. In patients with an acute coronary syndrome, there is some evidence that a target hemoglobin of 100 g/L may be superior, and thus a trigger of 70 g/L may be inappropriate.[5,6]

● Basic Immunohematology

In addition to understanding when to transfuse, the physician needs to appreciate the work performed by

Table 17.1 – Estimated Cost

Product	Cost* (CA$)
1 unit packed red blood cells	$300–400
5 units random donor platelets	$500
1 unit single donor platelets	$500–600
2 units FFP	$200
1 unit cryoprecipitate	$100
10 000 U erythropoietin (Eprex®)	$100
1 mg recombinant Factor VIIa (NiaStase®)	$1000
Tranexamic acid	< $10

the blood bank in order to provide the safest product possible. This knowledge goes a long way towards understanding why indiscriminate transfusion is potentially dangerous and expensive (Table 17.1). The two most clinically significant blood groups are the ABO and the rhesus (Rh) system. Administering ABO mismatched blood can cause potentially fatal major acute hemolytic reactions. The relative frequency of these antigens differs by ethnicity (Table 17.2).[14] Typing blood refers to determining the ABO and Rh group and takes about 5–10 minutes. Simultaneously a *screen* is performed for other alloantibodies (unexpected antibodies to red blood cells) in the recipient. Alloantibodies vary in frequency but, unlike the ABO system, require an immune stimulus to develop antibodies. As a result, at risk groups include multiparous women, transplant patients and patients who have received multiple transfusions. These patients may present difficulty finding compatible units for transfusion and have an increased incidence of transfusion reactions. The other donor blood group antigens that are potent antibody stimulators include Rh, Kell, Kidd and Duffy. Providing there are no recipient antibodies, blood can be typed, screened and crossmatched in as little as 45 minutes. The discovery of recipient antibodies or a prior history of antibodies necessitates a full crossmatch where patient serum is incubated with donor red cells. The presence of antibodies will frequently cause delays. If transfusion is urgently required, discussion is needed between the clinician and pathologist regarding the risk of giving suboptimal blood as compared to further

Table 17.2 – Blood Group Frequency and Ethnicity[14]

Blood Group	Caucasian	Asian	African	Native American
A	40	28	27	16
B	11	27	20	4
AB	4	5	4	< 1
O	45	40	49	79
Rh Positive	85	99	92	99
Rh Negative	15	1	8	1

delay. Ironically, in the absence of antibodies, it is often transport time to and from the blood bank rather than testing time that causes the longest delay.

Platelet Transfusion

A low platelet count (thrombocytopenia) can occur because of decreased production, accelerated destruction or increased sequestration in the spleen. Quantitative thrombocytopenia is typically defined as platelet counts below 150×10^9/L. Platelets are involved in both primary and secondary hemostasis. They function to "plug" a wound through adhesion and aggregation as well as by providing a surface for the progression of the coagulation cascade.

Serious spontaneous hemorrhage due to thrombocytopenia alone is unlikely with platelet counts above 10×10^9/L and thus this serves as the transfusion trigger unless additional risk factors are present. Unfortunately, these factors are common and include sepsis, fever, disseminated intravascular coagulopathy (DIC) and liver failure. It is recommended that the platelet count be raised to 50 $\times 10^9$/L for lumbar puncture, gastroscopy, insertion of central lines, liver biopsy or laparotomy, and to 100 $\times 10^9$/L for operations involving the orbits or central nervous system.[15] Conversely, platelet transfusions are contraindicated in thrombocytopenia caused by thrombotic thrombocytopenic purpura (TTP) or heparin induced thrombocytopenia and thrombosis (HITT), since this can exacerbate the thrombotic process from platelet microparticles. In view of these issues, it is important for physicians to attempt to determine the etiology of the thrombocytopenia prior to transfusion. In addition, platelet transfusion

may increase the platelet count for no more than a few hours in situations such as DIC, autoimmune thrombocytopenia, sepsis, hypersplenism or in those needing myelosuppressive medications. This implies that procedures should be performed as soon as the product is transfused, and should caution against empirically treating a number given the short-term benefit, the risk inherent in transfusion, the scarcity of the resource and the cost. Ensuring an adequate rise in platelet count following transfusion requires a platelet count to be measured 15 minutes to one hour following transfusion. Immune destruction will cause clearance of platelets within an hour but other peripheral destructive mechanisms will take longer. The post transfusion increment will help determine the etiology of the thrombocytopenia. In addition, it will provide evidence of both the magnitude and length of benefit to be expected if further transfusions are planned. If platelet transfusions offer no more than a few hours of increase in the platelet count, then standing orders are difficult to justify unless given immediately prior to life-saving invasive procedures.

Blood banks typically provide what are called "random" donor platelets, which are a pooled product derived from whole blood usually from five or six different donors. Each unit ideally raises the platelet count by $5–10 \times 10^9$/L. Single donor or apheresis platelets are typically reserved for patients with demonstrated platelet refractoriness or for those who require HLA matched products due to inventory pressures.[15] In terms of raising platelet count, a single unit of apheresis platelets is considered equivalent to 5–6 units of random donor platelets. Platelets are maintained at 22–24°C because colder temperatures activate the platelets in vitro and drastically reduce their ability to survive in the circulation. The warmer temperature, however, decreases the shelf life of platelets to under a week.

Plasma

Plasma has been described as the most misused of all the blood products.[1] As such, it is necessary to discuss its indications very deliberately. We are not treating the mere presence of a coagulopathy but rather using plasma to treat or prevent hemorrhage because organ failure can result. This is not semantics but rather emphasizes that the goal is not just to normalize an elevated INR or PTT. Physicians should strive to diagnose and reverse the causative pathology. Of note, in the absence of active or threatened bleeding, an elevated INR or PTT provides a useful indication of the degree of biochemical abnormality. Empiric therapy robs the physician of this valuable prognosticator. Individualized therapy mandates frequent bedside reassessments as well as coagulation and hematologic levels drawn both before and two to four hours post-transfusion.

Plasma is the preferred product when a multifactorial coagulation defect is present such as in liver dysfunction or sepsis (Table 17.3). In pre-surgical correction, plasma should be given immediately before it is needed, as the in vivo half-life may be as short as three hours. It is generally accepted that one should aim for an INR < 1.5 and a PTT < 50 pre-operatively. Interestingly, a small amount of plasma is contained within transfused platelets and PRBCs. Each unit of platelets contains roughly 50 ml of plasma, and transfusion of one blood volume of PRBCs can result in a 20–30% increase in coagulation factor levels.[1]

Canadian Blood Services produce three types of plasma that can be used for transfusion: "fresh frozen" plasma (FFP), cryosupernatant plasma (CSP) and frozen plasma 24 hours (FP24). The subtleties of when each product should be used are beyond the scope of this review. However this should again emphasize the essential work performed by the blood bank. Time to obtain plasma includes the aforementioned type, screen and crossmatch, as well as an additional 30–40 minutes of thawing time. Once thawed, plasma should be used within 24 hours. If not immediately used, plasma should be refrigerated at between 1 and 6°C in order to maintain clotting factors and to decrease the infection risk.

Table 17.3 – Indications for Plasma Infusion

1. Clinically significant bleeding in patients with liver disease and increased INR or PTT
2. Massive transfusion when associated with microvascular bleeding
3. DIC with active bleeding
4. Thrombotic thrombocytopenic purpura
5. Patients with coagulation factor deficiencies when factor concentrates are ineffective or unavailable

Recommendations for the dosing of plasma have unfortunately been quite variable in the past. The use of 6–8 units is the traditional order but this does not account for patient and other important variables. A more physiologic practice is to use 10–15 ml/kg. The premise for this is that 40% of the normal clotting factor levels is sufficient to normalize blood clotting. Assuming a blood volume of 70 ml/kg and a 45% hematocrit (therefore 55% plasma volume), the volume required to normalize clotting is 70 ml/kg × 55% × 40% or 15 ml/kg. Since most patients are not starting from clotting levels of 0%, the recommendation is 10–15 ml/kg. Although the majority of physicians are familiar with ordering in units, blood banks often prefer volume since individual plasma units can have volumes that vary (a typical unit is around 300 ml).

Cryoprecipitate

Cryoprecipitate (Cryo) contains fibronectin, fibrinogen, factor VIII, vWF antigen and factor XIII in 5–15 ml of plasma. Indications for Cryo include disproportionate hypofibrinogenemia and bleeds associated with uremia or von Willebrand's disease (Table 17.4). Although uremia and some forms of von Willebrand's disease are responsive to therapy with 1-deamino-8-d-arginine vasopressin (DDAVP), Cryo transfusions may be required. A unit of FFP or FP24 is roughly equivalent in fibrinogen to 2–3 units of Cryo.[1] In addition, there is enough factor VIII in FFP to maintain adequate levels without the need for Cryo. Infusion of cryoprecipitate will *not* normalize an increase in clotting tests due to the absence of the majority of coagulation factors. Its administration is only recommended following the documentation of a fibrinogen <1 g/L. Most clinicians would agree that the commonest reason to request Cryo is the tendency to give everything available in major hemorrhage or coagulopathy. Unfortunately the risk of disease transmission is increased because the typical dose of at least 5 units means exposure to multiple donors. Two concentrates that have the ability to decrease cryoprecipitate use, Haemate® P and fibrinogen, are not currently licensed for use in Canada. They require an Emergency Drug Release from Health Canada's Special Access Program.

● Minimizing Transfusion Volume

Transfusions are a life-saving act but have numerous risks and complications associated with their use. Decreasing the amount of blood given and optimizing the safety of the blood supply may however reduce the risks of transfusion. Physicians often overlook the simple effect of minimizing blood loss from laboratory phlebotomy. This has been estimated as up to 70 ml/day or 500–700 ml for an average stay in an intensive care unit.[1,8,16] Reducing standardized blood work, using pediatric blood tubes and using blood conservation devices can dramatically reduce transfusion.[16] Diagnosing and treating the underlying cause of the anemia might also remove the need for blood products. Causes of anemia can be divided into those associated with bleeding, premature destruction of red cells (hemolysis) or inadequate generation of new blood. A hemoglobin level and targeted investigations (e.g., peripheral smear, reticulocyte count, hematinic levels) should ideally

be drawn prior to the initiation of the transfusion. In a 70 kg adult, one unit of PRBCs should raise the hemoglobin level by 7–10 g/L.[17] A lesser increase suggests either an ongoing bleed, hemodilution from concomitant fluid infusions or hemolysis.

Combined therapy with folate and iron has been shown to decrease PRBC transfusion and is safe. Thus, routine hematinics such as ferrous sulphate (300 mg po tid), folic acid (5–10 mg iv or po od) and vitamin B_{12} (1 mcg x 1 dose IM), should be used before more expensive and controversial therapies are entertained. High cytokine levels decrease serum erythropoietin (Epo) production and function that can contribute to the development and persistence of anemia in the critically ill.[18] While it has been suggested that low Epo levels may offer the advantage of maintaining rheology and avoiding a hypercoagulable state, most authors presume that the failure of Epo to increase in the critical illness is maladaptive. As a result, Corwin et al.[19] and others[18] administered recombinant Epo to stimulate hemoglobin production. Exogenous Epo has yet to demonstrate improved mortality or a more rapid discharge in the critical care population. The cost of Epo is also prohibitive for routine use at roughly $1 per 100 units (Table 17.1) and with dose ranges from 80–120 units/kg/wk divided into three doses[20] up to 40 000 U once per week.[19] Up to 10 000 units per day has been tried in hemorrhaging Jehovah Witness patients due to the absence of alternatives, but this is done without the support of any randomized study, and with the realization that little effect will be seen for days. As such this review only recommends using Epo in the setting of chronic dialysis[20] or perhaps in those with particularly difficult crossmatches or a history of serious transfusion reactions. If Epo is used it should be given subcutaneously and must be supplemented with hematinics.

Antiplatelet therapies such as aspirin and clopidogrel should obviously be stopped following bleeds or thrombocytopenia. DDAVP is recommended for patients with inherited platelet storage defects or uremia.[15] DDAVP functions by releasing endothelial stores of von Willebrand's factor, increasing the activity of factor VIII and effecting platelet adhesion and aggregation. A typical dose is 0.3 mcg/kg or simply 20 mcg given subcutaneously. Rare cases of hyponatremia from the antidiuretic effect of DDAVP have been reported with repeated use but it is generally quite safe.[21] Tranexamic acid is a synthetic antifibrinolytic that inhibits plasmin thereby decreasing clot breakdown. Tranexamic acid has been shown to reduce transfusion requirements in some situations.[22] A typical dose is 10 mg/kg followed by an infusion of 1 mg/kg/hr. Aprotinin, a bovine polypeptide proteinase inhibitor that inhibits fibrinolysis has been effective in reducing blood loss during cardiopulmonary bypass and liver transplantation. Its cost and lack of widespread use in the general critical care population precludes widespread recommendation.[21,23] Although antifibrinolytics are often mistakenly viewed as a procoagulant, these drugs do not cause systemic clotting but rather decrease fibrinolysis systemically. Thus, clots will not spontaneously form but will continue to grow in size once they have been initiated.

Recombinant factor VIIa (NiaStase®) has been proposed as an adjunct therapy in life-threatening bleeds. Potential indications include bleeds associated with qualitative platelet defects or clotting factor deficiencies (including warfarin induced and secondary to liver failure); Jehovah's Witness patients; and those with posttraumatic, post-surgical bleeds and subarachnoid bleeds.[24–28] Recombinant factor VIIa binds to exposed tissue factor, and the complex activates factors IX and X with a subsequent "thrombin burst." Unlike other coagulation concentrates, recombinant factor VIIa should not cause systemic clotting because tissue factor is not exposed until tissue injury occurs. As a result it has been touted as a "magic-bullet" that activates clotting only at the site of damage and has the added advantage of preventing fibrinolysis of an immature clot.[28] It is currently only licensed for the management of bleeding in hemophilia A or B with inhibitors to factor VIII or IX. The dose in hemophilia is 90 mcg/kg, and up to three doses separated by two hours each may be required. Clinical trials are needed to help establish the indications and dose of this agent outside of hemophilic bleeds. In many jurisdictions, this agent can only be released following permission from a hematologist or hematopathologist. This is because of its prohibitive cost of roughly $500–$1000 per dose (Table 17.1). Although not recommended for routine use, it should be considered for life-threatening bleeds that have continued despite usual therapies (i.e., transfusion, antifibrinolytics and surgical hemostasis).

Much of the world is without access to reliable donor pools and suffers from natural disasters and wars that can preclude rudimentary refrigeration of the products that are obtained. Given the increasing demands on our blood supply and concerns regarding blood product safety, considerable efforts have been expended in an effort to introduce red cell substitutes. Unfortunately, these substitutes are neither widely available nor generally considered ready for routine clinical use.

Despite laudable efforts to decrease transfusion, the fact that massive hemorrhage is the number one cause of trauma-related death means that the need for blood transfusion is unlikely to fade. Bleeding may result from the trauma itself, but depletion and consumption of platelets and coagulation factors also contribute. In addition, hypothermia impairs hemostasis at all levels including quantitative and qualitative platelet defects, altered coagulation enzyme kinetics and disruption of the fibrinolytic equilibrium. Hypothermia and acidosis can result from a bleed and can also prevent cessation of that bleed. Without aggressive therapy this can increase the chances of a severe bleed progressing to intractable organ failure. Of note, a temperature below 33°C is equivalent to a significant factor deficiency and must therefore be reversed using heating blankets and fluid warmers. Since testing is always performed at a standardized temperature (i.e., test vials heated), temperature effects will not be apparent with typical lab tests. Prolonged operative time also increases the likelihood of hypothermia, DIC and acidosis.[26] Therefore, rather than providing definitive surgical correction, the goal of surgery in the unstable patient is to achieve rapid control of surgical bleeding and control of bacterial contamination. This may mean temporizing procedures such as a damage-control laparotomy. This is followed by rapid transportation to an Intensive Care Unit where the priority is to restore organ perfusion prior to further surgery.

Blood warmers may decrease the cardiac dysrhythmias that can be associated with rapid transfusion of a large volume of cold blood product. While routine use for transfusion is not absolutely necessary, they should be used if transfusion rates are above 100 ml/minute.[29] Blood warmers should be equipped with a visible thermometer and an audible alarm in order to avoid temperatures > 42°C which can cause hemolysis. Blood products should never be run under hot water or warmed with an unmonitored hot water bath or microwave oven due to the risk of hemolysis from uneven warming. Warmed blood that has not been administered cannot be re-refrigerated and issued at a later time because of the increased risk of both hemolysis and bacterial growth.

● Reducing Risk of Transfusion

Confirmation that the blood product has the correct name, ABO and rhesus blood group is the most vital step in the transfusion process. Without this, major transfusion reactions can occur with signs and symptoms that range from clinically undetected hemolysis, to back pain, chest tightness, chills and fever, and even fatalities. If a patient is sedated, intubated or already hemodynamically unstable, then signs of an adverse transfusion reaction may be difficult to recognize. Vigilance and a high index of suspicion is needed to differentiate whether any acute deterioration (cardiovascular collapse, oliguric renal failure, DIC or hypoxia) is from progression of the initial pathology or is due to a blood product. Any transfusion reaction except a mild allergic reaction, necessitates the immediate cessation of transfusion. Following patient stabilization, a clerical check should be performed along with submission of recipient and donor blood for repeat crossmatch and direct antiglobin testing. Additional testing in the case of a suspected acute hemolytic reaction includes submission of the patient's plasma and urine to determine if it contains free hemoglobin. Other biochemical indicators of hemolysis include an elevated bilirubin and a diminished haptoglobin.

When hemorrhage threatens imminent death without immediate transfusion, the options include type O Rh negative PRBCs or type O Rh positive PRBCs. Alternatively, type-specific but uncrossmatched PRBCs can be given. As outlined above, this third option requires a patient sample and a delay of approximately 5–10 minutes for the blood bank to determine their ABO and Rh. Many rural sites without blood banks have only type O Rh positive PRBCs due to the scarcity of O Rh negative donors. This presents little danger in the immediate transfusion period, but roughly 80% of those with a negative rhesus phenotype will generate antibodies and maintain these lifelong. Depending upon the patient's age, desire to have children or need for future transfusion, hematopathologists may need

to orchestrate follow-up rhesus immunoglobulin therapy for the recipient. In the elderly and in males, rhesus positive blood can usually be given with little concern. This allows preservation of Rh negative stores. For those with a history of previous transfusions there is still the risk of exposure to an unexpected red cell alloantibody.

Transfusion of PRBCs must be completed within four hours of issue from the transfusion service or satellite fridge. A unit that has been out of the blood bank for less than 30 minutes can be returned to inventory and used for transfusion in another patient. This time frame has been chosen because red cells that remained un-refrigerated for longer will likely exceed the maximum allowable temperature of 10°C. Both the four hour time period and 30 minute interval for return to inventory have been selected because of the concern of bacterial contamination.[30]

● Risks of Transfusion

Component therapy rather than whole blood is used in order to obtain an increased yield from a scarce resource. It also permits storage of each product under optimal conditions. However, the greater the number of products transfused, the greater the number of donors the recipient is exposed to.[30]

The risks of transfusion (Table 17.5) can be divided into three broad categories: risks associated with the blood itself (i.e., transfusion reactions), infectious risks and theoretical risks (including immunosuppression). Of note, many people focus on the risk of transmissible disease even though a transfusion reaction is much more likely. Furthermore, within the category of transmissible diseases, it is not widely appreciated that transmission of a bacteria is much more likely than a virus (Table 17.5). Screening for bacteria has yet to be widely implemented while nucleic acid testing for HIV, hepatitis C and now West Nile virus is well established. Despite extensive testing and research, there will always remain the likelihood of unknown risks from transfusion. These may originate from infectious agents yet to be identified or known diseases that cannot be screened for, such as variant Creutzfeld-Jacob disease.[31,32] The risk of immunosuppression from transfusion is unclear. Classically the effect was attributed to white blood cells that were found

Table 17.5 – Approximate Risks Associated with Transfusion in Canada[31,32]

Type of Reaction	1 unit of PRBC	5 units of platelets
Acute Hemolytic	1 in 12 500	extremely low
Fatal Acute Hemolytic	1 in 600 000	extremely low
Delayed Hemolytic	1 in 9000	extremely low
Febrile Non-hemolytic	1 in 500	1 in 15
Allergic Reaction (minor)	1 in 250	1 in 25
Anaphylaxis	1 in 25 000	1 in 1600
TRALI	1 in 70 000	1 in 8000
Bacterial Infection	1 in 28 000–140 000	1 in 2000–8000
CMV Infection	1 in 25 000	1 in 1600
Hepatitis B Infection	1 in 72 000	
Hepatitis C Infection	1 in 3 000 000	
HIV Infection	1 in 10 000 000	
Malaria Infection	1 in 4 000 000	
HTLV I and II	1 in 1 000 000	
Any Reaction	1 in 2300	1 in 800
Infectious Reaction	1 in 23 000	1 in 2300
Non-infectious Reactions	1 in 2500	1 in 1200

PRBC = packed red blood cell unit; TRALI = transfusion related acute lung injury; CMV = cytomegalovirus; HTLV = human T cell lymphoma virus. Allogeneic and autologous blood supplied by the Canadian Blood services is leukodepleted. Leukodepletion reduces the risk of HTLV transmission to close to zero. Transfusion risk data differ by jurisdiction (Canada, USA, UK) and year.

in PRBCs. Although blood in Canada is now white cell depleted, immunosuppressing effects may still be present secondary to cell fragments, cytokines and other substances that have been suspected of causing immunosuppression.

Transfusion related acute lung injury (TRALI) is a syndrome that may be under-reported due to the myriad causes of chest x-ray infiltrates and impaired gas exchange. TRALI presents like acute respiratory distress syndrome (ARDS), with non-cardiogenic pulmonary edema and hypoxemia and with or without fever or hypotension. It typically occurs between one and six hours following transfusion.[31] Its mechanism is still debated but anti-granulocyte antibodies, anti-HLA antibodies, cytokines and other biological response modifiers have been implicated.[33] TRALI is a diagnosis of exclusion and is managed in the same supportive manner as ARDS. Fortunately, it typically has a lower mortality and more rapid resolution. Regardless, for all of the above reasons, discussing the risks of blood transfusion has become part of obtaining a full informed consent. The acuity of critical illness frequently prevents such a discourse, but nonetheless this should remind us that blood products are no longer seen as benign or routine. Transfusions should therefore be considered with all of the caution associated with any therapies known to have a balance of risks and benefits.

● Conclusion

Winston Churchill said, "We are still confused but on a much higher level." His words seem particularly applicable to the modern-day treatment of the critically ill. Since donor pools are shrinking and demand is rising, those treating patients must remain active in the debate regarding the reasonable use of blood products. However, as long as the physician thoroughly assesses each patient, individually targets therapy and relies upon clinical acumen rather than empiric therapy, lives will still be saved by this kind of therapy and the pitfalls minimized.

Key Points

- Red cell transfusions are justified to maintain a hemoglobin > 70 g/L.
- Higher triggers are justified in actively bleeding patients and in those with acute coronary or cerebrovascular disease.
- Platelet transfusions are generally acceptable if levels are below 10×10^9/L.
- Consider platelet transfusions when levels are below 50×10^9/L if actively bleeding or before high risk procedures.
- Platelet transfusions are contraindicated in the setting of TTP, HUS or HITT.
- Plasma is indicated where coagulopathy exists and is contributing to bleeding.

- Cryoprecipitate is indicated in bleeds from hypofibrinogenemia, uremia or von Willebrand's disease.
- The simplest way to reduce transfusion is to adopt a transfusion trigger of 70 g/L.
- Iron and folate should be given in patients with suboptimal hematologic parameters.
- A reduction in transfusion may be achieved with DDAVP, tranexamic acid and aprotinin.
- Exogenous erythropoietin decreases transfusion but the high cost and lack of demonstrated benefit (decreased mortality) prevent general use.
- Recombinant factor VIIa may have a future role in treating coagulopathies.
- The risks of transfusion are still significant.

References

1. Nacht A: The use of blood products in shock. *Crit Care Clinics* 1992;8:255–89.
2. Marik PE, Sibbald WJ: Effect of stored-blood transfusion on oxygen delivery in patients with sepsis. *JAMA* 1993;269:3024–9.
3. Fridey J (ed): *Standards for blood banks and transfusion services.* 22nd ed. p. 51. American Association of Blood Banks, Bethesda, MD, 2003.
4. Goodnough LT, Brecher ME, Kanter MH, AuBuchon JP: Transfusion medicine. *N Engl J Med* 1999;340:38–47.
5. Wu WC, Rathore SS, Wany Y, et al: Blood transfusion in elderly patients with acute myocardial infarction. *N Engl J Med* 2001;345:1230–6.
6. Hebert PC, Wells G, Blajchman MA, et al: A multicenter, randomized, controlled clinical trail of transfusion requirements in critical care. *N Engl J Med* 1999;340:409–17.
7. Schonhofer B, Wenzel M, Geibel M, Kohler D: Blood transfusion and lung function in chronically anemic patients with severe chronic obstructive pulmonary disease. *Crit Care Med* 1998;26:1824–8.
8. Corwin HL, Parsonnet KC, Gettinger A: RBC transfusion in the ICU: Is there a reason? *Chest* 1995;108:767–71.
9. Wilkerson DK, Rosen AL, Gould SA, et al: Oxygen extraction ratio: A valid indicator of myocardial metabolism in anemia. *J Surg Res* 1987;42:629–34.
10. Office of Medical Applications and Research, National Institutes of Health: Perioperative red blood cell transfusion. *JAMA* 1988;260:2700–3.
11. Allen JB, Allen FB: The minimum acceptable level of hemoglobin. *Int Anesthiol Clin* 1982;20:1–22.
12. Heyland DK, Cook DJ, King D, et al: Maximizing oxygen delivery in critically-ill patients: A methodological appraisal of the evidence. *Crit Care Med* 1996;24:517–24.
13. Viele MK, Weiskopf RB: What can we learn about the need for transfusion from patients who refuse blood? The experience with Jehovah's Witnesses. *Transfusion* 1994;34:396–401.

14. Garratty G, Dzik W, Issitt PD, et al: Terminology for blood group antigens and genes: Historical origins and guidelines. *Transfusion* 2000;40:477–89.

15. British Committee for Standards in Hematology: Guidelines for the use of platelet transfusions. *BJH* 2003;122:10–23.

16. Peruzzi WT, Parker MA, Lichtenthal PR, et al: A clinical evaluation of a blood conservation device in medical intensive care patients. *Crit Care Med* 1993;21:501–6.

17. Petrides M (ed): *Practical guide to transfusion medicine.* p. 345–6. American Association of Blood Banks, Bethesda, MD, 2001.

18. Darveau M, Notebaert E, Denault A, Belisle S: Recombinant human erythropoietin use in intensive care. *Ann Phamacother* 2002;36:1068–74.

19. Corwin HL, Gettinger A, Rodriguez RM, et al: Efficacy of recombinant human erythropoietin in critically ill patients: A randomized controlled trial. *JAMA* 2002;288:2827–35.

20. IV. NKF-DOQI Clinical practice guidelines for anemia of chronic kidney disease: Update 2000. *Am J Kidney Dis* 2001;37(suppl 1):S182–238.

21. Wells P: Safety and efficacy of methods for reducing perioperative allogenic transfusion: A critical review of the literature. *Am J Therapeutics* 2002;9:377–88.

22. Laupacis A, Fergusson D: Drugs to minimize perioperative blood loss in cardiac surgery: Meta-analysis using perioperative blood transfusion as the outcome. *Anesth Analg* 1997;8:1258–67.

23. Bidstrup BP, Royston D, Sapsford RN, et al: Reduction in blood loss and blood use after cardiopulmonary bypass with high dose aprotinin. *J Thorac Cardiovasc Surg* 1989;97:364–72.

24. Poon MC, Katasarou O, Huth-Kuehne A, et al: Recombinant factor VIIa in congenital platelet bleeding disorders. *Blood* 2000;96(S1):256.

25. Martinowitz U, Kenet P, Lubetski A, et al: Possible role of recombinant activated factor VII in the control of hemorrhage associated with massive trauma. *Can J Anesth* 2002;49:S15–20.

26. Lynn M, Jeroukhimov I, Klein Y, Martinowitz U: Updates in the management of severe coagulopathy in trauma patients. *Intens Care Med* 2002;28:S241–7.

27. Erhardtsen E: Ongoing Novoseven® trials. *Intens Care Med* 2002;28:S248–55.

28. Hedner U, Erhardtsen E: Potential role for rFVIIa in transfusion medicine. *Transfusion* 2002;42:114–22.

29. Boyan CP, Howland WS: Cardiac arrest and temperature of banked blood. *JAMA* 1963;183:58–60.

30. British Committee for Standards in Hematology: The administration of blood and blood components and the management of transfused patients. *Transfusion Med* 1999;9:227–38.

31. Kleinman S, Chan P, Robillard P: Risks associated with transfusion of cellular blood components in Canada. *Transfusion Med Rev* 2003;17:120–62.

32. Chiavetta J, Escobar M, Newman A, et al: Incidence and estimated rates of residual risk for HIV, hepatitis C, hepatitis B and human T-cell lymphotropic viruses in blood donors in Canada, 1999–2000. *CMAJ* 2003;169:767–73.

33. Popovsky MA, Chaplin HC, Moore SB: Transfusion related acute lung injury: A neglected serious complication of hemotherapy. *Transfusion* 1992;36:589–92.

CHAPTER 18

VASOACTIVE MEDICATIONS

**DAVE NEILIPOVITZ AND
PIERRE CARDINAL**

You are treating a 45-year-old woman who presented to the hospital with a decreased level of consciousness. She was in severe respiratory distress and required intubation. Presently, she is hypotensive with a blood pressure of 70/45 and a heart rate of 145 despite repeated fluid boluses of over 6 litres of isotonic crystalloid solutions. Peripherally, she has very poor perfusion. You do not find any evidence of obstructive process such as a tension pneumothorax or cardiac tamponade. She is deteriorating in front of you. What should you do?

Vasopressors or inotropes? Dopamine or norepinephrine? These are questions physicians ask themselves when confronted with the need for vasoactive medications. Unfortunately, anxiety and confusion with these drugs can cause delays with potentially detrimental consequences. However, these medications can save lives so a rational approach is essential for critically ill patients.

Vasoactive medications primarily affect the cardiovascular system. The basic purpose of the heart and blood vessels is to supply the cells of the body with oxygen and other essential nutrients. In order to do this, the cardiovascular system must generate both pressure and flow. Which of these two factors is more important is debatable, but clearly both are necessary. Without pressure there is no flow, and pressure alone will not supply the cells. Ideally, fluid administration alone would be sufficient to improve both flow and pressure but this is not always so. Thus, the purpose of vasoactive medications is to improve either the pressure (i.e., blood pressure), the flow (i.e., cardiac output) or both. Although some drugs can raise both hemodynamic variables, most medications tend to preferentially increase one or the other. The choice of which vasoactive drug to use thus depends on which variable one is hoping to improve.

• Basic Principles and Physiology

A. Pressure

The blood pressure (BP) is the product of the cardiac output and the systemic vascular resistance (SVR). Thus, the BP can be increased by increasing either the SVR or the cardiac output. Since the SVR is primarily a reflection of the peripheral arterial tone, drugs that increase the arterial tone will raise the BP. Vasopressors are the medications that cause vasoconstriction of these arterial or resistance vessels by activating alpha 1 receptors. Drugs that increase the cardiac output, without decreasing the SVR, can raise the BP. Unfortunately, many drugs which increase the cardiac output do so by also lowering the SVR and thus can paradoxically lower the BP despite increasing the total blood flow.

B. Flow

The blood flow to the tissues is primarily a reflection of the cardiac output (CO). CO is calculated as a product of heart rate and stroke volume. Although moderate increases in the heart rate will initially raise the CO, rates above 120 bpm will have minimal benefit, and rates above 150 bpm actually cause it to decrease.[1] As the heart rate increases, the total time spent in diastole decreases, which thus reduces the filling of the ventricles (i.e., lowers the preload). Decreases in preload will in turn lower the CO (Starling's law of the heart). A disadvantage of raising the heart rate is that it increases myocardial oxygen consumption and can reduce the oxygen supply to the heart because the left ventricle is only perfused during diastole.[2] The increased demand and decreased supply can predispose patients to myocardial ischemia. Therefore, unless the heart rate is low, increasing the rate is not the preferred manner for increasing the CO. Rather, it is preferable to raise the CO by increasing the stroke volume.

The stroke volume is primarily influenced by preload, contractility and afterload. Preload refers to the amount of stretch exerted on the myofibrils of the heart at the end of diastole.[3,4] Simply, it is the amount of blood that fills the heart at the end of diastole and reflects venous return and blood volume. Starling's law of the heart describes how an increase in preload will increase the CO (Figure 18.1). Greater filling of the ventricle increases the force of cardiac contraction.[3-5] A point is, however, reached

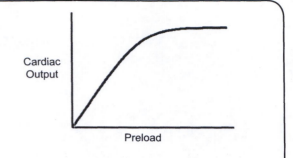

Figure 18.1 – Starling's Law of the Heart

Figure 18.1 illustrates the basis of Starling's law of the heart, whereby an increase in preload — namely the end diastolic volume of the ventricle — will increase the output of the ventricle. As can be seen, there is a point where further increases in preload do not increase the cardiac output. Although controversial, some believe that the cardiac output may start to decrease once preload becomes too high (see text for details).

where too much stretch occurs and the CO will start to decrease (though some physiologists debate this). The major advantage of augmenting the preload is that it increases the CO without raising myocardial oxygen consumption.[6]

Contractility refers to the amount of tension the heart generates during systole (i.e., the force of contraction) and the velocity of contraction (i.e., the rate at which the cardiac fibres form cross-bridges).[4] Many variables influence cardiac contractility and a full review of them is beyond the scope of this review. Aside from preload, the primary effect of these variables is their influence on intracellular calcium. A rise in the concentration of free intracellular calcium levels will increase the magnitude of cardiac contraction.

The final influence on CO is the afterload, which is primarily the force that opposes cardiac emptying during systole.[7] Again many variables influence afterload but a major component is the systemic vascular resistance (SVR). A rise in the SVR will increase the pressure in the aorta. As the pressure in the aorta increases, the amount of cardiac emptying during systole decreases thereby reducing CO (i.e., lower stroke volume). Although increasing the SVR raises the BP, the CO will be lowered by it. Conversely, the CO can be improved by reducing the SVR but this often occurs at the expense of lowering the BP.

Categories of Vasoactive Drugs

A simple approach to vasoactive drugs is to first classify them by their primary hemodynamic effects. Although some of these drugs can have multiple effects, they can be subdivided into one of three groups: a) vasopressors, b) inotropes or c) mixed.

A. Vasopressors

These are drugs that are primarily used to increase the BP. The majority of vasopressors work by stimulating the alpha 1 (α_1) adrenergic receptors but some act on the vasopressin receptors. These medications should be titrated to the BP. Although what is an adequate BP is influenced by many factors including pre-existing BP and coexisting medical problems, the minimal acceptable BP is usually at least a mean pressure usually above 65–70 mm Hg.[4,8] Since the exact role of the vasopressin analogues is presently unclear, the decision between using an α_1 agonist versus a vasopressin analogue at present depends upon availability and personal experience.

a. α_1 agonists — Norepinephrine and phenylephrine are the vasopressors that primarily work by stimulating the α_1 adrenergic receptors.[9–12] Stimulation of arterial α_1 receptors results in increased systemic vascular tone (higher SVR), which will increase the BP. Stimulation of α_1 receptors in the veins (capacitance vessels) causes venoconstriction, which increases venous return to the heart. Since a higher venous return increases preload, the CO and the BP will both increase. The CO may however decrease due to the increased afterload due to arteriolar vasoconstriction. The choice between these two vasopressors is guided by the gravity of the situation. Norepinephrine is generally considered to be the more potent drug and is therefore used when the hypotension is severe.[10]

b. vasopressin agonists — Vasopressin is the available drug that stimulates the V1 receptors to cause vasoconstriction and thereby raise the BP.[13] As with the α_1 agonists, the primary effect is to raise the SVR. At present, this drug should be considered to be experimental and thus indications for its use cannot be made.

B. Inotropes

These are medications which are primarily used to increase the CO. Inotropes are a more heterogenous group of medications since these drugs have several different mechanisms of action but ultimately these drugs raise the intracellular calcium levels. Ideally, these drugs would be titrated to the adequacy of peripheral blood flow. Unfortunately, there is presently no perfect monitor for this. In lieu of the perfect monitor, one should follow evidence of adequate end organ function (e.g., urine output, mentation, acid base status, etc.) or use an invasive monitor of CO (e.g., a Swan-Ganz catheter). The decision of which inotrope should be used is usually a choice between a beta agonist and a phosphodiesterase inhibitor. Each type has its advantages and disadvantages (Table 18.1) but presently there is no clear evidence that one type is better than the other.[14]

a. beta agonists — Dobutamine is an inotrope that primarily acts by stimulating (cardiac) beta 1 (β_1) receptors.[15–17] This increases heart rate but more importantly cardiac contractility and thus CO. Peripheral β_2 receptors are also stimulated which vasodilates the peripheral arterial vessels thereby reducing the afterload. The reduced afterload will increase the CO further but can lower the BP. The primary advantage of the beta agonists is that their duration of action is only a matter of minutes and thus their effects can be quickly reversed if their use worsens the situation (e.g., causes severe hypotension). The disadvantage of these drugs is that they can cause tachycardia, arrhythmias and increase myocardial oxygen consumption thus potentially causing myocardial ischemia. Dobutamine is contraindicated in patients with idiopathic hypertrophic subaortic stenosis or aortic stenosis.

b. phosphodiesterase inhibitors (PIs) — Milrinone and amrinone are PIs that selectively inhibit the type III phosphodiesterase enzyme.[4,13,18] This enzyme breaks down the second messenger cyclic AMP. Thus, PIs raise cyclic AMP levels, which raises intracellular calcium and ultimately increases myocardial contractility. The advantage of these drugs is that the rise in CO occurs with minimal increase in heart rate and without increasing myocardial oxygen consumption.[19] Additionally, PIs may improve relaxation of the heart (lusitropic effect), which will improve cardiac filling. The PIs are also called *inodilators*, which reflects their effects on both the

Table 18.1 – Comparison of Beta Agonists and Phosphodiesterase Inhibitors

	Advantages	Disadvantages	Example
Beta Agonist	- short acting, readily reversible	- increases myocardial O_2 use	- dobutamine
	- lower cost	- increases heart rate	- dopamine
		- arrhythmogenic	
Phosphodiesterase Inhibitors	- do not increase O_2 requirement	- long acting	- milrinone
	- improves relaxation of heart	- lowers blood pressure more	- amrinone
	- no direct heart rate effects	- costs more	
	- low arrhythmogenic potential		

heart and the peripheral blood vessels. Increases in cyclic AMP levels in the blood vessels will however cause vasodilation (analogous to β_2 stimulation). The decrease in arterial tone lowers the afterload, which further increases the CO but can decrease the BP (often substantially). Another disadvantage of the PIs is their relatively long duration of action (over 60 minutes). The effects of PIs, both beneficial and adverse, will therefore persist long after an infusion is discontinued. Due to the potential for severe hypotension, the loading dose recommended for milrinone (50 mcg/kg) should be given very slowly and reduced or even omitted unless the patient is hypertensive and volume overloaded.[20,21] Simply start the infusion at a low dose (0.25 mcg/kg/min) and titrate to the clinical effect (up to 0.75 mcg/kg/min). It is recommended that a vasopressor be prepared and available to treat an excessive fall in the BP.

c. cardiac glycosides — Digoxin is the most commonly used glycoside.[22] The primary mechanism is inhibiting the sodium-potassium-ATPase pump that raises intracellular sodium levels. Increases in sodium levels will raise the intracellular calcium concentration, which augments cardiac contractility. Cardiac glycosides also increase the parasympathetic tone, which decreases the heart rate.[23] Since the drug

must first accumulate in the cardiac myocyte to cause its inotropic effects, digoxin has a variable onset time. A further disadvantage is the very low therapeutic index associated with its use.[23] Thus, the utility of digoxin as an inotrope is very limited.

d. calcium — Calcium is a cation that is a short acting inotrope that transiently raises intracellular calcium levels to increase the CO via augmented contractility. Its brief duration of effect along with potential hypercalcemic toxicity with repeated use limits the role of elemental calcium as an inotrope.

e. glucagon — Glucagon is a polypeptide that is normally secreted by the pancreas and is important for blood glucose homeostasis. Exogenously administered glucagon can, however, also be used for its positive inotropic effects, which operate independently of adrenergic receptors.[24] Glucagon appears to activate adenyl cyclase as do the beta agonists but at a different receptor site. It is rarely used due to its considerable adverse effects and the fact that there are better inotropes available that have fewer side effects. The classic indication is beta blocker overdose. One can use a bolus dose of 1–5 mg IV or a continuous infusion of 5 mcg/kg/min following a loading dose of 50 mcg/kg.

C. Mixed

Dopamine and epinephrine are medications with both vasopressor and inotropic effects which occur in a dose dependent manner. The advantage of these drugs is that they can increase both the CO and the BP. Thus, in a patient whose underlying problem you are unsure of, these drugs are likely to address at least one of the underlying problems. A disadvantage of these drugs, however, is that it is difficult to preferentially increase one variable over the other (i.e., you are unlikely to focus your treatment to only increase BP or the CO rather than both). A further disadvantage is that these drugs tend to be more arrhythmogenic and raise the heart rate, which increases the risk of precipitating myocardial ischemia.[2]

a. dopamine — Dopamine is a mixed vasoactive drug that is unique in that in addition to its adrenergic receptor effects it can stimulate dopamine receptors.[25,26] Activation of the dopamine receptors vasodilates the splanchnic, renal and parts of the cerebral vasculature thereby increasing blood flow in these regions. Thus, the traditional use of dopamine was to use so-called renal dose dopamine to increase renal blood flow thereby decreasing the risk of renal failure. Unfortunately, the use of dopamine does not improve kidney outcomes and may paradoxically worsen them so its use for this purpose cannot be supported.[26-28] Although there is considerable variability, the hemodynamic effects reflect which receptors are predominantly stimulated, which in turn is dose dependent.

1. **Low Dose (renal dose)** – Below 2 mcg/kg/min the predominant effect is from stimulation of dopamine receptors in the splanchnic and renal vasculature. Low doses will cause diuresis and natriuresis.
2. **Moderate Dose (cardiac dose)** – The β_1 receptors usually begin to be stimulated above an infusion of 2 mcg/kg/min. At a moderate dose, dopamine primarily acts as an inotrope.
3. **High Dose (vasopressor dose)** – The α_1 adrenergic receptors begin to predominate above 7 mcg/kg/min, and once above 10 mcg/kg/min the β receptors and dopamine receptor effects are lost. Thus, at a high dose dopamine primarily acts as a vasopressor.

b. epinephrine — This mixed vasoactive drug will stimulate both alpha and beta receptors.[13,23] Although there is variability, the predominant hemodynamic effect again is dose dependent. Very low doses (1–2 mcg/min) will primarily stimulate β_2 receptors thus causing vasodilation, which may actually lower the BP (this dose can also be used to cause bronchodilation in the lungs). Low doses (around 4 mcg/min) begin to stimulate the β_1 receptors thus increasing the heart rate and contractility (i.e., an inotrope). Once the dose of epinephrine increases above 10–20 mcg/min, it predominantly stimulates the α_1 adrenergic receptors and thus acts as a vasopressor.[13]

● Drug Preparation and Administration

Tables 18.2–3 provide information on the preparation and dosing of the various vasoactive medications. Vasoactive drugs come in concentrated vials, which must be diluted prior to use. Although phenylephrine and ephedrine are vasopressors that can be used as intermittent boluses, most vasoactive drugs are given as an infusion. One or two vials are injected into 250–500 ml bags of saline or D5W. Avoid exposing the drugs to alkaline solutions (e.g., sodium bicarbonate) since this inactivates most vasoactive drugs. Although the drug solution can be dripped in at a rate that is titrated to the desired effect, it is better to use a volumetric infusion pump that accurately measures the administered dose.

Ideally, all vasoactive drugs are administered via a central line. In desperate situations, the drugs can be initiated via a peripheral line but should be switched to a central line as soon as possible. The danger with a peripheral line is the increased potential for the fluid to get into the interstitial tissue. Vasoactive drugs, especially vasopressors, can cause tissue ischemia and necrosis if this occurs. Interstitial drug may be treated by local infiltration, not intravascular, of phentolamine (dilute 5 mg into 10 cc of saline and inject several cc into the affected area).

● Application of Vasoactive Drugs

Although there are different strategies for the administration of vasoactive drugs, the suggested approach in Figure 18.2 is a relatively simple and effective. The first goal is to ensure that the patient

Table 18.2 – Preparation and Rates of Common Vasoactive Drugs

Drug	IV Push	Solution	Concentration	Infusion Range	Drug Effect
Epinephrine	5–20 mcg	1 mg / 250 cc	4 mcg/cc	0.1–1.0 mcg/kg/min	Mixed
Dopamine	N/R	200 mg / 250 cc	800 mcg/cc	0.5–25 mcg/kg/min	Mixed
Dobutamine	N/R	250 mg / 250 cc	1000 mcg/cc	0.5–30 mcg/kg/min	Inotrope
Phenylephrine	50–100 mcg	10 mg / 250 cc	40 mcg/cc	0.1–1.0 mcg/kg/min	Vasopressor
Norepinephrine	N/R	4 mg / 250 cc	16 mcg/cc	0.1–0.5 mcg/kg/min	Vasopressor
Ephedrine	5–10 mg	N/R	N/R	N/R	Vasopressor
Isoproterenol	N/R	1 mg / 250 cc	4 mcg/cc	0.1–0.5 mcg/kg/min	Inotrope
Milrinone	N/R	20 mg / 250 cc	80 mcg/cc	0.25–0.75 mcg/kg/min	Inotrope

N/R = not recommended

n.b. The above are suggested rates but doses must always be titrated to effect (see text for details).

Table 18.3 – Drug Effects of Common Vasoactive Drugs

Drug	Infusion Range	α 1	β 1	β 2	DA	CO	HR	SVR	MAP
Dopamine	0.5–3.0 mcg/kg/min	0	0	0	4+	⇑	⇑	⇓	0
	3–10 mcg/kg/min	1+	4+	2+	0	⇑⇑	⇑⇑	⇑	⇑
	> 10 mcg/kg/min	3+	1+	0	0	⇓ – ⇑	⇑	⇑⇑	⇑⇑
Dobutamine	0.5–30.0 mcg/kg/min	1+	4+	2+	0	⇑⇑	⇑	⇓	⇓ – ⇑
Epinephrine	0.03–0.15 mcg/kg/min	1+	4+	4+	0	⇑⇑	⇑⇑	⇑	⇑
	0.15–1.0 mcg/kg/min	4+	1+	1+	0	⇓ – ⇑	⇑	⇑⇑⇑	⇑⇑⇑
Isoproterenol	0.1–0.5 mcg/kg/min	0	4+	4+	0	⇓ – ⇑	⇑⇑⇑	⇓⇓	⇓⇓
Norepinephrine	0.1–0.5 mcg/kg/min	4+	1+	0	0	⇓ – ⇑	⇓ – ⇑	⇑⇑⇑	⇑⇑⇑
Phenylephrine	0.1–1.0 mcg/kg/min	3+	0	0	0	⇓ – ⇑	0 – ⇓	⇑⇑	⇑⇑

is adequately volume resuscitated at all times. The use of inotropes or vasopressors can be harmful in the presence of hypovolemia. Vasopressors can severely impair organ perfusion in the presence of hypovolemia. Inotropes will be ineffective since the heart cannot pump out blood if it is empty, regardless of how many inotropes are given. Adequacy of volume resuscitation is guided by the jugular venous pressure, central venous pressure (CVP) or the pulmonary artery occlusion pressure (i.e., wedge pressure). Regardless of how the patient responds to vasoactive drugs, the preload should be repeatedly assessed.

The first goal should be to improve the mean arterial pressure (MAP). The MAP is used since it is the best estimate of the driving pressure that supplies the various organ systems in the body. The goal should be to keep the MAP above a target value (usually above 60–65 mm Hg or even higher if there is a history of hypertension or high intracranial pressure).[4,8] The MAP can be increased by either increasing the CO (i.e., an inotrope) and/or by increasing the SVR (i.e., a vasopressor). Since many inotropes decrease the SVR, a vasopressor is the simplest drug to use to increase the MAP. Phenylephrine and norepinephrine are two drugs that act primarily as vasopressors. Dopamine and epinephrine at higher doses can, however, be used to increase the MAP.

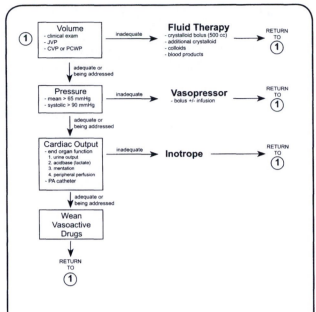

Figure 18.2 – Suggested Strategy for Vasoactive Drugs

Figure 18.2 presents a simple approach to the management of shock. The emphasis is to always optimize the volume resuscitation and to continuously re-evaluate the patient's need for fluid and vasoactive medications.

If, however, the problem is inadequate blood flow to the various organs despite restoration of the MAP, then the administration of an inotrope may be appropriate. The goal should be to obtain evidence of improvement in end organ function (e.g., increased urinary output, improved peripheral perfusion, etc.). One can also follow the CO as measured by a pulmonary artery (PA) catheter. The PA catheter does not replace the need to follow end organ function but rather compliments it. With the PA catheter, titrate the inotrope to keep the CO (or cardiac index) above a target value. The target value will depend upon the patient and the clinical situation. For example, a patient in heart failure may have the target cardiac index above 2.0 while a septic patient may require a cardiac index kept above 3.5 to improve end organ function. One must always correlate the measured values to the clinical situation.

The inotrope to select is usually either dobutamine or milrinone. If you are concerned that this may drop the BP, you could try dobutamine. If the patient tolerates dobutamine, it can be continued or replaced with milrinone, which is preferable if the increase in heart rate is risking myocardial ischemia or if the dobutamine is causing arrhythmias. Occasionally, an inotrope is used to improve CO along with a vasopressor to maintain an adequate BP. An alternative approach is to use low dose dopamine or epinephrine but one cannot ensure that their vasopressor effects will supersede their inotropic effects.

Key Points

- Blood pressure is the product of cardiac output and systemic vascular resistance.
- Blood pressure is primarily raised by the use of alpha 1 agonists.
- Inotropes that raise cardiac output are primarily either beta 1 agonists or phosphodiesterase inhibitors (PIs).
- Beta agonists are short acting but cause more tachycardia and arrhythmias.

- PIs are longer acting and cause more hypotension but fewer heart rate changes and arrhythmias.
- The first goal is usually to restore an adequate blood pressure.
- Inotropes are usually used to improve organ perfusion and thus improve end organ function.
- Vasoactive medications do not replace the need for adequate fluid resuscitation.

References

1. Canty JM Jr, Giglia J, Kandath D: Effect of tachycardia on regional function and transmural myocardial perfusion during graded coronary pressure reduction in conscious dogs. *Circ Res* 1990;82:1815–25.

2. Hjalmarson A: Significance of reduction in heart rate in cardiovascular disease. *Clin Cardiol* 1998;21(suppl 2):II3–7.

3. Sarnoff SJ, Berglund E: Ventricular function. I. Starling's law of the heart studied by means of simultaneous right and left ventricular function curves in the dog. *Circulation* 1954;9:706–18.

4. Kumar A, Parrillo JE: Chapter 20. Shock: Classification, pathophysiology, and approach to management. p. 371–420. In Parrillo JE, Bone RC (eds): *Critical care medicine: Principles of diagnosis and management*. Mosby, Toronto, 1995.

5. Gordon AM, Huxley AF, Julian FJ: The variation in isometric tension with sarcomere length in vertebrate muscle fibres. *J Physiol* 1966;184:170–92.

6. Suga H, Goto Y, Futaki S, et al: Systolic pressure-volume area (PVA) as the energy of contraction in Starling's law of the heart. *Heart Vessels* 1991;6:65–70.

7. Sonnenblick EH: Force-velocity relations in mammalian heart muscle. *Am J Physiol* 1962;202:931–9.

8. Schuster DP, Lefrak SS: Chapter 74. Shock. p. 891–908. In Civetta JM, Taylor RW, Kirby RR: *Critical care*. JB Lippincott, New York, 1988.

9. Dasta JF: Norepinephrine in septic shock: Renewed interest in an old drug. *DICP* 1990;24:153–6.

10. Smith LD, Oldershaw PJ: Inotropic and vasopressor agents. *Br J Anaesth* 1984;56:767–80.

11. Martin C, Papazian L, Perrin G, et al: Norepinephrine or dopamine for the treatment of hyperdynamic septic shock? *Chest* 1993;103:1826–31.

12. Bellomo R, Giantomasso DD: Noradrenaline and the kidney: Friends or foes? *Crit Care* 2001;5:294–8.

13. Section 6: Pharmacology II: Agents to optimize cardiac output and blood pressure. *Circulation* 2000;102(suppl I):I129–I35.

14. Benotti JR, McCue JE, Alpert JS: Comparative vasoactive therapy for heart failure. *Am J Cardiol* 1985;56:19B–24B.

15. Sonnenblick EH, Frishman WH, LeJemtel TH: Dobutamine: A new synthetic cardioactive sympathetic amine. *N Engl J Med* 1979;300:17–22.

16. Ruffalo RR Jr: The pharmacology of dobutamine. *Am J Med Sci* 1987;294:244–8.

17. Majerus TC, Dasta JF, Bauman JL, et al: Dobutamine: Ten years later. *Pharmacotherapy* 1989;9:245–59.

18. Benotti JR, Grossman W, Braunwald E, et al: Hemodynamic assessment of amrinone: A new inotropic agent. *N Engl J Med* 1978;299:1373–7.

19. Benotti JR, Grossman W, Braunwald E, et al: Effects of amrinone on myocardial energy metabolism and hemodynamics in patients with severe congestive heart failure due to coronary artery disease. *Circulation* 1980;62:28–34.

20. Baruch L, Patacsil P, Hameed A, et al: Pharmacodynamic effects of milrinone with and without a bolus loading infusion. *Am Heart J* 2001;141:266–73.

21. Kwak YL, Oh YJ, Shinn HK, et al: Hemodynamic effects of a milrinone infusion without a bolus in patients undergoing off-pump coronary artery bypass graft surgery. *Anaesthesia* 2004;59:324–31.

22. Smith TW, Haber E: Digitalis. *N Engl J Med* 1973;289:1063–72;1125–9.

23. Stoelting RK: Chapter 13. Digitalis and related drugs. p. 285–94. In *Pharmacology and physiology in anesthetic practice*. 2nd ed. JB Lippincott, Philadelphia, 1991.

24. White CM: A review of potential cardiovascular uses of intravenous glucagon administration. *J Clin Pharmacol* 1999;39:442–7.

25. Goldberg LI: Dopamine: Clinical uses of an endogenous catecholamine. *N Engl J Med* 1974;291:707–10.

26. Debaveye YA, van den Berghe GH: Is there still a place for dopamine in the modern intensive care unit? *Anesth Analg* 2004;98:461–8.

27. Kellum JA, Decker JM: Use of dopamine in acute renal failure: A meta-analysis. *Crit Care Med* 2001;29:1526–31.

28. Power DA, Duggan J, Brady HR: Renal-dose (low dose) dopamine for the treatment of sepsis-related and other forms of acute renal failure: Ineffective and probably dangerous. *Clin Exp Pharmacol Physiol Suppl* 1999;26(suppl):S23–8.

CHAPTER 19

HEMODYNAMIC MONITORING

DAVE NEILIPOVITZ,
JON HOOPER, AND
PETER BRINDLEY

A 55-year-old man presents to the hospital with severe septic shock. You have given 5 litres of crystalloid fluids but were forced to intubate the patient. Despite the fluid, the patient remained hypotensive and thus a vasopressor was initiated. Presently, the blood pressure is hard to detect by non-invasive techniques. You question whether the patient has been given enough fluid or whether he requires a higher vasopressor dose—or even if another medication such as an inotrope should be started. You wonder if hemodynamic monitors would help you answer these questions. Would they?

One of the most important principles when treating patients is a thorough and accurate physical exam. Unfortunately critical illness may make the interpretation of physical findings—and even a seemingly simple procedure such as blood pressure measurement—difficult. As such, technology is often applied to determine not only blood pressure but also filling pressures and cardiac output. Of course, these devices are not perfect. There are limitations to their accuracy as well as to the interpretation and application of the values obtained. The purpose of this chapter is to introduce the various hemodynamic measuring devices along with a discussion of potential pitfalls.

● Blood Pressure

Blood pressure enables perfusion of organs and tissue beds. Since hypotension is often a major problem in shock, it needs to be accurately measured. Blood pressure (BP) can be obtained indirectly or directly. Each method has advantages and disadvantages.

Auscultation is the simplest indirect method for measuring BP. A properly sized cuff is placed around the arm and inflated. The cuff is slowly deflated and auscultation of the Kortokoff sounds is used to determine systolic and diastolic pressures. The mean arterial pressure (MAP) can then be calculated as follows: MAP = DBP + 1/3(SBP – DBP). Although reasonably accurate in stable patients, auscultation may underestimate BP by as much as 20 mm Hg in low flow states. Therefore, direct measurements are preferred in critical care patients.[1]

The oscillometric method is another indirect method that is generally thought to be more accurate than auscultation. The various automatic oscillometric devices (e.g., Dinamap®) use plethysmography to detect pulsatile changes in an artery in order to measure mean and systolic pressures (the diastolic is then calculated).[2,3] Unfortunately, the oscillometric method can also be inaccurate in low flow states, at extremes of BP and in shivering patients and those with dysrhythmias.[2,4] Prolonged use or frequent cuff inflations can also cause tissue or nerve damage and direct methods are preferred in these settings.[5]

The present gold standard for assessing BP is direct measurement following insertion of an arterial catheter. Patients who may require arterial lines include those who are hemodynamically unstable (allows "beat to beat" BP observation), patients on vasoactive drugs and those requiring frequent blood sampling. Although arterial lines are considered to be more reliable than indirect measurements, they may cause complications such as needle trauma, hemorrhage, hematoma, potential infection and arterial thrombosis with distal ischemia.[6–10] Inaccurate values can also be recorded by arterial lines. As the pressure waves move peripherally in the arterial system, the systolic BP rises as a result of reflected waves from the periphery (systolic amplification).[11–13] Likewise, the diastolic BP decreases with increased distance from the aorta. For example, the radial systolic pressure may be higher than the aortic systolic pressure. The mean BP however is more robust and is therefore a more accurate reflection of central aortic BP (Figures 19.1). The transducer can also cause errors in the measurement of any parameter, be it the BP or central venous pressure (CVP). The transducer must be calibrated (often called zeroing) to the atmospheric pressure. Improper calibration can introduce errors in measurement. The transducer must be placed at the proper level (traditionally at the level of the right atrium). A transducer that is below this level will falsely elevate the measured value and if placed above will falsely lower it. The sensing device of the transducer, which converts the fluid wave into an electrical signal, can be wrongly amplified (hyper-

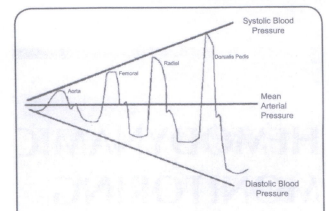

Figure 19.1a is a drawing illustrating the changes in blood pressure during progression from the aorta to the periphery. Note that the systolic increases, the diastolic decreases, and the mean arterial pressure remains relatively constant.

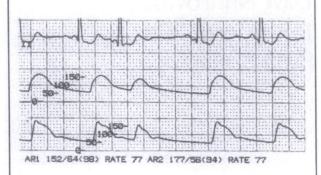

Figure 19.1b is an actual example of simultaneous femoral arterial tracing (middle trace) and radial arterial tracing (bottom trace).

Figures 19.1 – Blood Pressure Tracings, Changes from Aorta to Periphery

resonant) or attenuated (dampened). Amplification of the signal can lead to an overestimation of systolic and underestimation of diastolic BP. Attenuation can lead to an underestimation of systolic BP and overestimation of diastolic BP. However, in both cases the MAP is relatively preserved.[11–13] Figure 19.2 demonstrates normal and over-damped waveforms. The above signal alterations can also occur with any transduced pressure measurement, whether from an arterial line, a venous line or a pulmonary artery catheter.

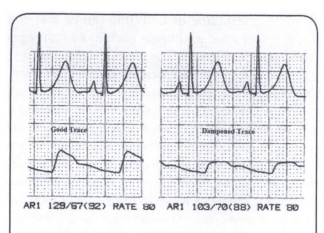

AR1 129/67(92) RATE 80   AR1 103/70(88) RATE 80

Figure 19.2 – Normal and Dampened Arterial Pressure Tracings

Arterial tracing in one patient. A dampened trace (right) was corrected to a normal trace (left). Note the relative preservation of mean pressure but decreasing of systolic and increasing of diastolic in dampened trace.

● Central Venous Pressure

A central venous catheter can be invaluable for rapid infusion of fluid, vasoactive drugs and various irritating substances (e.g., erythromycin, TPN). In addition, large central veins are often cannulated to measure venous pressure and guide fluid resuscitation in patients with precarious physiology. Administration of fluid can improve BP and cardiac output, but excess fluid can worsen pulmonary gas exchange. Thus, to help guide fluid therapy, the central venous pressure (CVP) is measured.

A properly positioned CVP catheter can accurately measure right atrial pressure. The typical CVP in healthy patients is 2–6 (mean 4) mm Hg when measured at end expiration. Caution should, however, be used when relating a measured pressure to presume a vascular volume.[14–16] The CVP can be affected by changes in pleural and pericardial pressures. In spontaneously breathing patients, the pressure will decrease during inspiration as a reflection of negative intrathoracic pressure. During positive pressure ventilation, however, inspiration will be associated with a rise in the pressure. Thus, the CVP values tend to be slightly higher in patients receiving positive pressure ventilation.

Aside from the measurement errors that can occur due to the transducer recording system (discussed above in BP section), other errors can affect the measured CVP values. The location of the venous catheter can affect the CVP reading. A femoral central venous catheter will usually give an accurate CVP reading except in the presence of raised intra-abdominal pressures.[17,18] A change in the compliance of the right atrium can also change the measured CVP without reflecting a change in fluid volume. Examples would include patients with pulmonary hypertension or right ventricular ischemia or infarction and those with pericardial disease. Greater caution is needed when using a CVP to estimate the preload of the left ventricle (see further discussion in the section on PACs).

Aside from crude numbers, observation of the CVP tracing can help identify various pathologies (Figure 19.3a).[19] In health, the *a* wave is associated with atrial contraction, the *c* wave is due to the closing motion of the tricuspid valve at the onset of systole, and the *v* wave reflects filling of the atrium during ventricular systole. The *x* descent corresponds to atrial relaxation and the vacuum effect, which occurs as the bottom of the atrium descends during ventricular contraction. The *y* descent occurs as the full atrium empties into the right ventricle following the opening of the tricuspid valve. Note that the waveform trace will vary with respiration. In atrial fibrillation *a* waves are missing, large "cannon" *a* waves can occur with atrioventricular dissociation (e.g., premature ventricular contraction, heart block) and large *v* waves suggest tricuspid regurgitation.

The proper technique for determining the CVP value is illustrated in Figure 19.3b. Ideally, the CVP value is determined by locating the pre-*c* wave value because this is the end-diastolic value for the ventricle (just before the tricuspid valve closes). If the *c* wave cannot be identified, the second best technique is to average the *a-c* wave. Identify the top of the *a* wave and the bottom of the x descent and take the middle of it as the CVP. The third technique, to identify the CVP value when the *a* or *c* waves are not visible, is to measure down to the *z* point from the ECG tracing (the end of the QRS complex). The third technique has more variability and thus is more subject to error. Regardless of how the CVP is measured, it should always be measured at end expiration to minimize the transmission of respiratory pressures to the cardiac chambers.

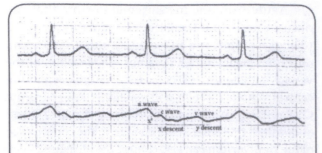

Figure 19.3a – The lower tracing is a typical central venous pressure (CVP) tracing with the corresponding ECG tracing (upper). The *a* wave is due to atrial contraction and corresponds to the *P* wave on the ECG. The delay between the *a* wave and the *P* wave reflects electromechanical dissociation. The *c* wave is due to closure of the tricuspid valve while the *x* descent reflects the drop in atrial pressure as the floor of the right atrium is pulled down during ventricular contraction. The *v* wave reflects venous return that fills until the tricuspid valve opens, which is the peak of the *v* wave. The *y* descent reflects rapid filling of the right ventricle after tricuspid valve opening (first phase of diastole). Note the small plateau after the *y* descent, which is the second phase of diastole and is followed by the third phase, atrial contraction.

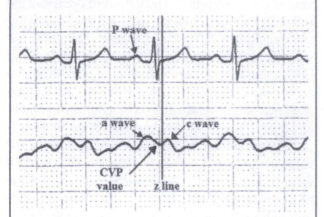

Figure 19.3b illustrates the three acceptable ways to read the CVP. The ideal technique is to locate the *pre-c* wave spot. The second technique is to average the *a-c* wave. The final technique is to measure down from the ECG tracing using the *z* line. The latter technique is especially useful when the *a* wave cannot be identified. Regardless of the technique, the measurement should always be performed at the end of expiration (see text for details).

Figures 19.3 – Typical Central Venous Pressure Tracing

The central line or CVP line can be inserted into several sites, and again each has advantages and disadvantages.[20,21] The femoral vein is easy to locate and the site is easily compressible if the artery is inadvertently punctured. It is a relatively safe site in patients with a coagulopathy. As discussed, the recorded CVPs are usually accurate if patients are kept supine and do not have raised intra-abdominal pressures. Unfortunately, femoral sites have been reported to have a higher incidence of line infections, are more likely to limit patient mobility and predispose patients to deep venous thrombosis in the cannulated vein.[20,21] The subclavian site is the least cumbersome for a patient and has the lowest infection rate.[20,21] Unfortunately, the subclavian site has the highest risk of pneumothorax during insertion and if the subclavian artery is inadvertently punctured it is not easily compressible. The internal jugular vein is frequently used due to a relatively low complication rate. However, injury to the carotid artery can compromise cerebral perfusion and/or hematomas in the neck can obstruct the airway.[22] The right internal jugular vein provides the most direct path to the heart, which assists the insertion of a pulmonary artery catheter or cardiac pacemaker. The external jugular vein is a central vein that is infrequently used, despite the risks of hematoma formation, pneumothorax and arterial injuries being relatively low. However, the mobility and tortuosity of the vein, along with a valve at the junction with the subclavian vein, can interfere with placement and thus it requires practice and patience to thread an external jugular line. Regardless of the upper extremity site chosen, attention should be paid to ensure that the CVP catheter tip is in the superior vena cava and not in the atrium as perforation here would cause cardiac tamponade. A chest x-ray should be performed post-central line insertion to rule out complications and to ensure the tip is well-positioned. The tip should not be seen below the right main stem bronchus.

● Pulmonary Artery Catheter

The pulmonary artery catheter (PAC) has been in widespread use since the 1970s.[23] Despite frequent use, there continues to be debate over its usefulness, accuracy and potential for harm.[24–27] As with any other instrument, the user should be aware of the many assumptions used in obtaining and interpreting data from the PAC.

The typical PAC provides three types of information: hemodynamic measurements, waveform tracings and special oxygen calculations. There are numerous potential uses but no absolute indication for PAC insertion. Regardless, the PAC never replaces the need for careful patient examinations and frequent reassessment. In general, however, a principle for PAC use should be that measuring intracardiac pressures, cardiac output, mixed venous gases or the various derived indices can improve the clinical situation. Typical clinical indications include the management of complicated myocardial infarction (e.g., cardiogenic shock), management of refractory shock and the assessment of various therapies used in critically ill patients (i.e., vasopressors, inotropes, PEEP, fluids).

A. Insertion of the PAC

The PAC is flow directed and is inserted aseptically through a 8.0 French single lumen central venous catheter. The catheter is 110 cm long and usually has two lumens (some have a ventricular infusion port). The distal port is used to measure pressures in the pulmonary artery whereas the proximal port, which is 30 cm from the distal tip, usually sits in the right atrium and can measure CVP. There is also a thermistor at the catheter tip for determining cardiac outputs and a balloon that can be inflated with air.

Once the tip of the PAC is passed through the end of the introducer catheter, the PAC is then floated (i.e., directed) through the right side of the heart by inflating the balloon and advancing the catheter. The air filled balloon acts like a sail as blood flow "pulls" the catheter through the heart. The rate of insertion should approximate the heart rate. As the catheter passes through the heart, the position of the tip is determined by observing changes in the waveform and the recorded vascular pressures (Figure 19.4). A typical CVP trace is initially seen, which is then followed in sequence by the right ventricle trace, pulmonary artery trace and finally the so-called "wedge" tracing. The wedge tracing occurs when the inflated balloon advances the catheter into a small distal branch of the pulmonary artery thereby obstructing flow distal to the balloon. It is essential that the waveforms be correctly interpreted. The PCWP should always be less than the pulmonary artery end diastolic pressure (PAEDP) and normally has a tracing similar to the CVP tracing. The catheter has markings of 10 cm intervals to determine how far it has been inserted. Knowledge of the usual insertion depths (Table 19.1) helps to identify if the catheter is coiling in the heart or if it has been inserted too far.

Occasionally the PAC will not pass through the right atrium into the right ventricle. This may be due to significant tricuspid regurgitation or a low cardiac output. Transient augmentation of the cardiac output with a bolus of calcium or ephedrine will sometimes

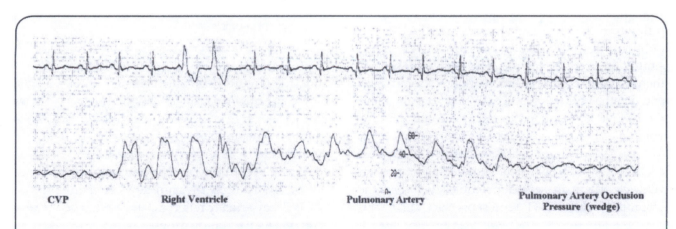

CVP   Right Ventricle   Pulmonary Artery   Pulmonary Artery Occlusion Pressure (wedge)

Figure 19.4 – Typical Waveform Tracings Seen with a Pulmonary Artery Catheter

Figure 19.4 shows the changes in waveform as the tip of the pulmonary artery catheter passes from the vena cava and right atrium (i.e., the central venous pressure or CVP) on to the wedge tracing. Note the rise in the diastolic component as the catheter passes from the ventricle into the pulmonary artery.

Table 19.1 – Approximate Insertion Depths of a Pulmonary Artery Catheter

Insertion Site	Right Atrium	Right Ventricle	Pulmonary Artery
Right Internal Jugular	20–25 cm	30–40 cm	45–55 cm
Left Internal Jugular	25–30 cm	35–45 cm	50–60 cm
Subclavian	15–20 cm	25–35 cm	40–45 cm
Femoral	40–45 cm	50–60 cm	65–75 cm
Right Cubital Fossa	50–55 cm	60–70 cm	75–85 cm
Left Cubital Fossa	55–60 cm	65–75 cm	80–90 cm

facilitate passage of the PAC. Occasionally, a PAC will enter the right ventricle but not pass into the pulmonary artery. Again augmenting the cardiac output may help. Other techniques to facilitate passage into the pulmonary artery include not using the Trendelenberg position and actually raising the left side up. Another trick is to spin the PAC while advancing it when it is in the right ventricle. Occasionally, filling the balloon with sterile saline and placing the patient left side down will help the catheter pass through the right ventricle into the pulmonary artery. Finally, fluoroscopy can be used to pass the PAC through the heart under direct vision.

B. Assumptions and Limitations of the PAC and CVP

The value measured from the distal port of the catheter when it is wedged has several names, including the pulmonary artery occlusion pressure (PAOP), the pulmonary capillary wedge pressure (PCWP) or just simply the wedge pressure. The wedge pressure is then thought to be a reflection of the left ventricular end diastolic filling pressure (LVEDP). Furthermore the LVEDP is presumed to reflect the end diastolic volume of the left ventricle (LVEDV) (Figure 19.5). The primary assumption is that there is a continuous column of blood from the tip of the catheter to the left ventricle. There are several potential sites where the assumption that PCWP represents the LVEDP (and subsequently the LVEDV) may lead to error (Figure 19.6).[28–30]

The greatest assumption made is that the LVEDP always reflects LVEDV. This relies upon a further assumption that the relationship between volume and pressure (i.e., the compliance) is always linear; this is

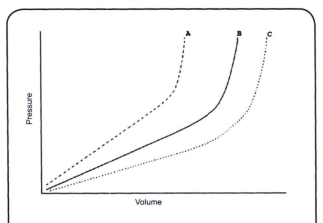

Figure 19.5 – Relationship of Left Ventricular Volume and Pressure

Figure 19.5 shows the relationship of left ventricular pressure and volume (i.e., the compliance). Curve A is a less compliant ventricle whereas C is a more compliant ventricle.

not true (Figure 19.5). Small changes in the LVEDV will cause minimal changes in LVEDP at low volumes but cause large changes at higher volumes. Since ventricular compliance is dynamic, a single PCWP may actually be associated with vastly different volumes depending on the ventricular compliance when the value is measured.[28,29] A change in the PCWP may actually reflect a change in left ventricular compliance (i.e., due to drugs or ischemia) rather than a volume change. Thus a wedge of 20 may reflect volume overload in some patients but not in others. Further, the ideal wedge value in a single patient can change over time as the compliance of the ventricle changes (i.e., the patient shifts to different compliance

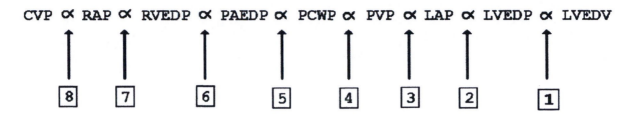

CVP = central venous pressure
RAP = right atrial pressure
RVEDP = right ventricle end diastolic pressure
PAEDP = pulmonary artery end diastolic pressure
PCWP = pulmonary capillary wedge pressure

PVP = pulmonary venous pressure
LAP = left atrial pressure
LVEDP = left ventricle end diastolic pressure
LVEDV = left ventricle end diastolic volume

Figure 19.6 – Assumptions and Potential Sites for Error with Central Hemodynamic Measurements

Figure 19.6 – Assumptions made when CVP or PCWP is assumed to represent the left ventricular volume:
1. compliance of left ventricle – altered by ischemia, infarction, hypertension, aortic valve disease, etc.
2. mitral valve – mitral stenosis or premature valve closure affects assumption
3. pulmonary venous disease – rare disorders of pulmonary venous occlusive disease
4. West zone III – if not there, measured pressure may represent alveolar pressure
5. pulmonary artery pressure – assumes there is no pulmonary hypertension present
6. pulmonic valve – assumed to be normal
7. tricuspid valve – assumed to be normal
8. central vein – no obstruction or interfering pressure (e.g., vena cava clot, elevated abdominal pressure)

curve). Therefore the entire clinical picture needs to be appreciated rather than just the wedge in isolation.

The next site of potential error is the mitral valve. At the end of diastole while the mitral valve is still open, the left atrial pressure should reflect LVEDP. This will not occur if there is obstruction at the mitral valve (mitral stenosis), in which case the measured PCWP may overestimate left ventricular filling. Conversely, in aortic regurgitation or with premature closure of the mitral valve, the LVEDP may be greater than the left atrial pressure. While very rare, if there is any obstruction in the pulmonary veins, the PCWP may overestimate the filling of the left ventricle.

It is also assumed that the catheter has "floated" to West zone III of the lung (Table 19.2). If the catheter tip is actually in West zone II or West zone I, then the measured value reflects alveolar pressure not capillary pressure. Fortunately the vast majority of catheters usually do go to West zone III, as it is the area with the most blood flow. A uniphasic tracing and a PCWP > PAEDP suggest inappropriate catheter placement.

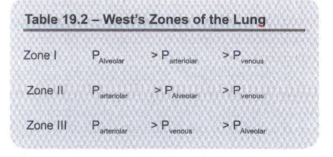

Table 19.2 – West's Zones of the Lung

Zone I	$P_{Alveolar}$	> $P_{arteriolar}$	> P_{venous}
Zone II	$P_{arteriolar}$	> $P_{Alveolar}$	> P_{venous}
Zone III	$P_{arteriolar}$	> P_{venous}	> $P_{Alveolar}$

Increases in alveolar pressure, position changes or decreases in the CO may change zone III physiology to zone II thereby creating inaccurate measurements. Pressures must also be measured at end expiration because that is when there is the least transmission of pleural pressure to the vasculature. A patient on a ventilator may have a combination of machine delivered breaths and spontaneous breaths making it difficult to determine end exhalation. Putting a hand on the patient's chest while watching the monitor will help determine what is inhalation and what is exhalation. It is best to try to obtain a reading during a "quiet" exhalation, but this may require sedating or paralyzing the patient. If pressures are not measured at end exhalation, an increase in pleural pressure from a forceful exhalation or PEEP, will elevate the PCWP. The amount of pleural pressure transmitted to the vasculature is difficult to estimate (and therefore compensate for) since it varies proportionally with lung compliance. A PEEP level below 10 cm H_2O is of minor concern. However, contrary to some recommendations, PEEP should not be removed in order to measure the PCWP, since this will acutely change the hemodynamics in patients and may potentially result in hypoxemia.

The proper technique for determining the PCWP value is similar to the measuring of the CVP but with some important differences: Unlike the CVP tracing, the *c* wave is not identifiable in the typical wedge tracing. Thus, the best technique to identify the PCWP value is to use the average of the *a-c* wave. The second technique to identify the PCWP value is to again use the *z* point from the ECG tracing but to add two small boxes (0.08 seconds) before measuring down to the PCWP tracing. The addition of the two small boxes accounts for the increased distance from the left ventricle to the pulmonary artery thus allowing time for the transmission of the waveform from the left ventricle to reach the recording site. As with CVP measurements, all PCWP measurements should be measured at end expiration to minimize the transmission of respiratory pressures to the cardiac chambers.

An "over-wedged" or uniphasic PAC tracing (Figure 19.7) is another source of error. This indicates that the catheter tip is too far in and the balloon is over inflated in the pulmonary artery. Not only will an over-wedged catheter give erroneous data, it also puts the patient at risk for pulmonary artery rupture and associated mortality. Pathologic *v* waves are another common potentially dangerous pitfall if they are not recognized, since the PAC has "wedged" but the tendency is to continue to advance the PAC (Figure 19.8). This is because giant *v* waves hide the usual change in waveform that indicates the catheter has reached the wedged position. Enlarged *v* waves are suggestive (but not diagnostic) of mitral regurgitation.[31–33] In the presence of enlarged *v* waves, the wedge tracing can be identified by watching for loss of the initial part of the pulmonary artery

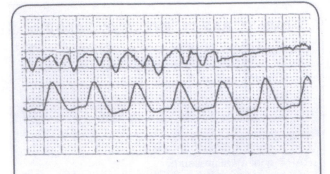

Figure 19.7 – Over-Wedged Tracing of a Pulmonary Artery Catheter

Figure 19.7 shows an over-wedged tracing of PA catheter (top trace) and an arterial line tracing (bottom trace). The appropriate management is to stop inserting, deflate balloon and withdraw to a safe distance.

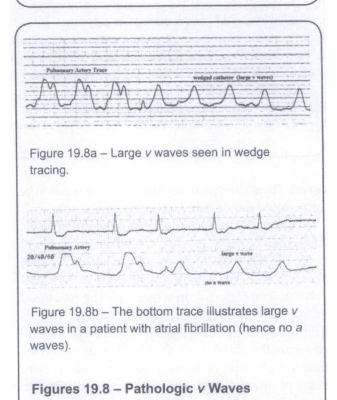

Figure 19.8a – Large *v* waves seen in wedge tracing.

Figure 19.8b – The bottom trace illustrates large *v* waves in a patient with atrial fibrillation (hence no *a* waves).

Figures 19.8 – Pathologic *v* Waves

tracing. As the initial deflection disappears, the large pathologic *v* waves remain. The presence of pathologic *v* waves can also be identified by correlating the wave tracings to the ECG. The *v* waves are found after the T waves where as the pulmonary artery trace is found between the QRS complex and the T waves.

Sometimes a PCWP cannot be measured. In that case, the PAEDP is sometimes used as an estimate of the PCWP (and thus also as an estimate of the left ventricular filling volume). Unfortunately, this is not reliable in any situation in which the pulmonary vascular resistance is elevated (i.e., hypoxia, emboli, acute or chronic lung diseases, tachycardia). Furthermore, using the CVP to estimate LVEDV has even more sources of potential error than for the PCWP. It assumes that the pulmonary valve is normal, that the tricuspid valve is normal and that there is no obstruction in the vena cavae. The use of a femoral CVP also assumes there is not an elevation of the intra-abdominal pressure. Hence, a CVP should only be used cautiously as an estimate of the filling of the left ventricle.[34]

C. Complications Associated with the Insertion and Interpretation of a PAC

Aside from the complications from insertion of any central venous catheter, there are several complications unique to the PAC.[35–38] Ventricular arrhythmias can occur when inserting the PAC. This is not uncommon but is, fortunately, typically non-sustained and stops once the catheter is in place, and therapy is rarely required. Right bundle branch block occurs in approximately 1% of patients.[35,36] Although the block is usually reversible, the insertion of a PAC in patients with a pre-existing left bundle branch block is relatively contraindicated since complete heart block can be precipitated in this setting. Perforation in the heart or the pulmonary artery is also very rare but can have devastating consequences. Pulmonary infarction due to persistent wedging can occur. Knotting of the catheter in the heart has occurred.[37,38] Typically, the catheter has been repeatedly advanced but has not successfully floated into the pulmonary artery. Instead, the catheter begins to coil in the heart. Removal of a knotted catheter is difficult and usually requires the assistance of an interventional radiologist. The position of the catheter should be routinely checked with a chest x-ray. If the PAC is coiled or the tip is too far in then the catheter should be partially withdrawn. The tip of the PAC should not be beyond the hilum of the lung. Regardless of the x-ray's findings, the depth of the catheter should always be assessed prior to inflating the balloon. If it appears to be in inordinately far, then it should be pulled back prior to inflating the balloon.

The balloon should always be inflated slowly while watching the tracing and inflation stopped as soon as the waveform changes. Obviously, one should never ever pull the catheter back with the balloon inflated. In addition, injury to the pulmonary artery or valve damage can occur secondary to the PAC. The longer the PAC remains in situ, the greater the likelihood that it will become infected or lead to thrombosis or thrombocytopenia.

D. Hemodynamic Measurements

In addition to hemodynamic measurements from the right atrial (RA), right ventricular (RV), pulmonary artery (PA) and pulmonary capillary wedge pressures (PCWP), the PAC is used to measure cardiac outputs using the thermodilution technique. A known amount of fluid (usually 10 ml of dextrose or saline) at a known temperature (usually room temperature) is injected through the proximal port into the right atrium. The thermistor at the end of the PAC measures the temperature change. The CO is inversely proportional to the integral of the time-temperature curve. Three outputs are typically measured and then averaged. A steady injection (over 2–4 seconds) performed at a similar point of the respiratory cycle (usually end expiration) will help minimize errors. Improper injectate volumes, tricuspid or pulmonic injectate regurgitation, intracardiac shunts or rapid infusions from peripheral intravenous lines will give inaccurate results.[39,40]

The PAC can be used to estimate other variables based on the aforementioned measured values along with other variables that are input (e.g., BP, weight, height, etc.). Table 19.3 lists the various calculated indices. As with all calculated scientific values, combining measured values introduces potential additional errors into the calculated value and thus should be used cautiously.

The cardiac outputs can be referenced to body surface area (BSA) by calculating the cardiac index (CI): CI = CO/BSA. The stroke volume (SV) is the volume ejected by the ventricles during systole. It is calculated by dividing the CO by the HR (SV = CO/HR). A "good" SV is approximately 1 ml/kg.

The systemic vascular resistance (SVR) is the calculated resistance across the systemic circulation (Figure 19.9). The SVR is frequently touted as an estimate of left ventricular afterload but unfortunately does not always accurately represent this. It is

Table 19.3 – Values Measured and Calculated using the Pulmonary Artery Catheter

Value	Acronym	Source or Formula	Normal Values
Cardiac Output	CO	directly measured	3.0–7.0 l/min
Stroke Volume	SV	SV = CO / HR x 1000	70–130 ml/beat
Central Venous Pressure	CVP	directly measured	0–6 mm Hg
Wedge Pressure	PCWP	directly measured	2–12 mm Hg
Cardiac Index	CI	CI = CO / BSA	2.5–4.5 l/min/m²
Stroke Index	SI	SI = SV / BSA	33–47 ml/m²/beat
Systemic Vascular Resistance	SVR	$SVR = \dfrac{(MAP - CVP) \times 80}{CO}$	800–1200 dyne·sec/cm⁵
Pulmonary Vascular Resistance	PVR	$PVR = \dfrac{(PAM - PCWP) \times 80}{CO}$	120–250 dyne·sec/cm⁵
Left Ventricular Stroke Work Index	LVSWI	LVSWI = (MAP – PCWP) × SI × 0.0136	45–60 g/beat/m²
Right Ventricular Stroke Work Index	RVSWI	RVSWI = (PAM – CVP) × SI × 0.0136	8–16 g/beat/m²
Right Atrial Pressure	RAP	directly measured	0–6 mm Hg
Right Ventricle Pressure			
Systolic	RVSP	directly measured	15–30 mm Hg
Diastolic	RVDP	directly measured	0–6 mm Hg
Pulmonary Artery Pressure			
Systolic	PASP	directly measured	15–30 mm Hg
Diastolic (end)	PAEDP	directly measured	5–13 mm Hg
Mean	PAM	directly measured	10–18 mm Hg

HR = heart rate measured by ECG monitoring

MAP = mean arterial pressure (input from arterial line or a non-invasive device)

BSA = Body Surface Area (nomogram or BSA = $\sqrt{\dfrac{\text{height in cm x weight in kg}}{3600}}$

calculated as follows: SVR = (MAP – CVP) × 80/CO. If the SVR is abnormally high or low, treatment changes should not be based solely on this number but rather the components that go into calculating the SVR should be examined. For example, a high SVR could be from arterial hypertension or a falling cardiac output (see below for an approach to the values). A similar calculation can be made for the pulmonary vascular resistance but this value is of limited use.

Left ventricular stroke work (LVSW) is the work performed by the ventricle to eject blood into the aorta. It is based upon the left ventricular pressure-volume curve (Figure 19.10). The area of the curve is approximated by assuming that the curve is a rectangle. The value is usually indexed to the body size and is touted as an estimation of the ventricular contractility function.

E. Waveform Tracings

Valuable information can be obtained from visualization of the actual waveforms.[19,41,42] Although a full review of abnormal waveforms is beyond the scope of this review.

F. Oxygen Calculations

Various oxygen calculations can be made using a typical PAC (Table 19.4). A blood gas sample is slowly withdrawn from the distal port (balloon is deflated) and simultaneously an arterial blood gas is taken. The sample from the distal port is the mixed venous gas. The oxygen saturation (Svo_2) from the mixed venous gas is normally 70–75%. A level below 60% is associated with inadequate oxygen delivery (poor oxygen delivery) whereas an increased Svo_2 may

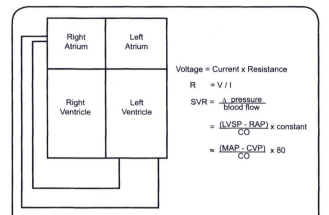

Figure 19.9 – The Systemic Vascular Resistance Calculation

The systemic vascular resistance (SVR) calculation is a proposed estimation of afterload. It is based upon a modification of Ohm's Law where voltage (V) is the product of current (I) times resistance (R). Voltage, or electrical potential difference, is replaced by the change in pressure, while current is replaced by total blood flow. The change in pressure is the difference between left ventricle systolic pressure (LVSP) and the right atrium pressure (RAP). The mean arterial pressure is used as an approximation of the LVSP while the RAP is approximated by the central venous pressure (CVP). The total blood flow is the cardiac output (CO).

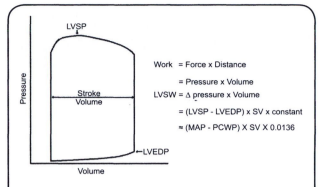

Figure 19.10 – The Left Ventricle Stroke Work Calculation

The left ventricular stroke work index (LVSWI) is a calculation based on the pressure volume curve of the left ventricle. The shape is assumed to be a rectangle with the area being the work performed by the left ventricle. The mean arterial pressure (MAP) is assumed to be a better estimate of the left ventricle systolic pressure (see Figure 19.1 for explanation). The pulmonary capillary wedge pressure is used to estimate the left ventricle end diastolic pressure (LVEDP) while the stroke volume (SV) is derived from cardiac output divided by the heart rate.

Table 19.4 – Oxygen Calculations

Calculation	Acronym	Formula	Normal Values
Oxygen Delivery	DO_2	$DO_2 = CI \times CaO_2 \times 10$	460–650 ml/min/m²
Oxygen Consumption	VO_2	$VO_2 = CI \times Ca\text{-}vO_2 \times 10$	95–170 ml/min/m²
Blood Oxygen Content	CaO_2	$CaO_2 = (0.134 \times Hgb \times SaO_2) + (0.0031 \times PaO_2)$	15–20 ml/dl
Oxygen Extraction	$a\text{-}vO_2$	$a\text{-}vO2 = (CaO_2 - CvO_2)/CaO_2$	0.23–0.32

be associated with sepsis, cirrhosis, and arterial-venous shunts. The size of dead space ventilation and physiologic shunt in the lungs can be calculated using the measured values. The amount of oxygen delivered to the periphery can also be calculated as follows: $DO_2 = CO \times$ (oxygen content), where oxygen content = $1.34 \times Hgb \times SaO_2$. The amount of oxygen consumed by the tissues is calculated as follows: $Vo_2 = CO \times 1.34 \times Hgb \times (SaO_2 - SvO_2)$.

G. Approach to PAC Hemodynamic Results

Unfortunately, there is no perfect approach to guide application of the PAC. Two important principles however must apply when interpreting the values obtained (Table 19.5). First, *treat the patient* not *the numbers*. The trend is far more important than the exact numeric value. Far too frequently, physicians aim for arbitrary targets or to normalize the numbers and in so doing either expose the patient to the side effects of the treatment required to obtain those parameters or simply forget to treat the whole patient. Although a patient may not have so-called normal numbers, the values may actually be adequate for that patient. For example, a cardiac index of 1.9 is low but if there are no signs of inadequate organ perfusion, then augmentation of the heart is likely not required. Conversely, a patient with a normal cardiac index may have signs of inadequate organ perfusion. Thus, algorithms that use specified values to direct patient therapy may inadvertently cause patient harm. For example, an algorithm that mandates giving furosemide if the PCWP > 20 may actually be the worst thing to do in a patient with aortic stenosis (although for many other patients it may be appropriate). The second important principle is to *look at all the PAC numbers* not just one or two values. Focusing on one or two values may cause one to miss critical information that could significantly alter patient treatment or lead to a potentially life-threatening omission. The so-called normal values for the different PAC measurements are listed in Table 19.6. However, these values are measured in young healthy patients and thus should be cautiously generalized to unhealthy patients (especially those on a mechanical ventilators). Figure 19.11 suggests a relatively simple alternate approach that can help direct therapy, stresses volume optimization and relies more on more accurate and directly measured values with less emphasis on calculated values.

Before the numbers of the PAC are actually reviewed, it is essential to appreciate background patient information. First and foremost is the clinical state of the patient. Is the patient in shock (i.e., no urine output, acidotic, shut down, etc.)? Suffering from pulmonary edema? Relatively stable? Etc. How one interprets the values must *always* be related back to the patient. As noted above, although the PAC numbers may appear to be reasonably normal, if the patient is in a profound state of shock then clearly they are inadequate. Furthermore, the patient who requires several vasoactive drugs to obtain PAC numbers similar to those of the patient who is on no drugs is likely to be far worse clinically. Thus, although the numbers may look reasonably good, if this is the result of several medications then there is room for improvement.

After the clinical situation of the patient is ascertained, some baseline measurements should be known since they influence the interpretation of the PAC numbers. The blood pressure, specifically the mean arterial pressure (MAP), is extremely important and is a product of the cardiac output (itself determined by stroke volume and heart rate) and the vascular resistance. As discussed in Chapter 15, an adequate pressure is required to perfuse the various organ beds. Inadequate blood flow to the organs needs to be quickly corrected, but severe hypotension is an emergency that needs immediate therapy. Thus,

Table 19.6 – Reportedly Normal Values for the Pulmonary Artery Catheter

Variable	Acronym	Normal Value
Cardiac output	CO	3.0–7.0 l/min
Cardiac index	CI	2.5–4.5 l/min/m²
Stroke volume	SV	70–130 ml/beat
Systemic vascular resistance	SVR	800–1200 dyne·sec/cm⁵
Pulmonary vascular resistance	PVR	120–250 dyne·sec/cm⁵
Left ventricular stroke work index	LVSWI	45–60 gm/beat/m²
Mixed venous saturation	MvO_2	70–75%
Oxygen delivery	DO_2	460–650 ml/min/m²
Oxygen consumption	VO_2	95–170 ml/min/m²

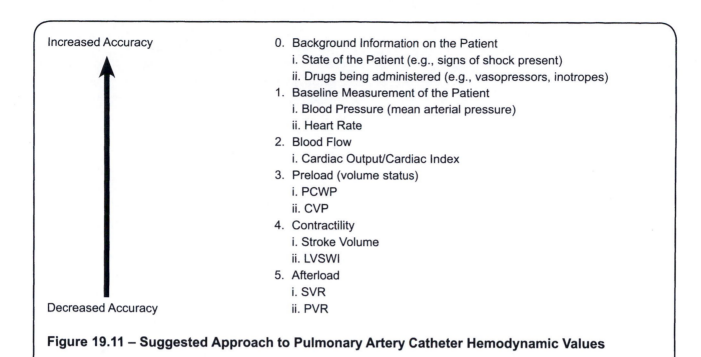

Increased Accuracy

0. Background Information on the Patient
    i. State of the Patient (e.g., signs of shock present)
    ii. Drugs being administered (e.g., vasopressors, inotropes)
1. Baseline Measurement of the Patient
    i. Blood Pressure (mean arterial pressure)
    ii. Heart Rate
2. Blood Flow
    i. Cardiac Output/Cardiac Index
3. Preload (volume status)
    i. PCWP
    ii. CVP
4. Contractility
    i. Stroke Volume
    ii. LVSWI
5. Afterload
    i. SVR
    ii. PVR

Decreased Accuracy

Figure 19.11 – Suggested Approach to Pulmonary Artery Catheter Hemodynamic Values

if it is critically low, typically a MAP below 55–60 mm Hg, then this usually must be corrected even before the rest of the PAC numbers are reviewed. However, the MAP influences how to proceed with the PAC numbers (e.g., an inadequate CO but associated high MAP would suggest the use of a vasodilator more than an inotrope). The heart rate is also important. Occasionally the value read by the machine is wrong, which will then alter numerous other values derived from it. More importantly, however, a patient who is relying on a high heart rate to maintain their CO is putting considerable strain on the heart, which may predispose them to myocardial ischemia.[43] Thus, alternative therapy should likely be used for such a patient (therapy to increase stroke volume rather than heart rate would be preferred to raise the CO).

A blood flow result is the next important value to assess. The CO or this value indexed to body size, namely the CI, should be evaluated. If clinically the blood flow is deemed inadequate to maintain perfusion to vital organs and the patient continues to deteriorate, then whatever value is measured is insufficient. The benefit of having the numeric value is that this value can serve as a reference or baseline to evaluate the subsequent effects of therapy. For example, a patient in profound shock had a CI of 2.2, and therapy was undertaken that increased the

CI to 2.6. Since the signs of shock can take a while to correct, the fact that the PAC value increased would give an earlier suggestion that therapy was working. Thus, if the measurement of blood flow is deemed insufficient, therapy to improve it is indicated. This has to be followed up with frequent reassessment and the physician must be prepared to re-evaluate the appropriateness of the therapy. Again this all hinges on the evolving clinical status of the patient. As mentioned, although heart rate influences the CO, since most patients are at risk for ischemia, increasing the heart rate to improve the CO is rarely indicated. Thus, therapy is usually directed at the other factors that influence the CO, namely the preload, contractility and afterload.

Preload refers to the amount of stretch exerted on the heart fibres at the end of diastole.[44] Essentially, it is the volume of blood that fills the heart at the end of diastole. Starling's law of the heart states that greater filling of the ventricle increases the force and the velocity of each cardiac contraction (Figure 19.12). Two important assumptions are that the heart rate and the afterload are constant. The primary advantage of augmenting preload is that it increases the CO with little increase in myocardial oxygen consumption.[45] As discussed above, the PCWP and CVP are used as estimates of the end diastolic blood volumes of the

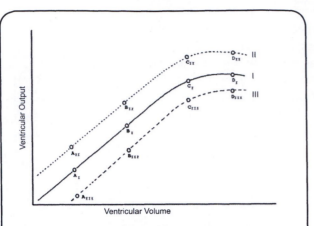

Figure 19.12 – Starling's Law of the Heart

Figure 19.12 – Ventricular output can be measured as cardiac index or stroke volume. The ventricular volume is the end diastolic volume (preload), which is approximated by the wedge pressure (PCWP). The assumptions made are that the heart rate and afterload levels are kept constant. Curve II represents an increase in the intrinsic myocardial contractility level (i.e., inotrope added). Curve III is a decrease in myocardial contractility level.

left and right ventricles respectively. Unfortunately, there is no magic number ideal for all patients. Again, the PCWP and CVP need to be correlated to the effect upon blood flow and the clinical state. For example, a patient in shock has a PCWP of 17 and a CI of 2.2. Most physicians will conclude that it is the CI that must be addressed and not the volume status. Using Figure 19.12, one does not know where the patient is on their Starling curve. Therefore, to clarify where the patient is on this imaginary Starling curve, additional points must be created. To do so, a fluid bolus of approximately 250 ml is given as quickly as possible (i.e., an instantaneous volume change). During the bolus, the patient should not have any changes in their medications or be stimulated (e.g., suctioned, turned). Drug changes or stimulation (which increases endogenous catecholamines) can alter the compliance of the ventricle, thus shifting the Starling curve (from curve I to curve II on Figure 19.12) thereby making PCWP comparisons inappropriate. Once the fluid bolus is completed, the PAC numbers are repeated. If the CI increases, then the patient has moved up the Starling curve. How far up the curve is however still unknown. The process is repeated until the PCWP

value increases but the CI does not (i.e., around point C_I). At this area, the patient has maximized their volume loading for that degree of ventricular compliance. The PCWP value around C_I is usually in the high teens but for some patients it is lower or considerably greater (e.g., a patient with severe aortic stenosis may have an optimal PCWP above 25). Thus, the actual PCWP value is not important but rather how it correlates to the patient's clinical state and how it changes with therapy. Once volume has been optimized, further improvements in the CI will require increases in contractility or changes in the afterload.

Contractility primarily refers to the intrinsic ability of the heart to generate the force and velocity for contraction.[46] Although it is extremely important, there are no readily available measures of contractility. The left ventricular stroke work index (LVSWI) has been touted as a useful contractility measure. In general, a result above 50 suggests excellent left ventricular contractility whereas a value below 20 is quite concerning. While the stroke volume is strongly influenced by preload and afterload, it can be thought of as a surrogate for contractility. As stated above, a good stroke volume is approximately 1 ml/kg. Inadequate values are first dealt with by volume augmentation. Using this approach, the physician has already optimized preload before tackling the contractility and afterload indices. Thus, the next step to increase the blood flow would be to increase contractility levels with an inotrope or to reduce afterload with an afterload reducing drug.

Afterload primarily refers to the forces that oppose cardiac emptying during systole.[47,48] Strictly speaking it refers to the wall stress of the ventricle.[48] Although many variables influence afterload, a major component is the systemic vascular resistance (SVR). As with contractility, there are no readily available measures of it. The SVR value is a calculated value using several of the directly measured PAC numbers. It makes several assumptions that may not be correct. It assumes that the highest back pressure resisting left ventricular emptying is the right atrial pressure (i.e., the CVP). The calculated SVR value also does not address myocardial wall tension. Despite these potential limitations, the SVR can be useful clinically. As with all the values, it must always be related back to the clinical state. Thus, it is important to remember that a high SVR does *not* automatically mean that drugs to reduce it are indicated. Sometimes these drugs might be contraindicated in patients with a high SVR (e.g., aortic stenosis). The values that are used to calculate the SVR, namely the MAP, CVP and the CO, have already been addressed in the above approach. Thus, whether or not the SVR index adds any additional information is debatable. Since there are several calculations and assumptions, it is preferable to use the directly measured indices to guide therapy.

The values that are characteristic of various pathologic conditions are listed in Table 19.7. Unfortunately, the majority of patients present with a mixed picture thereby complicating the interpretation of the values (e.g., a septic patient can have co-existing myocardial dysfunction). Thus, it is important to use a generalizable approach to the PAC values rather than a pattern recognition approach to the results.

● Summary

Despite numerous potential problems, the various hemodynamic devices can be extremely helpful in managing critically ill patients. A knowledge of their limitations and, hence, of when their use is or is not helpful is crucial for optimal patient care. Regardless of the values obtained, these devices supplement but never replace clinical judgment. Thus, although these devices can be invaluable in caring for sick patients, they must never supersede the need for an attentive and questioning physician.

Table 19.7 – Classic Pulmonary Artery Catheter Findings in Various Conditions

	RA	RV	PA	PCWP	BP	CI	SVR	SvO$_2$
Normal	0–6	25/0–6	25/6–12	6–12	120/80	> 2.5	1500	75%
Hypovolemic Shock	0–2	15–20/0–2	15–20/2–6	2–6	< 90/60	< 2.2	> 1500	< 65%
Cardiogenic Shock	6–10	30–50/8	50/20–30	> 15	< 90/60	< 2.2	> 1500	< 65%
Septic Shock	0–2	20–25/2	25/2–6	2–6	< 90/60	> 2.5	< 1200	70–80%
Pulmonary Embolism*	8–12	50/12	50/12–15	2–8	< 90/60	< 2.2	> 1500	< 65%
Tamponade	12–18	25/12–18	25/12–18	12–18	90/60	< 2.2	> 1500	< 65%

Table 19.7 – The values are for these pathologic disorders. The majority of patients present with several co-existing problems and thus the pattern may not be the same.

*Pulmonary embolism is massive in nature.

Key Points

- Arterial lines are the gold standard for BP.
- Mean arterial pressure is the most accurate and important BP measurement.
- There are many limitations and problems with the use of pulmonary artery catheters.
- Treat the patient not the numbers. The numbers are to be used as a guide to therapy, not to dictate therapy.
- Calculated values should be used with caution.

References

1. Cohn JN: Blood pressure measurement in shock: Mechanism of inaccuracy in auscultatory and palpatory methods. *JAMA* 1967;199:118–22.

2. Ramsey M III: Blood pressure monitoring: Automated oscillometric devices. *J Clin Monit* 1991;7:56–67.

3. van Montfrans GA: Oscillometric blood pressure measurement: Progress and problems. *Blood Press Monit* 2001;6:287–90.

4. Cleland MJ, Pham B, Miller DR: Influence of arrhythmias on accuracy of non-invasive blood pressure monitors. *Can J Anaesth* 1998;45:699–705.

5. Schaer HM: Peripheral nerve injury and automatic blood pressure measurement. *Anesthesiology* 1991;75:381.

6. Slogoff S, Keats AS, Arlund C: On the safety of radial artery cannulation. *Anesthesiology* 1983;59:42–7.

7. Wilkins RG: Radial artery cannulation and ischaemic damage: A review. *Anaesthesia* 1985;40:896–9.

8. Falk PS, Scuderi PE, Sheretz RJ, Motsinger SM: Infected radial artery pseudoaneurysms occurring after percutaneous cannulation. *Chest* 1992;101:490–5.

9. Mangar D, Laborde S, Vu DN: Delayed ischemia of the hand necessitating amputation after radial artery cannulation. *Can J Anaesth* 1993;40:247–50.

10. Band JD, Maki DG: Infections caused by arterial catheters used for hemodynamic monitoring. *Am J Med* 1979;67:735–40.

11. O'Rourke MF, Yaginuma T: Wave reflections and the arterial pulse. *Arch Intern Med* 1984;144:366–71.

12. MacDonald DA: *Blood flow in arteries.* Edward Arnold, London, 1974.

13. Fessler HE, Shade D: Chapter 6. Measurement of vascular pressure. p. 63–80. In Tobin MJ (ed): *Principles and practice of intensive care monitoring.* McGraw-Hill, Toronto, 1998.

14. Packman MI, Rackow EC: Optimum left heart filling pressure during fluid resuscitation of patients with hypovolemic and septic shock. *Crit Care Med* 1983;11:165–9.

15. Weisel RD, Vito L, Dennis RC, et al: Myocardial depression during sepsis. *Am J Surg* 1977;133:512–21.

16. Reuse C, Vincent JL, Pinsky MR: Measurements of right ventricular volumes during fluid challenge. *Chest* 1990;98:1450–4.

17. Alzeer A, Arora S, Ansari Z, et al: Central venous pressure from common iliac vein reflects right atrial pressure. *Can J Anaesth* 1998;45:798–801.

18. Ho KM, Joynt GM, Tan P: A comparison of central venous pressure and common iliac venous pressure in critically ill mechanically ventilated patients. *Crit Care Med* 1998;26:461–4.

19. Sharkey SW: Beyond the wedge: Clinical physiology and the Swan-Ganz catheter. *Am J Med* 1987;83:111–122.

20. Reed CR, Sessler CN, Glauser FL, Phelan BA: Central venous catheter infections: Concepts and controversies. *Intens Care Med* 1995;21:177–83.

21. Merrer J, De Jonghe B, Golliot F, et al: Complications of femoral and subclavian venous catheterization in critically ill patients: A randomized controlled trial. *JAMA* 2001;286:700–7.

22. Knoblanche GE: Respiratory obstruction due to hematoma following internal jugular vein cannulation. *Anesth Intens Care* 1980;8:94.

23. Swan HJC, Ganz W, Forrester JS, et al: Catheterization of the heart in man with use of a flow-directed balloon-tipped catheter. *N Engl J Med* 1970;283:447–51.

24. Gore JM, Goldberg RJ, Spodick DH, et al: A community-wide assessment of the use of pulmonary catheters in patients with acute myocardial: A prospective autopsy study. *Chest* 1985;88:567–72.

25. Zion MM, Balkin J, Rosenmann D, et al: Use of pulmonary artery catheters in patients with acute myocardial infarction. *Chest* 1990;98:1331–5.

26. Connors AF, Speroff T, Dawson NV, et al: The effectiveness of right heart catheterization in the initial care of critically ill patients. *JAMA* 1996;276:889–97.

27. Polanczyk CA, Rohde LE, Goldman L, et al: Right heart catheterization and cardiac complications in patients undergoing noncardiac surgery: An observational study. *JAMA* 2001;286:309–14.

28. Calvin JE, Driedger AA, Sibbald WJ: Does the pulmonary capillary wedge pressure predict left ventricular preload in critically ill patients? *Crit Care Med* 1981;9:437–43.

29. Morris AH, Chapman RH, Gardner RM: Frequency of technical problems encountered in the measurement of pulmonary artery wedge pressure. *Crit Care Med* 1984;12:164–70.

30. Raper B, Sibbald WJ: Misled by the wedge: The Swan-Ganz catheter and left ventricular preload. *Chest* 1986;89:427–34.

31. Pichard AD, Kay R, Smith H, et al: Large v waves in the pulmonary wedge pressure tracing in the absence of mitral regurgitation. *Am J Cardiol* 1982;50:1044–50.

32. Snyder RW 2nd, Glamann DB, Lange RA, et al: Predictive value of prominent pulmonary arterial wedge v waves in assessing the presence and severity of mitral regurgitation. *Am J Cardiol* 1994;73:568–70.

33. Fuchs RM, Heuser RR, Yin FC, Brinker JA: Limitations of pulmonary wedge v waves in diagnosing mitral regurgitation. *Am J Cardiol* 1982;49:849–54.

34. Forrester JS, Diamond G, McHugh TJ, Swan HJC: Filling pressure in the right and left sides of the heart in acute myocardial infarction. *N Engl J Med* 1971;285:190–3.

35. Shah KB, Rao TLK, Laughlin S, El-Etz AA: A review of pulmonary artery catheterization in 6245 patients. *Anesthesiology* 1984;61:271–5.

36. Morris D, Mulvihill D, Lew W, Wilbur W: The risk of developing complete heart block during bedside pulmonary artery catheterization in patients with left bundle branch block. *Arch Intern Med* 1987;147:2005–10.

37. Lipp H, O'Donoghue K, Resnekov L: Intracardiac knotting of a flow-directed balloon catheter. *N Engl J Med* 1971;284:220.

38. Slung HB, Scher KS: Complications of Swan-Ganz catheter. *World J Surg* 1984;8:76–81

39. Cigarroa RG, Lange RA, Williams RH, et al: Underestimation of cardiac output by thermodilution in patients with tricuspid regurgitation. *Am J Med* 1989;86:417–20.

40. Nishikawa T, Dohi S: Errors in the measurement of cardiac output by thermodilution. *Can J Anaesth* 1993;40:142–53

41. Tuman KJ, Carroll GC, Ivankovich AD: Pitfalls in interpretation of pulmonary artery catheter data. *J Cardiothor Anesth* 1989;3:625–41.

42. Gomez CMH, Palazzo MGA: Pulmonary artery catheterization in anaesthesia and intensive care. *Br J Anaesth* 1998;81:945–56.

43. Hjalmarson A: Significance of reduction in heart rate in cardiovascular disease. *Clin Cardiol* 1998;21(suppl 2):II3–7.

44. Sarnoff SJ, Berglund E: Ventricular function: I. Starling's law of the heart studied by means of simultaneous right and left ventricular function curves in the dog. *Circulation* 1954;9:706–18.

45. Suga H, Goto Y, Futaki S, et al: Systolic pressure-volume area (PVA) as the energy of contraction in Starling's law of the heart. *Heart Vessels* 1991;6:65–70.

46. Kumar A, Parrillo JE: Chapter 20. Shock: Classification, pathophysiology, and approach to management. p. 371–420. In Parrillo JE, Bone RC (eds): *Critical care medicine: Principles of diagnosis and management.* Mosby, Toronto, 1995.

47. Sonnenblick EH: Force-velocity relations in mammalian heart muscle. *Am J Physiol* 1962;202:931–9.

48. Pouleur H, Covell JW, Ross J Jr: Effects of alterations in aortic input impedance on the force-velocity-length relationship in the intact canine heart. *Circ Res* 1979;45:126–36.

SEPSIS

Objectives

1. Develop a working knowledge of sepsis.
2. Learn the important principles for managing patients with life-threatening infections.
3. Obtain a working knowledge of antibiotics.
4. Develop an approach to the management of fever.

CHAPTER 20

SEPSIS: NEW AND EMERGING THERAPIES

RICHARD HODDER

A 58-year-old male hospital worker, Mr. Schoque, complains of breathlessness and cough for three days. The presumed diagnosis is a community-acquired pneumonia. His past medical history consisted of hypertension and intermittent atrial fibrillation, for which he was taking coumadin, verapamil and propafenone. There was no known coronary artery disease nor diabetes mellitus. He had quit a 35-pack per year smoking history eight years ago and there was no recent travel nor obvious recent exposure to patients with cough and phlegm.

He had been his usual self until three days ago when he developed mild flu-like symptoms. Despite ibuprofen he got worse and one day ago, began to experience chills, fever, right-sided pleuritic chest discomfort and cough productive of purulent phlegm. He started treating himself with some azithromycin left over from a previous prescription for his wife, but the next day he felt significantly worse with persisting cough and fever, increasing chest pain, profound fatigue and progressive shortness of breath. He went to a walk-in clinic, but because he looked so ill, he was sent to the local emergency department where he was seen promptly and noted to be alternately agitated and drowsy.

Presently he is breathing at 42 bpm, has a heart rate of 120–140 (ECG: atrial fibrillation with no obvious ischemic changes) and blood pressure 100/40 mm Hg and is febrile at 39.1°C. Initial labs: WBC 23.3 $\times 10^9$/L (19.8 neutrophils, 2.8 bands, toxic changes); Hgb 105 g/L; platelets 237 $\times 10^9$/L; INR 3.2; CK 89 U/L; urea 9.3 mmol/L; creatinine 178 μmol/L; pH 7.36, Pco_2 32 mm Hg; Po_2 55 mm Hg and Sao_2 89% on an $Fio_2 = 0.40$ by mask. A chest radiograph confirmed right-sided pneumonia and pleural effusion (Figure 20.1).

What is wrong with Mr. Schoque? What are your immediate management goals for Mr. Schoque?

Sepsis is a syndrome of systemic inflammatory response related to infection. Sepsis is unfortunately a common, often fatal disorder whose incidence is increasing. The mortality rate associated with severe sepsis is around 50% in most studies.[1] The estimated costs related to sepsis are staggering. Fortunately, new strategies and therapeutic options will hopefully improve the management of these challenging patients. The goal of this chapter is to review sepsis and the pathophysiology underlying it. A critical appraisal of the different strategies for sepsis is presented along with an introduction to emerging therapies.

Epidemiology of Sepsis and Septic Shock

Despite advances in our knowledge of disease states and despite technical and pharmacological advances in intensive care, the mortality rate from severe sepsis and septic shock remains unacceptably high in most centres (Figure 20.2).[1,2] In part this reflects our current inability to effectively monitor and modulate dysfunction of the microvasculature, which is the real battleground for sepsis,[3–8] and in part it reflects a certain persisting inability to recognize sepsis in its early stages, in order that definitive and preventive therapies could be started in a more timely fashion than is usually the case. Recently, an international consensus statement on evidence-based management of severe sepsis, the Surviving Sepsis Campaign, has been published[9] and its recommendations will be listed throughout this chapter.

Sepsis Nosology

In 1992, in an attempt to standardize sepsis research and to address the problem of delayed recognition of sepsis-induced systemic inflammation, the concept of *systemic inflammatory response syndrome* (SIRS) was put forward.[10,11] In general terms, SIRS was defined as the presence of two or more of the following features of systemic inflammation: fever or hypothermia, leukocytosis or leukopenia, tachycardia, and tachypnea or a supranormal minute ventilation (Figure 20.3). According to this scheme, *sepsis* is considered to exist when there is SIRS plus a documented infection; *severe sepsis* indicates sepsis plus documented organ failure (see Table 20.1 for

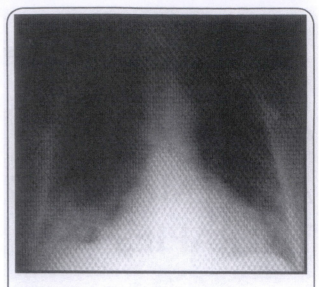

Figure 20.1 – Chest X-ray of Case Presentation

Chest radiograph of 58-year-old man with community-acquired pneumonia and sepsis.

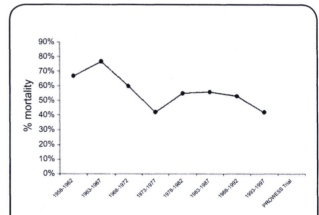

Figure 20.2 – Changing Mortality from Sepsis

Graph demonstrating how mortality rates secondary to sepsis have changed over the last 50 years.

source: Adapted from Friedman et al.[1]

definitions of organ failure);[12] and *septic shock* indicates severe sepsis plus hypotension (or an elevated lactate in the absence of hypotension).

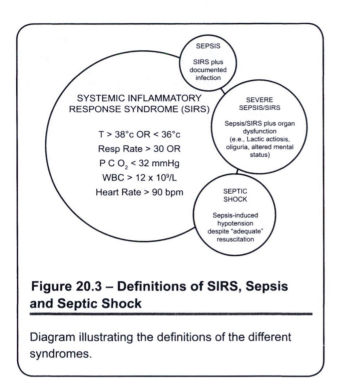

Figure 20.3 – Definitions of SIRS, Sepsis and Septic Shock

Diagram illustrating the definitions of the different syndromes.

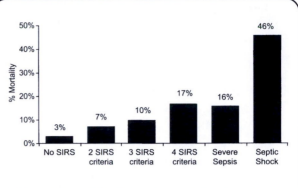

Figure 20.4 – Mortality from SIRS, Sepsis and Septic Shock

Graph demonstrating the mortality rates secondary to the different syndromes related to SIRS.

source: Adapted from Rangel-Frausto et al.[19]

SIRS really describes the clinical manifestations of a pro-inflammatory "cytokine storm," and it is important to realize that this syndrome can also be caused by non-infectious processes such as burns, acute pancreatitis, ischemia, drug reactions and overdose, etc. Because SIRS is not specific for sepsis, and in particular because it does not identify patients at risk for severe sepsis, the SIRS concept has recently been criticized as being too non-specific to be clinically useful.[13–17] For example, some patients with sepsis might not manifest SIRS criteria, due to the existence of co-morbid disease, or due to the influence of treatment such as antipyretics, vasopressors or beta-blockers etc. In addition, SIRS criteria might conceivably even be met by a healthy individual exercising heavily on a hot day. Notwithstanding these valid concerns, the SIRS concept seems to be robust[13] and recently it has been used effectively as an entry criterion in a significant and positive trial on early goal-directed treatment of severe sepsis and septic shock.[18] In addition, there is other evidence supporting the clinical validity of the SIRS concept, in that mortality appears to increase with increasing numbers of SIRS criteria and the progression from SIRS to septic shock (Figure 20.4).[19] Recently, the SIRS concept has again been endorsed to facilitate early recognition of sepsis, by the Surviving Sepsis Campaign.[9]

Because the clinical manifestations of systemic inflammation can be protean, it has been suggested that immunologic or biochemical markers of widespread inflammation may be more consistent than the clinical signs embodied in the SIRS paradigm.[13] By measuring markers such as the cytokine IL-6 or procalcitonin (produced by unknown extrathyroidal tissues in sepsis) or C-reactive protein (produced by the liver in response to tissue damage, etc.), it may be possible to identify the systemic inflammatory response to injury and sepsis earlier and with more precision, although currently no large prospective studies have been done to support this contention. In particular, a role for frequent serum procalcitonin levels has been suggested, as elevated levels of this hormone seem to be quite sensitive and specific for the presence of sepsis.[20] Such an approach would be very useful, however, because traditional markers of infection may be misleading, making early diagnosis of infection often difficult. Early confirmation of sepsis is clearly important, because we know that prompt treatment of sepsis with appropriate antibiotics is associated with lower mortality.[21,22] Early and accurate exclusion of infection would also be very helpful in limiting inappropriate or unnecessary antibiotic therapy that can have harmful consequences, such as antibiotic resistance, C. difficile colitis, and cost. Clearly, additional work needs to be done in this area in order that we may refine our ability to recognize (and thus treat) sepsis in a more timely fashion. Various criteria that may help in the early recognition of sepsis[13] are listed in Table 20.1. Although none of these markers are specific for an inflammatory response to infection, their presence may help reinforce the clinician's impression that "this patient looks septic," and thus has a high risk of death. For example, both hypothermia[23] and an altered mental status[24] have been shown to be associated with an increased risk of death from sepsis. Being aware of these warning signs may therefore facilitate efforts at definitive diagnosis and an earlier aggressive intervention to stop septic shock before it begins. Let's return to the case of Mr. Schoque described earlier.

Clearly, Mr. Schoque is sick and according to the SIRS nosology, he has everything: SIRS (fever, leukocytosis, tachypnea and respiratory alkalosis, tachycardia); probable sepsis as a cause for his SIRS (history of purulent phlegm and a chest radiograph consistent with right-sided pneumonia); severe sepsis based on evidence of organ dysfunction (respiratory failure, renal failure), and shock (despite a BP of 100/60 mm Hg).

The real question is why didn't he come to the Emergency Department sooner? At this stage, even the ED ward clerk acknowledged that he "looked septic" and that aggressive measures were indicated. Your immediate treatment goals for him are several: Although he should be referred to an ICU, your first goal is to begin resuscitation immediately (remember… "time is tissue," "time is life"). Prompt intubation and ventilation should be done because of his breathing distress and respiratory failure. You should also establish IV access for initial fluid resuscitation and prepare for central venous access in the likely event that he will need vasopressor support. Attempts to at least provide better rate control for his chronic atrial fibrillation (likely amiodarone with or without IV magnesium in preference to beta blockers in view of his hypotension) should be made. Attempts to diagnose the etiology of his pneumonia (cultures of blood, urine, endotracheal aspirate or bronchoscopy specimens) along with initiation of empiric IV antibiotics are essential. Finally, you must reassure both Mr. Schoque and his worried family.

Once these goals are underway, what are your specific treatment goals at this stage? Further, how will you monitor your success at achieving these goals?

● Pathophysiology of Sepsis and Septic Shock

Severe sepsis continues to have a high mortality rate as a consequence of three inter-related processes: 1) an activity of host innate immunity and inflammatory response; 2) sepsis-associated coagulopathy; and 3) dysregulation of the microvasculature. The ways in which these processes interact are complex, and there are also marked variations in the host response to infection that remain largely unexplained so that we still do not understand why some septic patients live and why some progress to death. For example, in meningococcal sepsis, young, apparently otherwise healthy individuals can develop fatal multi-organ failure and die within a matter of hours, despite appropriate antibiotic therapy and good supportive care. Indeed, the host response is arguably more important than the site of infection or type of micro-organism in determining the presentation and course of sepsis.

The situation is often complex. Patients with negative blood cultures but presumed infection and patients with serious inflammatory conditions not caused by infection (e.g., pancreatitis) have biochemical and physiologic changes, rates of organ failure and survival rates similar to those of patients with confirmed infection. In cases of confirmed infection, no single pathogen predominates, and over time, the spectrum of causative organisms will vary in response to the selective pressure exerted by antibiotic therapy.

Normally, a potent, complex immunologic/ inflammatory cascade ensures a prompt protective response to microbial invasion in humans, and conversely, a deficient immunologic defense may allow infection to become established. For example, mortality in patients with septic shock who cannot mount a febrile response (approximately 10% of patients) is about double the mortality in febrile septic patients.[23,25] It is important, therefore, that clinicians be aware of the many manifestations of sepsis (Table 20.1), because many septic patients (e.g., elderly, uremic patients) do not become febrile. A brief review of some of the relevant issues follows.

A. Vital Role of Innate Immunity

A person's innate immunity has an important role in the pathogenesis of sepsis. One of the initial

Table 20.1 – Diagnostic Criteria for Sepsis

Infection

A pathological process induced by a micro-organism

Documented or suspected along with some of the following:

General Parameters

- Fever (core temperature > 38.3°C)
- Hypothermia (core temperature < 36°C)
- Heart rate > 90 bpm or > 2 standard deviations (SD) above the normal value for age
- Tachypnea > 30 bpm
- Altered mental status
- Significant edema or positive fluid balance (> 20 ml/kg over 24 hrs)
- Hyperglycemia (plasma glucose > 7.7 mm/L) in the absence of diabetes

Inflammatory Parameters

- Leukocytosis (white blood cell count > 12 × 10⁹/L)
- Leukopenia (white blood cell count < 4 × 10⁹/L)
- Normal white blood cell count with > 10% immature forms
- Plasma C reactive protein > 2 SD above the normal value (an acute phase reactant produced by liver during tissue damage)
- Plasma procalcitonin > 2 SD above the normal value (produced by unknown extrathyroidal tissues in sepsis)

Hemodynamic Parameters

- Arterial hypotension (systolic blood pressure < 90 mm Hg, mean arterial pressure < 70 mm Hg, or a systolic blood pressure decrease > 40 mm Hg in adults or < 2 SD below normal for age)
- Mixed venous oxygen saturation > 70%
- Cardiac index > 3.5 l/min/m²
- Organ dysfunction parameters
- Arterial hypoxemia (PaO_2/FiO_2 < 300)
- Acute oliguria (urine output < 0.5 ml kg/min/h for at least 2 hrs)
- Creatinine increase 44 mol/L
- Coagulation abnormalities (international normalized ratio > 1.5 or activated partial thromboplastin time > 60 sec)
- Ileus (absent bowel sounds)
- Thrombocytopenia (platelet count < 100 × 10⁹/L)
- Hyperbilirubinemia (plasma total bilirubin > 70 mmol/L)

Tissue Perfusion Parameters

- Hyperlactatemia (> 3 mmol/L)
- Decreased capillary refill or mottling

---

responses to a localized bacterial infection, such as pneumonia or an intra-abdominal abscess, is the release of endotoxins or exotoxins. This induces tissue macrophages to generate cytokines, which are pleomorphic immunoregulatory polypeptides that may have both beneficial and harmful effects in sepsis.[26,27] T-helper lymphocytes can secrete both pro-inflammatory and anti-inflammatory cytokines. In particular, CD4 cells with Th-1 properties secrete pro-inflammatory cytokines such as TNF-α, interferon-γ, and certain interleukins (IL) such as IL-1, 2, 8. These cytokines have several effects, including the promotion of leukocyte adhesion to endothelial cells, the release of proteases and arachidonate metabolites, and activation of clotting (see below). Interleukin-8, a neutrophil chemotaxin, may have an especially important role in perpetuating tissue inflammation. On the other hand, CD4 cells with Th-2 properties secrete anti-inflammatory cytokines such as IL-4 and IL-10, which are perhaps counter-regulatory and inhibit the generation of tumor necrosis factor, augment the action of acute-phase reactants and immunoglobulins, and inhibit T-lymphocyte and macrophage function. The factors that determine whether CD4-T cells have Th-1 or Th-2 properties are not clearly known, but may include the type of pathogen, the size of the innoculum and the site of infection. Thus although these early-response cytokines play an important part in host defense by attracting activated neutrophils to the site of infection, the entry of these cytokines and bacterial products into the systemic circulation can also bring about widespread microvascular injury, leading to multi-organ failure. The arachidonic acid metabolites thromboxane A_2 (a vasoconstrictor), prostacyclin (a vasodilator), and prostaglandin E_2 are also involved in the septic response and participate in the generation of the fever, tachycardia, tachypnea, ventilation-perfusion abnormalities and lactic acidosis characteristic of sepsis.

Both an overactive and underactive immune response may be harmful to the host. One theory has been that severe sepsis represents an uncontrolled inflammatory response or a runaway "cytokine storm" and that this excessive or poorly regulated inflammatory response may harm the host through a maladaptive release of endogenously generated inflammatory compounds.[26] Lewis Thomas[28] popularized this notion when he wrote: "The micro-organisms that seem to have it in for us turn out to be rather more like bystanders. It is our response to their presence that makes the disease. Our (endogenous) arsenals for fighting off bacteria are so powerful that we are more in danger from them than the invaders." That this may in part be true is evidenced by several studies showing an association between circulating levels of inflammatory cytokines such as tumor necrosis factor alpha (TNF-α) and interleukin-6 and increased mortality from sepsis.[29,30] This philosophy formed the basis for numerous clinical trials aimed at blocking various mediators of the inflammatory cascade, including corticosteroids,[31]

antiendotoxin antibodies,[32,33] tumor necrosis factor (TNF) antagonists[34,35] and other agents such as ibuprofen.[36] The situation is complex, however, and all of these trials of anti-inflammatory mediators were unable to demonstrate a reduction in mortality from severe sepsis and septic shock. In part, this may be due to the fact that the central role of microvascular coagulation in the pathogenesis of septic shock was not addressed in these trials and it may also reflect the fact that, as mentioned, cytokines have multiple and sometimes conflicting properties, depending on the time course of sepsis and other factors.

If an exaggerated inflammatory response to infection can be harmful, so to can the lack of an acute-phase response be associated with a high mortality rate and may reflect an abnormal, immunosuppressive phase of sepsis.[37] This theory holds that much of the morbidity and mortality of severe sepsis may be related to immunosuppression from a failure of the immune system.[38,39] Proponents of this view maintain that the body's normal stress response is activation of anti-inflammatory mechanisms and that, outside of affected tissues, these systemic anti-inflammatory responses predominate. They postulate that because immune cells and cytokines can have both pathogenic and protective roles, therapies designed to block these mediators may worsen outcome. Some patients with sepsis do seem to have features consistent with immunosuppression, including a loss of delayed hypersensitivity, an inability to clear infection, a reduced ability to secrete TNF-α and IL-1 and a predisposition to nosocomial infections compared to controls.[26] Therefore, in some cases, or at certain times, immune stimulant therapy might be helpful. In one trial for example, survival was increased and the adverse sequelae of sepsis-associated immunosuppression were reversed with the administration of interferon-γ in patients with sepsis, perhaps secondary to restoration of macrophage TNF-α production.[40]

Because the role of the inflammatory cascade in the response to infection may be both helpful and harmful, it is not surprising that mediator antagonist trials have produced conflicting results. On the one hand for example, a TNF antagonist was associated with increased mortality from sepsis,[35] while in another trial, subgroup analysis revealed patients who had improved survival when treated with a TNF anagonist.[41] Similarly, although use of the cyclooxygenase inhibitor ibuprofen to suppress production of inflammatory prostanoids reduces temperature, heart rate, minute ventilation and lactic acidosis, it has not been shown to result in a lower mortality rate,[36] except perhaps in those few septic patients who are hypothermic.[23]

Even fighting microbes is more complex than simply prescribing antibiotics. Indeed, the current approach of prescribing high dose, broad spectrum antibiotics to fight sepsis may actually also do harm by suppressing normal flora remote from the infected site. Modern antibiotics are so successful that their use has provoked adaptive changes by the pathogens themselves. In this regard, understanding how micro-organisms defend themselves is leading to new insights in how sepsis may be treated in the future.[42,43]

Cells of the innate immune system recognize micro-organisms and initiate responses through pattern recognition receptors on the host–pathogen interface called "toll-like receptors" (TLRs). TLR polymorphisms have been identified in humans and may make certain persons more susceptible to infection and therefore death from sepsis. For example, expression of TLR4 seems to confer tolerance to endotoxin, so that failure of this mechanism in some individuals could lead to a devastating overaction of inflammatory cascades. Both gut endothelial cells and hepatocytes can express TLRs, and both are key sites in the early events of septic shock. How this information will affect future therapy is not clear. For example, the use of soluble TLRs specific for particular organisms might be helpful, if they can be given early enough. Blocking certain TLR activity might help, on the one hand, but could also neutralize beneficial components of the host response and lead to overwhelming sepsis from other organisms. Knowledge about TLRs may also lead to better ways of administering antibiotics. For example, indiscriminant use of antibiotics can change the type of bacterial lipid A to which the host is exposed. This could be important because some types of lipid A are antagonist to TLR4 (a good thing), whereas others are agonist for TLR4 (a bad thing).

Apoptotic cell death may trigger sepsis-induced anergy. Although the conventional belief was that cells die by necrosis, recent work has shown that cells can die by apoptosis—genetically programmed cell death. In apoptosis, cells "commit suicide" by the activation of proteases that disassemble the cell. Large numbers of lymphocytes and gastrointestinal epithelial cells die by apoptosis during sepsis.

Apoptotic cells induce anergy, or anti-inflammatory cytokines that impair the response to pathogens, whereas necrotic cells cause immune stimulation and enhance antimicrobial defenses. Autopsy studies in persons who have died of sepsis have disclosed a profound, progressive, apoptosis-induced loss of cells of the adaptive immune system.[44] The potential importance of abnormal apoptotic-induced loss of immune cells is seen from animal studies showing improved survival when lymphocyte apoptosis is prevented.[26] It is interesting to note that a potential mechanism of lymphocyte apoptosis may be stress-induced endogenous release of glucocorticoids, which might provide an argument against the role of low dose glucocorticoid therapy in sepsis (see below).

Thus it appears that the response to sepsis is both complex and dynamic and that optimal therapy may also require a temporal component, so that the most appropriate therapy will be determined by the particular phase of the septic response (Figure 20.5). For example, before sepsis develops, augmentation of the immune response might offer the best opportunity for prevention. Once infection is established, very brief administration of highly organism-specific antibiotics to kill micro-organisms and limit damage to the body's normal flora would be appropriate. If the SIRS response is exaggerated, then anti-inflammatory and anticoagulant therapies might help rescue and preserve function of the microvasculature. On the other hand, if the host immune response is impaired, then brief administration of agents that could inhibit proximal mediators of inflammation might help block progression to multiple organ failure. Other novel aspects of sepsis therapy will depend upon increasing knowledge of the complex interactions of inflammatory and coagulation cascades, the

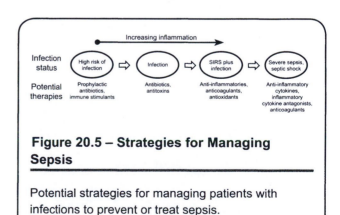

Figure 20.5 – Strategies for Managing Sepsis

Potential strategies for managing patients with infections to prevent or treat sepsis.

pathophysiology of the microcirculation in sepsis and even upon individual genetic predispositions to severe sepsis and response to specific therapies.

B. Relationship of Inflammation and Coagulation in Sepsis

The coagulation cascade (Figure 20.6) has emerged as an important player in the response to sepsis, particularly in the microvasculature.[45] Indeed, simultaneous activation of the inflammatory response and the coagulation cascade following tissue injury is a phylogenetically ancient survival strategy. For example, the horseshoe crab, which has remained relatively unchanged over the past 250 million years, has evolved a rapid response to injury designed to repair and protect its exoskeleton that involves activation of its sole circulating blood element, the amebocyte. The amebocyte simultaneously performs the dual functions of both platelets (to promote coagulation to mechanically plug up damage to the exoskeleton) and phagocytic cells (to phagocytose invading micro-organisms). These basic co-operative interactions between clotting and inflammation are well preserved in vertebrates today and have evolved into the platelets, neutrophils, macrophages and other antigen-presenting cells active in humans.

Abnormal, uncontrolled coagulation can, however, be harmful and several procoagulant mechanisms have been associated with decreased survival among patients with sepsis.[46] It appears that sepsis mortality is higher in patients who have elevated levels of plasminogen activator inhibitor type 1(PAI-1), an inhibitor of normal fibrinolysis, as well as decreased levels of the natural circulating anticoagulants antithrombin III and protein C.[47] Endotoxins and early-response cytokines generate an environment that favours coagulation by means of a number of mechanisms, including activation of the extrinsic coagulation pathway through the expression of tissue factor (Figure 20.7). There are also important molecular links between the procoagulant and inflammatory mechanisms in the pathogenesis of organ failure in patients with sepsis. Furthermore, some components of the coagulation system have the capacity to be inflammatory. For example, the generation of thrombin can activate receptors on platelets and the vascular endothelium, which can lead to inflammation and tissue injury. Thus, there are several synergistic pathways by which inflammatory and procoagulant mechanisms can initiate and perpetuate organ injury in patients with sepsis.

The above observations form the basis for the theory that activated protein C might be an effective therapy in patients with sepsis (Figure 20.8). First, most patients with severe sepsis have diminished levels of activated protein C, in part because the inflammatory cytokines generated in sepsis down-regulate thrombomodulin and the endothelial-cell protein C receptor, components of the coagulation

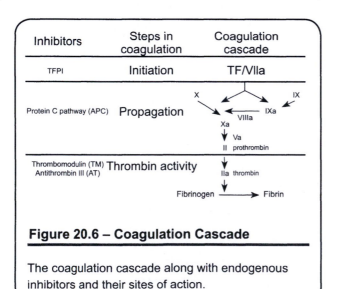

Figure 20.6 – Coagulation Cascade

The coagulation cascade along with endogenous inhibitors and their sites of action.

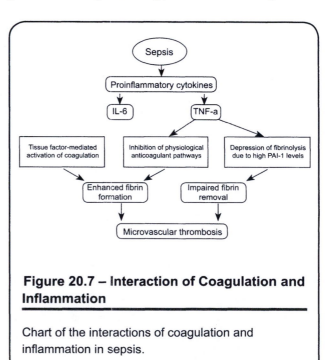

Figure 20.7 – Interaction of Coagulation and Inflammation

Chart of the interactions of coagulation and inflammation in sepsis.

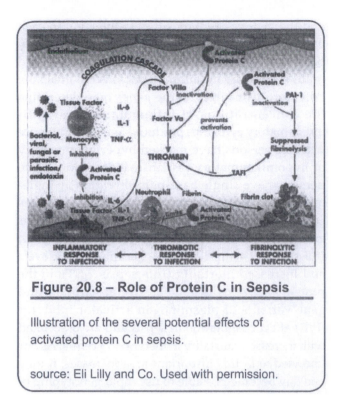

Figure 20.8 – Role of Protein C in Sepsis

Illustration of the several potential effects of activated protein C in sepsis.

source: Eli Lilly and Co. Used with permission.

system that are necessary for the conversion of inactive protein C to activated protein C. Second, activated protein C inhibits activated factors V and VIII, thereby decreasing the formation of thrombin. Third, activated protein C stimulates fibrinolysis by reducing the concentration of plasminogen activator inhibitor type 1. Fourth, activated protein C reduces interactions between neutrophils and endothelial cells and decreases tissue ischemia, in part by reducing the endothelial expression of the adhesion molecule E-selectin. Because there is an intimate relationship between the inflammatory cascades and the coagulation cascades, one might postulate that one requirement for an effective sepsis therapy would be to have both anti-inflammatory and anticoagulant properties.[45] Activated protein C is such a therapy, as in vitro data indicate that APC exerts a direct anti-inflammatory effect by inhibiting pro-inflammatory cytokine production, including TNF-α, from monocytes and limiting rolling of monocytes and neutrophils on the injured endothelium via selectins. The recent observation that mortality from severe sepsis and septic shock was reduced in response to therapy with recombinant human activated protein C (APC) confirms this hypothesis.[48,49] In this trial, APC use was associated with a reduction in plasma D-dimer levels, evidence that the procoagulant effects

of sepsis were reduced by this therapy. There was also a reduction in the circulating levels of IL-6, indicating that treatment attenuated the inflammatory cascade as well.

C. Microvasculature Dysfunction in Sepsis

The microcirculation is a complex and integrated system that supplies and distributes oxygen throughout the tissues.[3,50] Red blood cells (RBCs) not only deliver oxygen but also sense local oxygen gradients and, within the microcirculation, are distributed both passively, by rheologic factors including RBC deformability and vessel geometry, and actively, by arteriolar tone. The microcirculation is regulated by many neuroendocrine and paracrine pathways that integrate in a complex fashion to preserve microcirculatory flow. Nitric oxide is an important modulator of this process, by regulating arteriolar tone, RBC deformability, monocyte and platelet adhesion to endothelial cells and blood volume. Sepsis results in abnormal microvascular oxygen transport, as capillary blood flow stops in some areas, but the microvasculature fails to compensate (Figure 20.9). The result is a mismatch of oxygen delivery and demand, which affects the critical oxygen delivery and oxygen extraction ratio. During sepsis, nitric oxide is overproduced in an attempt to protect microvascular blood flow, but this also contributes to the systemic hypotension of sepsis. On the other hand, attempts to maintain

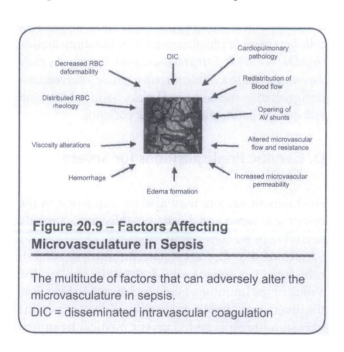

Figure 20.9 – Factors Affecting Microvasculature in Sepsis

The multitude of factors that can adversely alter the microvasculature in sepsis.
DIC = disseminated intravascular coagulation

systemic blood pressure in sepsis are associated with inadequate perfusion of the microcirculation in sepsis. Therapy for septic shock must ultimately seek to improve tissue perfusion through the restoration of an evenly distributed microcirculation. Current therapy for septic shock is mainly "macroscopic" and aimed at optimization of cardiac function and arterial hemoglobin saturation. Therapy with activated protein C likely improves microcirculatory flow through its anti-inflammatory and anticoagulant properties. Future trends in therapy may emphasize a greater role for vasodilators, including nitric oxide, in order to target improved microcirculatory flow. The use of dobutamine in the algorithm of a recent successful trial of early goal-directed therapy in septic shock is of interest in this regard.[18] Therapy targeted to the microcirculation will require some means to monitor this circulation more accurately (e.g., using sublingual microcirculation as an index), and at least one clinical index has been proposed for this purpose.[50]

Future therapy may also have to take into account mitochondrial dysfunction in sepsis: In addition to dysfunction of the microvasculature in sepsis, there is evidence of a cellular block to oxygen consumption by certain tissues in response to severe infection. This has been termed "cytopathic hypoxia"[6] and is not felt to be due to a problem with oxygen delivery on the basis of diminished microvascular perfusion, but rather to an acquired intrinsic defect in cellular respiration. This defect may have several causes, including inhibition of cytochromes by nitric oxide, inhibition of mitochondrial respiratory complexes and depletion of cellular stores of nicotinamide adenine dinucleotide (NAD+/NADH). Future therapies for sepsis may therefore need to include pharmacologic interventions designed to preserve normal mitochondrial function and energy production in septic patients.

D. Genetic Predispositions for Severe Sepsis

Host genetic factors may also be important in the response to sepsis and death from infection is strongly heritable in human populations.[51,52] Thus, genetic variations that disrupt innate immune sensing of infectious organisms could possibly explain the ability of the immune system to respond to infection, the diversity of the clinical presentation of sepsis, the variation in response to current medical treatment and the genetic predisposition to infection in each individual. Such genetic variations may help identify patients at high risk for the development of sepsis and multi-system organ failure in response to infection. Polymorphisms in cytokine genes may determine the concentrations of inflammatory and anti-inflammatory cytokines produced and may influence whether persons have marked hyperinflammatory or hypoinflammatory responses to infection. Some persons have single base-pair alterations (single-nucleotide polymorphisms or SNPs) in genes controlling the host response to microbes. For example, an SNP in the TNF-β gene (lymphotoxin) is associated with higher circulating TNF-α levels and increased mortality from sepsis. SNPs in the protein C gene reduce its rate of transcription, and gene variants of plasminogen activator inhibitor (PAI) affect coagulation in sepsis and are associated with increased mortality in meningococcemia. As our knowledge in this important area increases, it may one day become possible to use rapid genotyping of patients in order to help prioritize various available therapies and so individualize sepsis management.

Let's return to the case of the unfortunate Mr. Schoque described earlier.

After a wait of two hours in the ED, while an ICU bed was made available for him, Mr. Schoque was transferred to ICU where, because of impending respiratory collapse, he was quickly intubated and a central venous catheter and arterial line were placed. On arrival in the ICU his BP was 90 systolic and upon intubation it fell quickly to 70 mm Hg systolic, requiring a 1 L saline bolus plus an infusion of norepinephrine at 15 mcg/min to achieve a mean arterial pressure (MAP) of 55 mm Hg. STAT gram stain of the endotracheal aspirate demonstrated abundant polymorphs and abundant gram-positive diplococci (which would later turn out to be penicillin resistant). He was given loading doses of cefotaxime and azithromycin (later changed to cefotaxime plus levofloxacin).

Despite another litre of pentaspan and 1.5 litres of normal saline over the next two hours, CVP was 16 mm Hg and MAP remained at 55 mm Hg while receiving infusions of norepinephrine at 20 mcg/min and phenylephrine at 100 mcg/min with a heart rate of 65–80 bpm, still atrial fibrillation. Temperature was 38.6°C, his fingers and toes looked mottled and his urine output dropped to 5 ml/hour. Lab data at this stage revealed: WBC = 3.4 × 10⁹/L (an ominous fall), Hb 85 g/L; platelets 95 × 10⁹/L; INR 3.8; creatinine 208 μmol/L; BS = 7.2 mmol/L; lactate = 6 *mmol/L; and an arterial blood gas with a pH 7.24, P_{CO_2} 40 mm Hg; P_{O_2} 75 mm Hg; Sa_{O_2} 91% on an Fi_{O_2} = 0.80 and PEEP = 12 cm H_2O. A pulmonary artery catheter was placed revealing the following: CI = 10.2 ml/min/m²; PAP = 35/15 mm Hg; PAOP = 12 mm Hg; mixed venous Sv_{O_2}% = 64%.*

What is his risk of dying? At this point would you (and Mr. Schoque) be content with only continued aggressive supportive care, or would you want to initiate any additional therapies?

● Therapy of Sepsis and Septic Shock

The apparent decline in the mortality rate in some subgroups of patients with severe sepsis, despite growing microbial resistance and in the absence of specific therapy (Figure 20.2), suggests that improved basic supportive measures are in fact beneficial (nevertheless, our Mr. Schoque has an expected mortality risk of about 35% based on data from the control arm of the APC trial).[48] Timely provision of enteral nutrition prevention of nosocomial infections, stress ulcers, skin breakdown and deep venous thrombosis and judicious use of sedation perhaps play a more important part in the outcome than was once appreciated. The Surviving Sepsis Campaign[9] mentioned earlier, has provided an evidence-based summary of the current state of the art of sepsis management. Although many of the recommendations carry only a consensus opinion level of evidence, these guidelines are useful and if they can be effectively implemented in a widespread fashion, may lead to further improvements in the mortality from severe sepsis and septic shock. (Levels of evidence used: Grade A – supported by at least 2 large randomized controlled trials (RCT) with clear results; Grade B – supported by 1 large RCT with clear results; Grade C – supported by small RCTs with uncertain results; Grade D – supported by at least 1 non-randomized, contemporaneous trial; Grade E – supported by non-randomized, historical controls, case series, uncontrolled trials or expert opinion). The steering committee for this project plans a targeted implementation strategy in certain centres that will also include an attempt at evaluation/validation of these concepts. Selected key recommendations from this consensus statement will be briefly discussed below.

A. Early Recognition of Sepsis

Having a so-called "high index of suspicion" for the presence of severe sepsis is important, because early and aggressive resuscitation can save lives.[18] In the early goal-directed trial of Rivers et al.,[18] an important entry criterion was the presence of SIRS in patients presenting to the Emergency Department. Table 20.1 lists other criteria that are useful in making an earlier diagnosis of severe sepsis (Recommendation 20.1).

Recommendation 20.1 – Early Recognition of Sepsis

The presence of SIRS in a compatible clinical setting is an early warning sign that sepsis may likely be present and should not be ignored. An elevated serum lactate identifies tissue hypoperfusion, even in patients who are not hypotensive.
Grade B

B. Initial Resuscitation

The first step in management of the patient with septic shock is to assess and support the airway, respiration and perfusion. Supplemental oxygen should be supplied to all patients with sepsis, and oxygenation monitored using continuous pulse oximetry. Intubation may be required for airway protection because encephalopathy and a depressed level of consciousness may complicate sepsis. The next priority is to assist ventilation and augment oxygenation. Respiratory failure frequently complicates sepsis due to the development of acute respiratory distress syndrome (ARDS). Subsequently, measures are taken to restore the blood pressure to levels that perfuse core organs. Circulatory failure is present by definition in patients with septic shock. Early and complete resuscitation of the circulation is a prerequisite for preventing or limiting multiple organ dysfunction. Note that the blood pressure cuff may be unreliable in hypotensive patients. Thus, an arterial catheter may be inserted if blood pressure is labile or if restoration of arterial perfusion pressures is expected to be a protracted process. However, vital moments should not be expended in attempts to insert an arterial line to the exclusion of the prompt management of shock. Regardless of the method used to measure blood pressure, numeric evidence of hypotension is corroborated with clinical evidence of organ hypoperfusion in order to assess the severity of shock and its response to treatment. Signs of sepsis and organ failure are listed in Table 20.1. Although lactate measurement is useful for diagnosis, it lacks precision as a measure of tissue metabolic status and so is not recommended as a parameter to follow the progress of sepsis or response to therapy. The consensus panel judged central venous and mixed venous oxygen saturation to be equivalent and a better parameter to follow. Either intermittent or continuous measurements of oxygen saturation were judged to be acceptable. In mechanically ventilated patients, a higher target central venous pressure of 12–15 mm Hg is recommended to account for the increased intrathoracic pressure.

Since sepsis results in hypermetabolism, tissue O_2 needs are typically elevated. Thus, it has been suggested that augmenting oxygen delivery (Do_2) into the supernormal range should theoretically reverse tissue hypoxia and improve patient outcomes. However, this hypothesis has not been consistently supported by available clinical trials, probably because these trials were instituted in septic patients who where already in the ICU and thus relatively late in the course of their sepsis and already suffering from a runaway cytokine storm.[53–55]

Until recently, the clinical utility of early, aggressive Do_2 optimization had not been systematically tested. Now, however, in a randomized, controlled trial of 263 patients comparing treatment targeted at maintaining a central venous oxygen saturation ($ScvO_2$%) > 70% versus standard supportive care, Rivers and colleagues demonstrated that early, goal-directed therapy can result in reduced mortality from severe sepsis and septic shock.[18] Treatment was begun early in the Emergency Department where patients with severe sepsis or septic shock were identified and a step-wise algorithm combining fluid resuscitation, vasopressors, red cell transfusion and inotropes was followed (Figure 20.10). Treatment goals for patients in the control group included mean arterial pressure (MAP) > 65 mm Hg, central venous pressure (CVP) > 8 mm Hg and urine output > 0.5 ml/kg per hour. Therapy directed toward these goals for the initial six-hour period of the resuscitation was able to reduce 28-day mortality rate by 16% (46.5% mortality in the standard care group versus 30.5% mortality in the early goal-directed group). One of the key goals of this trial was to achieve resuscitation as defined above within the

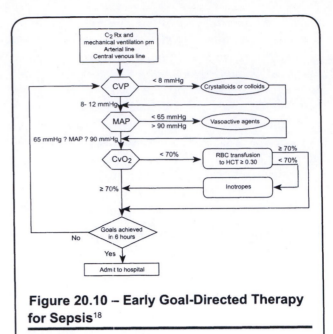

Figure 20.10 – Early Goal-Directed Therapy for Sepsis[18]

Suggested algorithm for the use of goal-directed therapy in sepsis and septic shock.

source: Adapted from Rivers et al.[18]

first six hours of therapy. The standard group on the other hand, did not have this time demand placed upon them, analogous to the early failed trials of pushing oxygen delivery mentioned above. Other novel elements of this resuscitation scheme included a liberal RBC transfusion strategy (aiming for a hematocrit > 0.30) and the use of inotropes in order to achieve a $ScvO_2$% > 70%. Transfusion of RBCs in this setting does not conflict with the current practice of restricted transfusion in critically ill patients, as the TRICC trial[56] dealt with sick but stable patients, whereas the septic patients being resuscitated in the Rivers trial were quite unstable. As noted earlier, it is speculative, but intriguing, that an inotrope with vasodilator properties such as dobutamine may have had a special effect on the microcirculatory flow.

Vasopressors are second line agents in the treatment of severe sepsis and septic shock. Intravenous fluids are preferred so long as they increase cardiac output and/or blood pressure without seriously impairing gas exchange. However, vasopressors are useful in patients who remain hypotensive despite adequate fluid resuscitation or who develop cardiogenic pulmonary edema. A variety of agents with different profiles of peripheral and cardiac actions are available. Phenylephrine, a pure alpha-adrenergic agonist, may be particularly useful when tachycardia or arrhythmias preclude the use of agents with beta-adrenergic activity (e.g., acute coronary ischemia). In general, agents that augment peripheral vascular resistance, such as dopamine, norepinephrine, epinephrine or phenylephrine, are required for initial stabilization. However, large trials comparing outcomes with different vasopressors have not been performed, and therefore there is no definitive evidence of the superiority of one vasopressor over another. Limited experience with vasopressin (an antidiuretic hormone) suggests that infusion of this agent at 0.01–0.04 U/min may be useful in vasodilatory septic shock, perhaps because about one third of patients with septic shock demonstrate a relative vasopressin deficiency, albeit for unknown reasons.[57–59] Although commonly used in septic shock, this is still considered an experimental therapy, which is currently being investigated in a multicentre trial by the Canadian Critical Care Trials Group (Recommendation 20.2).

Recommendation 20.2 – Initial Resuscitation

The resuscitation of a patient in severe sepsis or sepsis induced tissue hypoperfusion (hypotension or lactic acidosis) should begin as soon as the syndrome is recognized and should not be delayed pending ICU admission. During the first six hours of resuscitation, the goals of initial resuscitation of sepsis induced hypoperfusion should include all of the following as one part of a treatment protocol:

1. Central venous pressure: 8–12 mm Hg
2. Mean arterial pressure = 65 mm Hg
3. Urine output = 0.5 ml/kg/hr
4. Central venous (superior vena cava) or mixed venous oxygen saturation = 70%

Grade B

C. Composition of Resuscitation Fluids

Hypotension in sepsis results from a loss of plasma volume into the interstitial space, decreases in vascular tone, and myocardial depression (which may limit an appropriate compensatory increase in the cardiac output). Intravenous fluids, packed red blood cells and vasoactive agents are often required, depending upon the patient's intravascular volume and cardiac status and the severity of shock.

Rapid, large volume infusions of intravenous fluids are usually indicated as initial therapy in patients with septic shock, unless there is coexisting clinical or radiographic evidence of congestive heart failure. Relative intravascular hypovolemia is usual in septic shock and may be severe; some patients require 10 litres of crystalloid within the first 24 hours. Fluid therapy should be administered in well-defined, rapidly infused boluses, rather than by high hourly infusion rates alone. Volume status, tissue perfusion, blood pressure, and the presence or absence of pulmonary edema must be assessed before and after each bolus. Intravenous fluid challenges can be repeated until blood pressure, tissue perfusion and oxygen delivery are acceptable, pulmonary edema ensues or the pulmonary capillary wedge pressure exceeds 18–20 mm Hg. Careful monitoring is essential in this approach because patients with sepsis can develop pulmonary edema at wedge pressures below 18 mm Hg (non-cardiac pulmonary edema).

Although prospective studies of choice-of-fluid resuscitation in patients with septic shock only are lacking, meta-analysis of clinical studies comparing crystalloid and colloid resuscitation in general and surgical patient populations indicate no clinical outcome difference between colloids and crystalloids and would appear to be generalizable to sepsis populations.[60,61] A recent large scale trial comparing resuscitation with albumin versus crystalloids also found no difference in all-cause, 28-day mortality in critically ill patients.[62] As the volume of distribution is much larger for crystalloids than for colloids, resuscitation with crystalloids requires more fluid to achieve the same end points and results in more edema. For similar reasons, some have advocated including hypertonic saline or hetastarches as part of the resuscitation fluid recipe.[63,64] Additional putative advantages of hypertonic saline resuscitation include less capillary edema and improved RBC rheology due to hemodilution, all of which could enhance tissue oxygen delivery. Large RCTs are needed to test these hypotheses (Recommendation 20.3).

Recommendation 20.3 – Composition of Resuscitation Fluids

Fluid resuscitation may consist of natural or artificial colloids or crystalloids. There is no evidence based support for one type of fluid over another.
Grade C

D. Diagnosing the Etiology

Obtaining blood cultures peripherally and through a vascular access device is an important strategy. If the same organism is recovered from both cultures, the likelihood that the organism is causing the severe sepsis is increased. In addition, if the culture drawn through the vascular access device is positive much earlier than the peripheral blood culture (i.e., > 2 hours earlier), it may offer support for the idea that the vascular access device is the source of the infection. Diagnostic studies should be performed promptly to determine the source of the infection and the causative organism. Imaging studies and sampling of likely sources of infection should be performed when indicated. Similarly, diagnostic studies may identify a source of infection that must be drained to maximize the likelihood of a satisfactory response to therapy. However, some patients may be too unstable to warrant certain invasive procedures or transport outside of the ICU. Bedside studies, such as ultrasound, may be useful in these circumstances (Recommendation 20.4).

Recommendation 20.4 – Making an Etiologic Diagnosis of Sepsis

Appropriate cultures should always be obtained before antimicrobial therapy is initiated. To optimize identification of causative organisms, at least two blood cultures should be obtained with at least one drawn percutaneously and one drawn through each vascular access device, unless the device was recently (< 48 hrs) inserted. Cultures of other sites such as urine, cerebrospinal fluid, wounds, respiratory secretions or other body fluids should be obtained before antibiotic therapy is initiated as the clinical situation dictates.
Grade D

E. Antibiotic Therapy

There is evidence that administering appropriate antibiotic therapy within the first 24 hours of the diagnosis of sepsis can lower mortality.[22] Therefore, prompt infusion of antimicrobial agents is a logical strategy. Establishing a supply of premixed antibiotics in an emergency department or critical care unit for such urgent situations is an appropriate strategy for enhancing the likelihood that antimicrobial agents will be infused promptly, although this may be too costly to be practical. Initial empirical anti-infective therapy should include one or more drugs that have activity against the likely pathogens (bacterial or fungal) and that penetrate into the presumed source of sepsis. The choice of drugs should be guided by the susceptibility patterns of micro-organisms in the community and in the hospital (Recommendation 20.5).

Recommendation 20.5 – Antibiotic Therapy

Intravenous antibiotic therapy should be started within the first hour of recognition of severe sepsis, after appropriate cultures have been obtained.
Grade E

F. Recombinant Human Activated Protein C

As discussed above, a number of coagulation abnormalities have been noted in septic shock, and it is logical that drugs with anti-inflammatory and anticoagulant properties might be useful therapeutic agents to prevent and treat severe sepsis. This has been confirmed in a large multicentre trial of recombinant human activated protein C (drotrecogin alfa) for patients with known or suspected severe infection and evidence of shock.[48] This trial randomly assigned 1690 patients to receive a 96-hour infusion of drotrecogin alfa or placebo, beginning within 24 hours of presentation. The 28-day mortality rate was significantly lower in the drotrecogin-treated group (24.7% versus 30.8%). Overall risk of bleeding was low and there were no significant differences in bleeding complications between groups. Based upon post hoc analysis of the study data, treatment was of greater benefit in the most acutely ill patients, as identified by an APACHE II score > 25. An analysis of secondary end points suggested that the incidence of multiple organ dysfunction was lower in patients treated with drotrecogin alfa and that therapy was associated with more rapid recovery of cardiac and pulmonary function. This agent (Xigris™) is now commercially available and in Canada, at least, is being used under strict guidelines. The suggested dosing regimen is 24 mcg/kg per hour for 96 hours, with an estimated cost in Canada in excess of CA$10 000 per course of therapy, depending upon the patient's weight. The role of drotrecogin alfa in the treatment of adults with less severe disease has not been determined (Recommendation 20.6).

> ### Recommendation 20.6 – Recombinant Human Activated Protein C (APC)
>
> APC is recommended for patients at high risk of death (Acute Physiology and Chronic Health Evaluation (APACHE) II = 25; sepsis induced multiple organ failure; septic shock; or sepsis induced acute respiratory distress syndrome [ARDS]) and with no absolute contraindication related to bleeding risk or relative contraindication that outweighs the potential benefit of APC.
> **Grade B**

G. Low-Dose Corticosteroids

As discussed above, because the pathogenesis of sepsis involves an intense and potentially deleterious host inflammatory response, corticosteroids have been investigated as therapeutic agents in sepsis. Early trials of corticosteroid therapy were largely negative and limited by the lack of a standard definition of either sepsis or septic shock, variable dosing regimens, heterogeneous patient populations and late introduction of therapy.[31] A 1995 meta-analysis identified 10 prospective, randomized, controlled trials of various corticosteroid regimens in the treatment of sepsis and/or septic shock, only one of which demonstrated positive findings.[65] The majority of these negative studies used high-dose steroids (dexamethasone 1–6 mg/kg or methylprednisolone 30 mg/kg) for short periods of time, usually one day. In contrast, later studies have employed physiologic stress dose corticosteroids (hydrocortisone 100 mg tid) given for longer periods of time. These regimens were associated with a shorter duration of vasopressor dependence but no improvement in mortality. Based on these observations, a controlled trial of 300 adults who met standard criteria for septic shock randomly assigned patients to treatment with hydrocortisone (50 mg iv q6h) and fludrocortisone (50 mcg po od) or placebo for seven days.[66] In an attempt to clarify the prognostic value of endogenous adrenocortical function, a high-dose cosyntropin test (250 mcg) was administered to all patients at the time of enrollment. Most patients (229 of 300, 76%) had relative adrenal insufficiency, defined as

an increase in plasma total cortisol of ≤ 9 mcg/dL following cosyntropin challenge. The benefits of corticosteroid supplementation were limited to these patients, referred to as non-responders. Among the 229 non-responders, corticosteroid therapy was associated with a significantly lower 28-day mortality (53% versus 63%). Non-responders who received corticosteroids were also significantly more likely to have vasopressors withdrawn within 28 days than were untreated non-responders (57% versus 40%). Therapy was not associated with an increased incidence of adverse events.

On the basis of these findings, it is reasonable to consider an evaluation of adrenal function in conjunction with corticosteroid supplementation in patients with vasopressor-dependent septic shock that persists despite adequate fluid repletion. However, the definition of adrenal insufficiency used in this trial is not standard, and total rather than free plasma cortisol was measured. Complications including hyperglycemia may result from the use of corticosteroids in this setting. Corticosteroids should be discontinued in patients with an increase in plasma cortisol of > 9 mcg/dL following cosyntropin challenge. If cosyntropin challenge is not practical, empiric use of low dose corticosteroids may be tried, but should be stopped after 7 days if no apparent clinical benefit is seen (persisting vasopressor-dependent shock) (Recommendation 20.7).

> ### Recommendation 20.7 – Low Dose Corticosteroids for Vasopressor Dependent Septic Shock
>
> Intravenous corticosteroids (hydrocortisone 200–300 mg/day for seven days in three or four divided doses or by continuous infusion) are recommended in patients with septic shock who, despite adequate fluid replacement, require vasopressor therapy to maintain adequate blood pressure.
> **Grade C**

H. Tight Control of Blood Glucose

Hyperglycemia, caused by insulin resistance in the liver and muscle, is a common finding in ICU patients, including septic patients. Until recently, this has been considered an adaptive response, providing glucose for the brain, red cells and wound healing, and generally has only been treated when blood glucose increased to > 12 mmol/L. However, there are several potentially harmful consequences of hyperglycemia, including impaired neutrophil and macrophage activity, a procoagulant effect, altered cardiovascular tone and worsening of neuronal damage. These observations suggest that hyperglycemia may not always be adaptive and that it should be treated to avoid the onset of specific complications.

The hypothesis that hyperglycemia (> 6.1 mmol/L) predisposes to specific ICU complications has been tested in a prospective, randomized, controlled trial.[67] This large single-centre trial of postoperative surgical patients showed significant improvement in survival when continuous infusion insulin was used to maintain glucose between 4.4 and 6.1 mmol/L. Exogenous glucose was begun simultaneously with insulin with frequent monitoring of glucose (every hour) and intensity of monitoring greatest at the time of initiation of insulin. Thirty-five of the 765 patients (4.6%) in the intensive insulin group died in the ICU, compared with 63 patients (8.0%) in the conventional therapy group. Although the APACHE II scores of the patients in this trial were quite low, there is no reason to think that these data are not generalizable to all severely septic patients. This hypothesis is currently being tested by the Canadian Critical Care Trials Group. Post hoc data analysis of the trial data revealed that achieving a goal of < 8.3 mmol/L also improved outcome when compared with higher concentrations. The control of the blood glucose concentration appears to be more important than the amount of insulin infused. In patients with severe sepsis, a strategy of glycemic control should include a nutrition protocol with the preferential use of the enteral route (Recommendation 20.8).

Recommendation 20.8 – Tight Control of Blood Glucose

Following initial stabilization of patients with severe sepsis, maintain blood glucose < 8.3 mmol/L. Studies supporting the role of glycemic control have used continuous infusion of insulin and glucose. With this protocol, glucose should be monitored frequently after initiation of the protocol (every 30–60 min) and on a regular basis (every 4 hrs) once the blood glucose concentration has stabilized.
Grade D

Now back to our patient.

The good news is that Mr. Schoque recovers. Mr. Schoque was devastatingly ill when last we visited him and because he was so ill, the full gamut of ICU therapy was given to him. Because he had persisting vasopressor-dependent septic shock, he was enrolled in the vasopressin in septic shock trial. That he was likely getting active vasopressin was evidenced by an initial improvement in MAP to 70 mm Hg despite a reduction in phenylephrine to only 5 mcg/min. However, this improvement was short-lived and the next day he was again back on high dose vasopressor therapy and only maintaining a MAP = 60 mm Hg. His renal failure progressed and he required continuous renal replacement therapy.

A 250 mcg cosyntropin test was administered and he was empirically started on hydrocortisone 50 mg iv q6h. Within six hours of starting corticosteroids, his MAP improved to 78 mm Hg and vasopressors were weaned significantly. Simultaneously with the corticosteroid therapy, an APC infusion was started, because of concern that he was not improving consistently and continued to manifest multi-organ failure (ARDS, renal failure, inability to feed enterally, altered level of consciousness, cool blue extremities despite a CI of 8 ml/min/m^2, persisting lactate acidosis and low ScvO$_2$% in the range of 55–65%). There were no signs of clinical bleeding and platelets were stable at 45 × 10^9/L.

Forty-eight hours after beginning APC and corticosteroids, he was much improved and continued to improve steadily from that point onward. Five days later he was hemodynamically stable and off all pressors and his ScvO$_2$% was 75%. Continuous dialysis was successfully stopped three days later and he was extubated five days after that. Four weeks after being discharged home he was still weak but returning to normal daily activities and happy in the fact that he had practically no memory of his ICU stay.

I. Future Therapies for Sepsis

Much research is being done to provide more fundamental approaches to sepsis management.[13] One possible development to watch for over in the next few years is a possible role for therapeutic and prophylactic IV immunoglobulin therapy in sepsis.[68] Prophylaxis with IV immunoglobulin can significantly reduce the incidence of infection in post surgical ICU patients, but to date, a mortality benefit has not been shown. It has, however, despite a lack of definitive evidence, become a standard therapy for Group A streptococcal (GAS) toxic shock syndrome and necrotizing fasciitis (work on developing a vaccine for GAS is also progressing fairly well). A number of other novel therapies for sepsis are under investigation, including recombinant human platelet activating factor; anti–factor IX monoclonal antibody and nitric oxide and oxygen free-radical molecular scavengers. High volume hemofiltration is also being studied.[69–72] A small number of patients with refractory septic shock were treated with 35L of ultrafiltration over a four-hour period and about 50% showed an acute response and had a reduced 28-day mortality.[69] Additional trials are needed.

Given the uncertainties and lack of precision of the current clinical SIRS approach to classification of sepsis, as our knowledge about sepsis pathophysiology expands, a new paradigm for sepsis, such as the PIRO scheme (Figure 20.11) may improve our ability to research and perhaps treat sepsis.[13–17]

It is also interesting to speculate about what sepsis therapy will be like in the far distant future.[73,74] Our ability to do bedside genotyping, together with the advent of novel molecular therapies, might conceivably reduce mortality from sepsis to 5% or lower. Fifty years hence, the following approaches may be routine.[73]

Maybe there will be rapid point-of-care diagnostics based on identification of bacterial products. Bedside genomics may allow identification of genetic polymorphisms, which will facilitate identification of antibiotic resistance genes and of patients who are likely (or unlikely) to respond to specific therapies. An improved understanding of host–microbial symbiosis might lead to the new concept that patients might die from the "absence" of infection. A new approach in which highly microbe-specific antibiotics are given for only 6–12 hours to kill pathogens selectively while preserving indigenous flora might be developed. "Probiotic" therapies may use bacteria as drug delivery systems—for example, to deliver anti-inflammatory cytokines such as IL-10 or to administer bacteria that promote neutrophil apoptosis. Strategies to monitor and prevent microvascular coagulation could become the new standard of care. Finally, it may be realized that blood pressure–driven therapy compromises microvascular blood flow, and vasodilator therapy may be the gold standard in the new age of "permissive hypotension." The goal of direct visualization of microvascular flow may now guide therapy.

To consider how therapy for our Mr. Schoque might look 50 years hence, I have applied some speculative thoughts on this topic from John Marshall:[73]

Mr. Schoque—fifty years hence… Mr. Schoque and his family are known to have a TRL2 receptor polymorphism resulting in a hyperactive immune response to gram-positive organisms. He had been previously counselled about gene therapy to alter this, but had refused.

Following his initial resuscitation in the ED, this BP = 70/40 mm Hg, and this alarms the ICU staff, who immediately start vasodilator therapy to lower the BP to a more respectable 40–50/20 mmHg; he has a gratifying response as determined by intravital MR microscopy, which confirms excellent blood flow to all vital vascular beds. A single large dose of penicillin is administered along with a potent anti-inflammatory anticoagulant (iv ASA) and adjuvant heparin. He was fed an E. coli strain engineered to produce recombinant human IL-11 to protect the gastrointestinal epithelium and IL-10 to augment gut anti-inflammatory activity. Aeromonas sp. was added to the fluid being used for liquid ventilation in order to accelerate neutrophil apoptosis in the lung. All goes well and he is discharged home in 48 hours and continues to do well. His family has consented to genetic counselling. Maybe in fifty years.

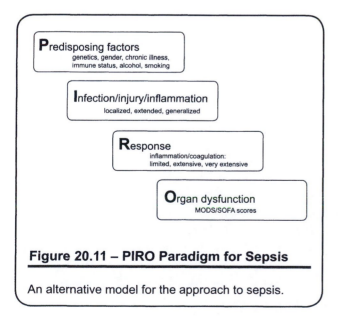

Predisposing factors
genetics, gender, chronic illness, immune status, alcohol, smoking

Infection/injury/inflammation
localized, extended, generalized

Response
inflammation/coagulation:
limited, extensive, very extensive

Organ dysfunction
MODS/SOFA scores

Figure 20.11 – PIRO Paradigm for Sepsis

An alternative model for the approach to sepsis.

Key Points

- Sepsis is a common problem whose incidence is increasing.
- Cytokines play a pivotal role in the pathophysiology of sepsis.
- Sepsis causes both uncontrolled inflammatory response and immune suppression.

- Early recognition and aggressive therapy likely improve sepsis outcomes.
- Management of sepsis requires a multi-modal approach to care.

References

1. Friedman G, Silva E, Vincent JL: Has the mortality of septic shock changed with time? *Crit Care Med* 1998;26:2078–86.
2. Dellinger RP: Cardiovascular management of septic shock. *Crit Care Med* 2003; 31:946–55.
3. Bateman RM, Sharpe MD, Ellis CG: Bench-to-bedside review: Microvascular dysfunction in sepsis: Hemodynamics, oxygen transport, and nitric oxide. *Crit Care* 2003;7:359–73.
4. Ware LB, Matthay MA: Measuring microvascular blood flow in sepsis: A continuing challenge. *Lancet* 2002;360:1187–8.
5. Vincent JL: Microvascular endothelial dysfunction: A renewed appreciation of sepsis pathophysiology. *Crit Care* 2001;5(suppl 2): S1–S5.
6. Fink MP: Bench-to-bedside review: Cytopathic hypoxia. *Crit Care* 2002;6:491–9.
7. Marshall JC: Inflammation, coagulopathy, and the pathogenesis of multiple organ dysfunction syndrome. *Crit Care Med* 2001;29(7 suppl):S99–106.
8. Amaral A, Opal SM, Vincent JL: Coagulation in sepsis. *Intens Care Med* 2004;30:1032–40.
9. Dellinger RP, Carlet JM, Masur H, et al: Surviving Sepsis Campaign guidelines for management of severe sepsis and septic shock. *Crit Care Med* 2004;32:858–73.
10. Bone RC: The sepsis syndrome: Definition and general approach to management. *Clin Chest Med* 1996;17:175–81.
11. Bone RC, Sibbald WJ, Sprung CL: The ACCP-SCCM consensus conference on sepsis and organ failure. *Chest* 1992;101:1481–3.
12. Marshall JC, Cook DJ, Christou NV, et al: Multiple organ dysfunction score: A reliable descriptor of a complex clinical outcome. *Crit Care Med* 1995;23:1638–52.
13. Levy MM, Fink MP, Marshall JC, et al: 2001 SCCM/ESICM/ACCP/ATS/SIS International Sepsis Definitions Conference. *Crit Care Med* 2003;31:1250–6.
14. Angus DC, Burgner D, Wunderink R, et al: The PIRO concept: P is for predisposition. *Crit Care* 2003;7:248–51.
15. Gerlach H, Dhainaut JF, Harbarth S, et al: The PIRO concept: R is for response. *Crit Care* 2003;7:256–9.
16. Vincent JL, Wendon J, Groeneveld J, et al: The PIRO concept: O is for organ dysfunction. *Crit Care* 2003;7:260–4.
17. Vincent JL, Opal S, Torres A, et al: The PIRO concept: I is for infection. *Crit Care* 2003;7:252–5.
18. Rivers E, Nguyen B, Havstad S, et al: Early goal-directed therapy in the treatment of severe sepsis and septic shock. *N Engl J Med* 2001;345:1368–77.
19. Rangel-Frausto MS, Pittet D, Costigan M, et al: The natural history of the systemic inflammatory response syndrome (SIRS): A prospective study. *JAMA* 1995;273:117–23.
20. Balc IC, Sungurtekin H, Gurses E, et al: Usefulness of procalcitonin for diagnosis of sepsis in the intensive care unit. *Crit Care* 2003;7:85–90.
21. Yu DT, Black E, Sands KE, et al: Severe sepsis: Variation in resource and therapeutic modality use among academic centers. *Crit Care* 2003;7: R24–R34.
22. Garnacho-Montero J, Garcia-Garmendia JL, Barrero-Almodovar A, et al: Impact of adequate empirical antibiotic therapy on the outcome of patients admitted to the intensive care unit with sepsis. *Crit Care Med* 2003;31:2742–51.

23. Arons MM, Wheeler AP, Bernard GR, et al: Effects of ibuprofen on the physiology and survival of hypothermic sepsis. Ibuprofen in Sepsis Study Group. *Crit Care Med* 1999;27:699–707.

24. Sprung CL, Peduzzi PN, Shatney CH, et al: Impact of encephalopathy on mortality in the sepsis syndrome. The Veterans Administration Systemic Sepsis Cooperative Study Group. *Crit Care Med* 1990;18:801–6.

25. Clemmer TP, Fisher CJ, Bone RC, et al: Hypothermia in the sepsis syndrome and clinical outcome. The Methylprednisolone Severe Sepsis Study Group. *Crit Care Med* 1992;20:1395–1401.

26. Hotchkiss RS, Karl IE: The pathophysiology and treatment of sepsis. *N Engl J Med* 2003;348:138–50.

27. Zeni F, Freeman B, Natanson C: Anti-inflammatory therapies to treat sepsis and septic shock: A reassessment. *Crit Care Med* 1997;25:1095–100.

28. Thomas L: Germs. *N Engl J Med* 1972;287:553–5.

29. Casey LC: Role of cytokines in the pathogenesis of cardiopulmonary-induced multisystem organ failure. *Ann Thorac Surg* 1993;56(suppl):S92–S96.

30. Casey LC, Balk RA, Bone RC: Plasma cytokine and endotoxin levels correlate with survival in patients with the sepsis syndrome. *Ann Intern Med* 1993;119:771–8.

31. Bone RC, Fisher CJ, Clemmer TP, et al: A controlled clinical trial of high-dose methylprednisolone in the treatment of severe sepsis and septic shock. *N Engl J Med* 1987;317:653–8.

32. Ziegler EJ, Fisher CJ, Sprung CL, et al: Treatment of gram-negative bacteremia and septic shock with HA-1A human monoclonal antibody against endotoxin: A randomized, double-blind, placebo-controlled trial. The HA-1A Sepsis Study Group. *N Engl J Med* 1991;324:429–36.

33. Bone RC, Balk RA, Fein AM, et al: A second large controlled clinical study of E5, a monoclonal antibody to endotoxin: Results of a prospective, multicenter, randomized, controlled trial. The E5 Sepsis Study Group. *Crit Care Med* 1995;23:994–1006.

34. Abraham E, Wunderink R, Silverman H, et al: Efficacy and safety of monoclonal antibody to human tumor necrosis factor alpha in patients with sepsis syndrome: A randomized, controlled, double-blind, multicenter clinical trial. TNF-alpha MAb Sepsis Study Group. *JAMA* 1995;273:934–41.

35. Fisher CJ, Agosti JM, Opal SM, et al: Treatment of septic shock with the tumor necrosis factor receptor: Fc fusion protein. *N Engl J Med* 1996;334:1697–1702.

36. Bernard GR, Wheeler AP, Russell JA, et al: The effects of ibuprofen on the physiology and survival of patients with sepsis. *N Engl J Med* 1997;336:912–8.

37. Wheeler AP, Bernard GR: Treating patients with severe sepsis. *N Engl J Med* 1999;340:207–14.

38. Munford RS, Pugin J: Normal responses to injury prevent systemic inflammation and can be immunosuppressive. *Am J Respir Crit Care Med* 2001;163:316–21.

39. Munford RS, Pugin J: The crucial role of systemic responses in the innate (non-adaptive) host defense. *J Endotoxin Res* 2001;7:327–32.

40. Docke WD, Randow F, Syrbe U, et al: Monocyte deactivation in septic patients: Restoration by IFN-gamma treatment. *Nat Med* 1997;3:678–81.

41. Reinhart K, Karzai W: Anti-tumor necrosis factor therapy in sepsis: Update on clinical trials and lessons learned. *Crit Care Med* 2001;29(7 suppl):S121–S125.

42. Opal SM, Huber CE: Bench-to-bedside review: Toll-like receptors and their role in septic shock. *Crit Care* 2002;6:125–36.

43. Hopkins P, Cohen J: Toll-like receptors: The key to the stable door? *Crit Care* 2002;6:99–101.

44. Hotchkiss JR, Swanson P, Freeman B, et al: Apoptotic cell death in patients with sepsis, shock and multiple organ dysfunction. *Crit Care Med* 1999;27:1230–51.

45. Opal SM, Esmon CT: Bench-to-bedside review: Functional relationships between coagulation and the innate immune response and their respective roles in the pathogenesis of sepsis. *Crit Care* 2003;7:23–38.

46. Matthay MA: Severe sepsis: A new treatment with both anticoagulant and antiinflammatory properties. *N Engl J Med* 2001;344:759–62.

47. Lorente J, Garcia-Frade L, Landin L, et al: Time course of hemostatic abnormalities in sepsis and its relation to outcome. *Chest* 1993;103:1536–42.

48. Bernard GR, Vincent JL, Laterre PF, et al: Efficacy and safety of recombinant human activated protein C for severe sepsis. *N Engl J Med* 2001;344:699–709.

49. Bernard GR: Drotrecogin alfa (activated) (recombinant human activated protein C) for the

treatment of severe sepsis. *Crit Care Med* 2003;31(1 suppl):S85–S93.

50. Spronk P, Zandstra D, Ince C: Bench-to-bedside review: Sepsis is a disease of the microcirculation. *Crit Care* 2004;8:2894.

51. Walley KR, Russell JA: Genetic predictors of adverse outcome from sepsis, ARDS and SIRS. *Critical Care Rounds* 2002;3:1–6.

52. Villar J, Maca-Meyer N, Perez-Mendez L, et al: Bench-to-bedside review: Understanding genetic predisposition to sepsis. *Crit Care* 2004;8:180–9.

53. Bishop MH, Shoemaker WC, Appel PL, et al: Prospective, randomized trial of survivor values of cardiac index, oxygen delivery, and oxygen consumption as resuscitation endpoints in severe trauma. *J Trauma* 1995;38:780–7.

54. Gattinoni L, Brazzi L, Pelosi P, et al: A trial of goal-oriented hemodynamic therapy in critically ill patients. SvO2 Collaborative Group. *N Engl J Med* 1995;333:1025–32.

55. Hayes MA, Timmins AC, Yau E, et al: Elevation of systemic oxygen delivery in the treatment of critically ill patients. *N Engl J Med* 1994;330:1717–22.

56. Hebert PC, Wells G, Blajchman MA, et al: A multicenter, randomized, controlled clinical trial of transfusion requirements in critical care. Transfusion Requirements in Critical Care Investigators, Canadian Critical Care Trials Group. *N Engl J Med* 1999;340:409–17.

57. Patel BM, Chittock DR, Russell JA, et al: Beneficial effects of short-term vasopressin infusion during severe septic shock. *Anesthesiology* 2002;96:576–82.

58. Tsuneyoshi I, Yamada H, Kakihana Y, et al: Hemodynamic and metabolic effects of low-dose vasopressin infusions in vasodilatory septic shock. *Crit Care Med* 2001;29:487–93.

59. Sharshar T, Blanchard A, Paillard M, et al: Circulating vasopressin levels in septic shock. *Crit Care Med* 2003;31:1752–8.

60. Choi PT, Yip G, Quinonez LG, et al: Crystalloids vs. colloids in fluid resuscitation: A systematic review. *Crit Care Med* 1999;27:200–10.

61. Cook D, Guyatt G: Colloid use for fluid resuscitation: Evidence and spin. *Ann Intern Med* 2001;135:205–8.

62. The SAFE Study: A comparison of albumin and saline for fluid resuscitation in the intensive care unit. *N Engl J Med* 2004;350:2247–56.

63. Schortgen F, Brochard L, Burnham E, et al: Pro/con clinical debate: Hydroxyethylstarches should be avoided in septic patients. *Crit Care* 2003;7:279–81.

64. Oliveira RP, Velasco I, Soriano F, et al: Clinical review: Hypertonic saline resuscitation in sepsis. *Crit Care* 2002;6:418–23.

65. Lefering R, Neugebauer EA: Steroid controversy in sepsis and septic shock: A meta-analysis. *Crit Care Med* 1995;23:1294–1303.

66. Annane D, Sebille V, Charpentier C, et al: Effect of treatment with low doses of hydrocortisone and fludrocortisone on mortality in patients with septic shock. *JAMA* 2002;288:862–71.

67. Van den BG, Wouters P, Weekers F, et al: Intensive insulin therapy in the critically ill patients. *N Engl J Med* 2001;345:1359–67.

68. Laupland K: Polyclonal intravenous immunoglobulin for the prophylaxis and treatment of infection in critically ill adults. *Can J Infect Dis* 2002;13:100–6.

69. Honore PM, Jamez J, Wauthier M, et al: Prospective evaluation of short-term, high-volume isovolemic hemofiltration on the hemodynamic course and outcome in patients with intractable circulatory failure resulting from septic shock. *Crit Care Med* 2000;28:3581–7.

70. Honore PM, Matson JR: Hemofiltration, adsorption, sieving and the challenge of sepsis therapy design. *Crit Care* 2002;6:394–6.

71. Honore PM, Matson JR: Short-term high-volume hemofiltration in sepsis: Perhaps the right way is to start with. *Crit Care Med* 2002;30:1673–4.

72. Honore PM, Matson JR: Extracorporeal removal for sepsis: Acting at the tissue level: The beginning of a new era for this treatment modality in septic shock. *Crit Care Med* 2004;32:896–7.

73. Marshall JC: The International Sepsis Forum's controversies in sepsis: How will sepsis be treated in 2051? *Crit Care* 2002;6:465–7.

74. Abraham E: The International Sepsis Forum's controversies in sepsis: How will sepsis be treated in 2051? *Crit Care* 2002;6:277–8.

CHAPTER 21

CRITICAL POINTS IN INFECTIOUS DISEASES

DON BURKE

A 18-year-old male arrives in your emergency room in respiratory distress. He had been complaining of a sore throat for the last two days, which worsened into a bad headache, an unusual rash and breathing difficulties this evening. Presently, he is combative and confused and you are unable to get vitals due to his agitated state.

An important element in the approach to treating patients who are acutely ill from an infection, begins with looking at the host. Having knowledge of the antibiotics is often not as important as understanding the person infected. The first aspect to look at, once you have initiated proper oxygen and hemodynamic support, is the immune status of the patient. A simple way to break it down is by looking at whether they have a problem with neutrophils, with humoral immunity or with cell-mediated immunity. Each of these scenarios can have different disease patterns and different approaches to treatment. Research has shown that patients treated with the wrong antibiotic (or with no antibiotic) within the first eight hours have a higher mortality. Hence, your first shot has to be reasonably accurate.

● Neutrophil Function

After leaving the bloodstream, neutrophils migrate predominantly to two sites: the subepithelium of the skin and the submucosa of the gut. Hence, patients who have neutropenia or other neutrophil defects are at risk for serious infections with either skin or gut organisms. The absolute neutrophil count (ANC) is determined by adding the percentage of polymorphonuclear leukocytes (PMNs) and bands, then multiplying by the total white blood cell count. An ANC of < 1000 cells/mm^3 in a patient in whom the white blood cell count (WBC) count is expected to drop further is considered neutropenic. The most life-threatening of the gut and skin flora are Staph aureus, Strep species (especially group A Strep or viridans Strep species) and Pseudomonas. These organisms produce toxins that allow rapid spread. Look for painful mottling, cellulitis features or ecthyma gangrenosum (hemorrhagic spots surrounded by halos of normal skin with a purple rim, classically due to disseminated P. aeruginosa), or erythroderma with desquamation.

A very important life-threatening complication that could occur in a patient who received chemotherapy is neutropenic enterocolitis. Previously called typhlitis, it usually presents with abdominal pain (often right lower quadrant), fever and diarrhea. Although this could be the same presentation as for Clostridium difficile colitis or ischemic colitis, the treatment is very different.

There are two principles that are considered truisms in the empiric treatment of someone with a neutrophil defect: Always use bactericidal agents (not bacteriostatic) and always cover initially for P. aeruginosa. Furthermore, in someone with prolonged neutropenia, think about fungi as a reason for occult fevers or worsening clinical status. The two most clinically important fungi to consider are Candida and Aspergillus species. It is important to note that fungal blood cultures are notoriously unreliable and that 50% of patients with metastatic fungal disease will have repeatedly negative blood cultures up to the time of death. As a corollary, the vast majority of patients who *do* have positive fungal blood cultures (especially for species like C. albicans or C. tropicalis) already have disseminated fungal disease at the time of the positive blood cultures.

● Humoral Immunity

Humoral immunity includes both antibodies and complement. The importance of this system of defense is for opsonization; i.e., to coat an organism such that it is easier for a phagocyte to ingest. The alternative is to poke holes into the organism with complement alone. For example, if you are exposed to an organism such as pneumococcus or meningococcus, which your immune system has never been exposed to before (and so has no preformed antibody against) and which is difficult for your phagocytes to ingest because of a polysaccharide capsule, then you need some way of attacking the organism before it causes damage.

This is where complement comes in. The cell wall constituents of the bacteria activate C3 esterase, which in turn activates the complement system by splitting C3 into C3b. This initiates both the inflammatory process as well as the terminal cascade to create a membrane attack complex, which is important for killing organisms such as meningococci.

The importance of a spleen in humoral immunity is threefold. First, it acts as a filter for bacteria that have an antibody attached. Second, it is an important reservoir for B-lymphocytes, which become activated to plasma cells to make more antibody. Third, the alternate complement pathway is housed in the spleen. Hence, without a functioning spleen, the host suffers a significant setback with respect to humoral immunity.

Organisms that can rapidly cause fulminant disease in the patient who is asplenic or hyposplenic are entities such as Haemophilus influenzae, Streptococcus pneumonia, Neisseria, Babesia or Plasmodia species, Capnocytophaga (from dog saliva), as well as other encapsulated bacteria such as Klebsiella and Staphylococcus.

● Cell-Mediated Immunity

The significance of cell-mediated immunity is that most of the bacteria that cause problems for the host when this system is defective, are *intracellular* organisms. Examples of these include Mycobacteria, Listeria, Legionella, Salmonella and less commonly (but potentially dangerous in the HIV patient), Nocardia, Rhodococcus and Bartonella (formerly Rochalimaea, which causes several syndromes including bacillary angiomatosis, cat-scratch disease and peliosis hepatis). Such patients are also at higher risk of more fulminant disease with several fungi (Cryptococcus, Blastomycosis, Histoplasmosis, Candida and Aspergillus). The viruses that are particularly worrisome in the host with cell-mediated immune dysfunction are the DNA viruses (Herpes simplex, Epstein Barr, Cytomegalovirus, Varicella-Zoster). Such patients are also at increased risk of severe disease with certain protozoa (Cryptosporidium, Toxoplasmosis, Pneumocystis) and certain parasites (e.g., Strongyloides).

It sometimes is not apparent that a certain patient will have a particular type of immune deficit, but most patients who present with unexpectedly fulminant disease do, in fact, have some type of immune deficit that wasn't appreciated. Knowing certain patterns helps in dealing with this. For instance, advanced age increases the degree of cellular deficit. Women in the third trimester of pregnancy have a transient loss in cellular immunity, which reconstitutes approximately 90 days after delivery. This explains why such pregnant patients can have overwhelming Varicella or Listeria infections.

Steroids and HIV infection both decrease the total number of T lymphocytes capable of making the necessary lymphokines (required to initiate the cellular immunity pathway); whereas drugs like cyclosporine do not affect the total *number* of lymphocytes, but rather decrease their capacity to make lymphokines. Lymphoid malignancies, corticosteroids, chronic alcohol intoxication and certain multi-drug chemotherapy regimens can cause a mixed immune deficit involving more than one cell line.

● Disease Patterns

Equipped with some essential knowledge of the immune function, one looks for certain patterns of recognition. For instance, the triad of cavitary lung disease, brain abscesses and skin lesions in someone with a cell-mediated immune deficiency would make one think of Nocardia or Rhodococcus. Bilateral cavitary lung disease in a patient on higher dose chronic steroids (> 15 mg prednisone equivalent per day for > 4 weeks) would make one consider Legionella or Mycobacteria tuberculosis early in the differential.

Systemic fungal infections can be divided into those that occur in healthy persons versus those that are usually only seen in compromised hosts. The former include blastomycosis, cryptococcosis, histoplasmosis, paracoccidioidomycosis and coccidioidomycosis while the latter include aspergillosis, pneumocystosis, candidosis and mucormycosis.

Amongst bacterial infections, consider gram-positive cocci as potential pathogens when there is a clinical picture typical of pyrogenic exotoxins, with diffuse, blanching erythroderma (like a sunburn), high fever, shock or exfoliation of skin (especially on the extremities). Because of the ability of these exotoxins of Staph aureus and group A Strep to intensely stimulate T-cell proliferation (with subsequent production of a variety of immune-activating cytokines), they have been designated *superantigens*. Treatment options would thereby include therapies that would either inhibit cytokine production (e.g., steroids, activated protein C, high-dose clindamycin) or bind toxin (e.g., immune globulin) in conjunction with conventional antibiotics.

Consider gram-negative organisms when you see evidence of purpuric skin lesions or DIC in the presence of shock, suggesting endotoxemia. Ecthyma gangrenosum (purplish-red skin lesions surrounded by near-normal skin with a red rim) should make you think of Pseudomonas aeruginosa until proven otherwise, and antibiotic coverage should include two drugs that cover for this organism (preferably an anti-pseudomonal beta-lactam along with either an aminoglycoside or ciprofloxacin) until culture and sensitivity results come back.

Diabetics, burn patients and patients with loss of colonic mucosal integrity often have polymicrobial infections. Therefore, start with broad coverage and narrow it down if culture results become available. If a patient should present with two separate gram-negative organisms in blood cultures, or Strep mitis or bovis, always think of some serious disease in their colon (e.g., cancer, Strongyloides infection).

● Helpful Considerations

Try to avoid central lines unless the drugs being administered are particularly hard on peripheral veins, or the patient has very poor peripheral access. Infectious and other complications with peripheral IVs are generally easier to detect and to rectify than with central venous catheters.

Another point to consider is drug fever. A "pearl" is that, with rare exceptions, the presence of eosinophilia usually does *not* imply a progressive or inadequately treated bacterial infection. In fact, eosinophils are usually suppressed in the presence of bacterial infections. Therefore, consider an adverse drug reaction as a possible culprit. Watch for a pattern to the fever curve (since bacteria never follow patterns), as it may correlate with the timing of a drug.

Although deep vein thrombosis and atelectasis are commonly cited as causes of occult fever or elevated WBC counts, these elevations are usually mild and not consistent. If the patient has a continually rising

WBC count or progressive fever, consider more serious etiologies such as abscess (especially is there was a recent surgery), antibiotic resistance (especially with organisms such as Serratia, Pseudomonas, Acinetobacter, Citrobacter or Enterobacter) or C. difficile infection (especially if the platelet count is also climbing rapidly).

Monotherapy is adequate when treating neutropenic fever with no obvious focus and no organism isolated. Adding an aminoglycoside only increases the toxicity but has not been shown to improve outcome in this setting. Also, remember to use only bactericidal drugs in neutropenia (so macrolides, sulfa drugs and tetracyclines are out). Furthermore, aminoglycosides have poor penetration into lung parenchymal tissue and tend to be inactivated at the low pH of microabscesses.

However, in the setting where an aminoglycoside is being used, know that, for anti-Pseudomonal potency as well as for cost of drug, the order (from least to most) is: gentamicin < tobramycin < amikacin. Once-a-day dosing of aminoglycosides is easier to do and is probably less toxic to the kidneys and creates a better kill-potential (especially for the post-antibiotic effect) than with conventional q8h dosing. Furthermore, it requires less monitoring, in that you don't have to check peak levels, just check a trough level prior to the fourth or fifth dose (to know that the kidneys are getting rid of the drug).

Never give two beta-lactams together, as you could get competitive inhibition when both drugs are competing together for the same receptor (thereby cancelling out the effectiveness of each drug.). Also, try to avoid, if possible, a tetracycline with a beta-lactam for serious infections (like meningitis), since the tetracycline decreases cell turnover and there is, therefore, less cell wall synthesis (which the beta-lactam needs to kill the organism).

If a patient is clearly improving on an existing regimen, you will want to have good reason for changing it (unless you are simplifying the regimen or the patient is on superfluous or redundant therapy). In anaerobic lung infections, use clindamycin over metronidazole since the latter does not cover anaerobic gram-positive cocci well (which are seen in oral flora). Metronidazole is typically better for anaerobes below the diaphragm and clindamycin for those above the diaphragm. One exception to this is a brain abscess (which usually originates from gut anaerobes). Furthermore, metronidazole exhibits concentration-dependent killing (i.e., higher doses = better kill); hence the initial loading dose in serious anaerobic infections. Remember also that if metronidazole is given to an infected patient who recently ingested alcohol (not uncommon), the disulfiram-like reaction can confuse the clinical picture.

● Specific Scenarios

A. Severe Pneumonia

Often you will be called to assess a patient either in the emergency department or on the ward who is hypoxic and has significant dyspnea. Obviously you will need to address the ABC's (as always) to restore their airway patency (suction secretions), improve their oxygenation and reduce their work of breathing while maintaining their intravascular volume status. Then you will have to address the underlying problem.

The most common method of entry of micro-organisms into the lower respiratory tract is micro aspiration of oropharyngeal secretions. Gross aspiration of gastric contents is a much less common cause of pneumonia. Furthermore, it has been shown that anaerobes play a very small role in pneumonia even when there is gross aspiration. In fact, if the patient is edentulous, then *anaerobic* pneumonia is actually rare.

What differs between hospitalized and community-acquired pneumonia is what the host's upper respiratory tract is colonized with at the time they get sick as well as their premorbid state (healthy vs. multiple medical problems). Hence, for community acquired pneumonia, bacteriostatic drugs probably will suffice, whereas for the already hospitalized patient, try to stick with cidal antibiotics, at least until you have a better understanding of the host. Certain organisms do not require previous colonization but can reach the lungs by direct inhalation (Legionella, Mycobacterium tuberculosis) or by hematogenous spread (Staph aureus).

Sputum samples should be obtained if the cough is productive, but often the samples are unreliable. Induced sputum is probably most valuable for diagnosing Pneumocystis carinii (PCP) or M. tuberculosis. A bronchoscopic specimen is more reliable if a protected brush or bronchoalveolar lavage (BAL) is used, especially in an immunocompromised host. Although blood culture results yield positive results in only 10% of patients, the information from this is extremely valuable. It is worthwhile to tap any effusion that layers > 10 mm on a lateral decubitus film as the positive predictive results are high.

Although the urinary antigen test is reasonably sensitive for Legionella pneumophilia serogroup 1 only, the vast majority of Legionella that you will encounter is of this serogroup. Sputum samples that grow Legionella often have few polymorphonuclear leukocytes (PMNs), such that the lab may discard the sample as "poor quality." Therefore, if you have a reasonable suspicion for Legionella, ask the lab to hold the specimen anyway. A direct fluorescent antibody stain can be done on the sample, which detects all subtypes.

Recommended empiric therapy should include coverage for Strep. pneumonia, Haemophilus influenzae, aerobic gram-negative rods (especially E. coli and Klebsiella) and Legionella (especially if the pneumonia is severe).

B. Occult Sepsis

At times you may be called to assess a patient on the ward who has been declining clinically with no obvious source of infection. They may only have fever and leukocytosis and possibly a metabolic acidosis. Considering the patient's recent course of events in the hospital will often steer you in the right direction. An old adage in infectious diseases is "Go where the surgeons have gone." Namely, consider some bacterial contamination of a surgical site as a likely culprit. Physical examination (e.g., abdominal tenderness) may be less helpful if the patient has been on post-op analgesics or is quite elderly.

It takes approximately seven days for visible signs of an intra-abdominal abscess to be present on CT in post-operative patients. Therefore, do not be dissuaded in your clinical suspicion due to negative findings prior to one week.

In a patient with cirrhotic ascites, always consider primary peritonitis as a potential etiology. Such patients may look sick but have few if any abdominal findings. It is safe to obtain a small amount (50 cc) of fluid with a fine needle, even if the patient has a coagulopathy. You can increase your culture yield by adding at least 10 cc of ascitic aspirate to each blood culture bottle. Treat if PMNs > 250/mm^3; usually the pathogen is a single enteric aerobe or a gram-positive

coccus; it is almost never an anaerobe, so you won't need anaerobic coverage.

The large majority of central line infections are due to coagulase negative staphylococci; however, this is also the commonest contaminant. Two ways for a central line to become infected are: 1) spread from the skin site (the usual way); or 2) hematogenous spread with secondary catheter colonization (more often Staph aureus). To determine which has occurred, send both the tip and the cuff (the part of the catheter that travels under the skin) in separate culture containers. If both are growing the same organism, then the insertion site is more than likely the source. If the tip is positive but the cuff negative, consider another occult source of bacteremia. For non-tunnelled central lines, treat for five to seven days if the catheter has been removed; but for two weeks if for some reason the catheter cannot be removed. If it is Candida, the line needs to come out (tunnelled or not).

Unless there has been a recent surgery or procedure on the urinary system, it is unusual for Staph aureus or Staph epidermidis to cause an isolated UTI. Hence, if one of these organisms is detected in the urine culture, be suspicious that the organism got there via the blood stream, so look for another, occult source of staphylococcal bacteremia (e.g., endocarditis).

C. Serious Skin and Soft Tissue Infections

Organisms of greatest concern in this setting are group A Strep (pyogenes) and Clostridia species because of their ability to produce superantigens (exotoxins) that significantly accelerate the immune response with cytokine production and the rapid onset of sepsis. Other organisms of concern such as Vibrio vulnificus and Bacillus cereus typically affect people with impaired bacterial clearance (e.g., cirrhotics, asplenics). Certain strains of Strep are able to elaborate collagenases that allow the organism to dissect rapidly along tissue planes.

Look carefully for areas of ischemic blotches or mottling because the underlying blood supply to the skin is lost. These areas are typically painful for the patient, but not necessarily to the touch (as they may have anesthesia in the affected area as the superficial nerve supply is taken out by the underlying infection). The overlying skin may be indurated or even crepitant to palpation. These are grave findings and are not seen in usual cellulitis. In group A Strep fasciitis, the overlying skin may look unremarkable early on. However, the patient will have considerable pain and the tissue will feel firmer to the touch.

This should be considered a surgical emergency, as rapid surgical debridement is the mainstay of therapy, along with aggressive IV antibiotics. The surgeon will need to make an incision and blunt-probe to determine involvement of the fascial plane. Furthermore, you will need a STAT gram stain (and culture) to determine the etiology (Strep, Staph, Clostridia or polymicrobial). Necrotizing fasciitis that develops in ischemic tissue is generally polymicrobial, so antibiotic coverage must be broad (e.g., imipenem or meropenem).

A common misconception is that if gas is seen on CT or MRI, it implies an anaerobic infection. *Any organism associated with necrotizing fasciitis can produce gas.* Another point is that, although Staphylococcus aureus is commonly isolated from polymicrobial necrotizing infections, it is seldom a cause of monobacterial fasciitis. Staph aureus usually causes abscesses, but *can* cause a scalded skin syndrome, which is confined to the epidermis.

Because high-dose clindamycin can suppress toxin production by way of protein synthesis inhibition, it is often added to the regimen (900 mg iv q8h). Furthermore, high-dose intravenous immunoglobulin (IVIG, 1–2 g/kg) has also been shown to be effective, which is felt to be related to toxin binding.

D. Serious Central Nervous System Infections

Generally, the most helpful parameter on the cerebrospinal fluid (CSF) after a lumbar puncture (LP) is the gram stain. Unfortunately, this is negative most of the time. Therefore, the next more vital piece of data is the cell count and differential. The three main patterns one sees with an infectious process are: PMN predominant, lymphocyte predominant with normal CSF glucose and lymphocyte predominant with low CSF glucose. Brain, subdural and epidural abscesses can cause a variable CSF profile, but in these scenarios one should not be doing an LP to make a diagnosis anyway.

The first group comprises most of the common bacteria that cause meningitis. The second group mostly consists of viruses. The third group essentially comprises the fungal and tuberculous forms. However, this latter group is also represented by partially treated bacterial meningitis and carcinomatous meningitis.

The first steps in the approach to someone with suspected meningitis is to obtain two blood cultures as fast as possible then start IV antibiotics in large doses, then get the head CT, then do the LP. Hence, therapy is started even before you have LP results. Because of the resistance patterns of pneumococcus, it is best to start with a high-dose third generation cephalosporin (e.g., ceftriaxone 2 g q12h or cefotaxime 2 g q4h). If your region has any incidence of high level penicillin-resistant pneumococci, it is safest to add vancomycin, but in this setting, use 750 mg iv q6h to obtain higher CSF levels (since vanco has variable penetration across the blood-brain barrier). Avoid imipenem, even if you suspect anaerobes (e.g., a brain abscess), because this drug can lower the seizure threshold in someone who is predisposed to seize. Be aware that high doses of penicillin (4 million units q4h) can also significantly lower the seizure threshold. Therefore, avoid NSAIDs and any other drug that will lower seizure thresholds or inhibit penicillin clearance.

CT can be helpful in the location of disease. Fungi, M. tuberculosis and Listeria tend to infect the base of the brain, hence the increased incidence of cranial nerve deficits and hydrocephalus. Rhodococcus and Nocardia can cause multiple brain abscesses, but usually in someone with a deficient cell-mediated immunity, and usually in conjunction with lung and skin manifestations. If a brain abscess is seen (especially with any mass effect), avoid doing an LP because of the risk of herniation.

Recent data now show what had been assumed all along: that steroids appear beneficial even in adults with meningitis. A study done recently in Europe on 301 adults with meningitis showed virtually a 50% decrease in morbidity and mortality in patients given dexamethasone 10 mg iv q6h for four days. The key is that the first dose of steroids has to go in either before or at the time of the first dose of antibiotics. The idea is to decrease the overwhelming cytokine response as a result of bacterial cell wall lysis from the cidal antibiotics. The cytokine release from immune cells in response to bacterial cell wall debris is believed to be what causes the significant inflammation and swelling that occurs in meningitis. Dexamethasone suppresses the host's inflammatory response to the organism.

Remember that aminoglycosides have almost no penetration into the CSF, so it is best to avoid them in meningitis: the risk-benefit ratio is too small. There is concern, however, that steroids will decrease the meningeal inflammation that drugs like vancomycin and third generation cephalosporins need in order to adequately cross the blood-brain barrier. This is why we use much larger doses of these drugs to treat meningitis. Also, most of these concerns arise from animal models.

One of the few scenarios where two beta-lactams are used together is if you suspect Listeria (some risk factors are malignancy, alcoholism/cirrhosis, diabetes, third trimester of pregnancy and impaired cellular immunity). Since Listeria monocytogene is resistant to third generation cephalosporins, one needs to add either ampicillin or penicillin to the regimen. Furthermore, if you do suspect Listeria, ask the micro lab to hold the CSF cultures for a full seven days, since there may be delayed isolation. Also, given the fact that Listeria is an intracellular pathogen, it is recommended that treatment continue for three weeks to ensure eradication.

● Closing

As a final helpful hint, don't be afraid to admit when you're stuck and could use some help. Acceptance of one's limitations and willingness to ask for help in a patient's care is a sign of strength, not weakness. We all have areas that we are not as strong in. Asking for advice from a colleague can often help you to re-examine the situation yourself. One of the purposes of this course is to help you recognize how we can all, at times, become fixated on a particular problem, and fail to see "the forest for the trees." Sometimes the mere process of describing a difficult case to a colleague can make you consider things you would not have thought of otherwise.

● Summary

Always use bactericidal antibiotics (beta-lactams, fluoroquinolones, vancomycin, aminoglycosides, rifampin) for significant infections in neutropenic hosts. If fever persists for more than three days of broad antibacterial therapy, consider empiric antifungal therapy—if the neutropenia is expected to last more than five to seven days.

If a patient has no spleen and is septic, think of the encapsulated organisms (Pneumococcus, Meningococcus, Haemophilus influenzae, Klebsiella, Staph aureus). The same applies if they have a splenic dysfunction (sickle cell disease, cirrhosis, leukemia/lymphoma).

Remember the common cell-mediated immune dysfunction categories: malignancy, diabetes, immunosuppressive therapy, third trimester pregnancy and cirrhosis. In these scenarios, consider organisms like Listeria, Legionella, Mycobacteria and Salmonella (along with the usual pathogens).

Dose-dependent (or concentration-dependent) killing occurs with antibiotics such as aminoglycosides, fluoroquinolones, metronidazole and amphotericin-B, meaning that their ability to kill an organism is dependent upon the dose being well above the minimum inhibitory concentration (MIC) of the organism, hence the rationale for using once daily dosing of gentamicin or tobramycin (5–7 mg/kg/day) when treating serious gram-negative bacterial infections and, in particular, Pseudomonas aeruginosa.

Time-dependent killing occurs with antibiotics such as the beta-lactams (e.g., all penicillins, cephalosporins, and carbapenems like imipenem and meropenem), vancomycin, clindamycin, oxazolidinone (linezolid), macrolides (e.g., erythromycin, clarithromycin, azithromycin) and tetracyclines. For such drugs to be effective, levels have to be above the MIC for an extended period, but once they are above the MIC, being even higher does not improve killing potential. This is the rationale for using penicillin (or more recently, vancomycin) continuous infusions. This also explains why, for treating non-central nervous system infections, 1 gram of ceftriaxone daily is as efficacious as 2 grams. Doubling the dose only doubles the cost of the treatment.

If a patient starts to look sick two to three days postoperatively, think of a surgical wound infection or an anastomotic leak (e.g., from a bowel resection). When patients have fevers from atelectasis or a deep vein thrombosis (DVT), they are generally low grade and the patient doesn't really look sick. If the WBCs continue to rise, consider that something is definitely wrong.

When toxin-producing gram-positive organisms (e.g., Staph, group A Strep and Clostridia) are suspected, as is seen with skin and soft tissue infections causing sepsis, add clindamycin at 900 mg iv q8h (or 600 mg iv q6h) to help decrease toxin production. Although clindamycin achieves high concentrations in most tissues (including lung), it has very poor penetration into the central nervous system and can potentiate the paralyzing effect of neuromuscular blocking agents.

If you suspect meningitis, get blood cultures and start treatment immediately, then investigate further (CT, LP). This tends to go against the grain of the usual approach to infections but is necessary due to the rapid lethality of meningitis. Also, if steroids are to be given, start before or at the time the antibiotics are started. If there is any concern of penicillin-resistant pneumococcus, add vancomycin at high doses (3 grams/day). Recently recommended dexamethasone doses are in the range of 10 mg iv q6h for four days.

In a central nervous system infection that involves cranial nerve defects, consider organisms that infect the basal portions of the brain, such as Listeria, fungi and Mycobacteria. Rhodococcus and Nocardia can present with multiple scattered brain abscesses which can resemble embolic phenomena; however, infectious agents that spread to the brain via the latter route usually involve the "watershed" area of the gray-white matter junction. Toxoplasmosis often presents with a mass effect, similar to a brain abscess. If there is any suggestion of a mass effect, either clinically or by CT scan, do *not* do a lumbar puncture, for fear of herniation.

Key Points

- Management of infected patients requires a basic understanding of immune defenses.
- Disease patterns can help focus diagnosis.
- Adjust antibiotics based on probable organism and dose appropriate for site of infection.

- Dose-dependent killing of bacteria occurs with aminoglycosides, fluoroquinolones, metronidazole and amphotericin-B.

CHAPTER 22

FEVER IN CRITICALLY ILL PATIENTS

JOHN KIM

> You are asked to assess a febrile 40-year-old man who was admitted to the hospital several days prior for elective knee surgery. The patient has very vague complaints but does complain of some leg pain and has a new cough. Examination is unremarkable aside from a temperature of 39°C. The nurse wants to know what you would like to do?

Fever is a common problem in critically ill patients. It is estimated that one-third of all medical patients will experience a fever at some point during their hospitalization.[1] The figure is even higher in the critically ill population. Studies indicate an incidence of fever as high as 70% within 24 hours of admission to an intensive care unit (ICU).[2,3]

The presence of fever in critically ill patients often leads to a battery of diagnostic tests and the institution of broad-spectrum antibiotic therapy because of the spectre of infection. Fever, however, has multiple causes aside from infection. A "shotgun" approach—that is, investigating every fever for all causes—not only represents a significant financial cost but may also increase patient morbidity through increased blood loss and other risks inherent in invasive diagnostic procedures. Therefore, the clinical setting is crucial in guiding management. A rational approach to both investigation and management of fever is essential when dealing with critically ill patients who are febrile.

The goal of this chapter is to review the current understanding of the pathophysiology of fever, as well as the etiology of fever in critically ill patients. A discussion of the various recommendations for investigating and managing fever in critically ill patients will also be presented.

● Pathophysiology of Fever

The mean body temperature in healthy individuals is 36.8 degrees Celsius (°C) but the normal range can vary from 35.6°C to 38.2°C.[4] For this reason, fever is defined by the Society of Critical Care Medicine as a core temperature greater than 38.3°C.[5] The site of measurement for core temperature is important when defining fever. Accurate and reproducible measurements of body temperature are essential in assessing febrile patients. The gold standard of core temperature is mixed venous blood found in the pulmonary artery.[6–8] Clearly, the placement of a pulmonary artery catheter for temperature measurement alone is inappropriate. Infrared ear thermometry usually produces measurements a few tenths of a degree Celsius lower than actual core temperature (accuracy requires the external auditory canal to be clear and patent).[9–12] Conversely, rectal thermometry often produces measurements a few tenths of a degree Celsius higher than core temperature.[9–12] The intake of fluids or food, as well as the temperature of inhaled gases, can influence oral temperature measurements.[9] Axillary temperatures often underestimate body temperature and have poor reproducibility.[9] For these reasons, while mixed venous blood thermometry is the gold standard, both rectal and ear thermometry are viewed as acceptable alternatives.[5]

Fever production is a complex interaction of multiple endogenous pyrogens. Of the numerous proposed pyrogens, most notable are the interleukins (IL), namely IL-1 and IL-6, the interferons and tumor necrosis factor alpha (TNF-α).[13] The introduction of exogenous stimuli, such as viruses and various toxins, induces white blood cells (WBCs) to produce endogenous pyrogens. These pyrogens act on the anterior hypothalamus at the level of the organum vasculosum of the laminae terminalis (OVLT).[14] The OVLT is a key element in regulating body temperature. The exact mechanism by which the OVLT produces fever or how the pyrogens stimulate the OVLT is unclear. The OVLT synthesizes prostaglandins, most notably PGE_2, in response to pyrogen exposure. Speculation is that interaction with the cyclooxygenase (COX) enzymes in the neural vasculature leads to the formation of fever. Non-steroidal anti-inflammatory drugs (NSAIDs) and acetaminophen inhibit COX enzymes, thus potentially explaining each agent's anti-pyretic effect. Acetaminophen's effect is limited to neural COX enzymes, explaining why it does not produce a systemic anti-inflammatory response.

Fever is a physiologic response found in invertebrates, amphibians, reptiles and mammals.

Lizards exposed to infection will seek out warmer climates to raise their body temperature.[15] The fact that fever is so well preserved along multiple evolutionary lines suggests some benefit to the host. In vitro studies demonstrate that fever causes an increase in antibody production, T-cell activation, production of cytokines and enhanced neutrophil as well as macrophage function.[16–19] Animal studies suggest that the presence of fever leads to increased survival,[20,21] and that lowering body temperature actually reduces survival.[22] Furthermore, fever reduces the mean inhibitory concentration (MIC) of antibiotics, thus translating to an increase in antimicrobial activity with fever.[23]

Fever is responsible for the production of the heat shock response. This complex reaction produces heat shock proteins (HSPs), a class of proteins postulated to be essential for cell survival. The DNA and protein structure of HSPs are similar in many diverse organisms thereby suggesting they have a vital role in cell survival during times of stress. HSPs provide cells and organisms with thermotolerance by controlling translocation, cell repair and apoptosis.[24] The hypothesis is that HSPs exert their protective effect by being activated by a sublethal heat stress (i.e., fever). Once active, the HSPs then protect the cell from a subsequent lethal heat stress. HSPs may also confer this protection not only against subsequent lethal heat stresses but also against entirely different types of stress that may be equally or more lethal (e.g., endotoxin). Thus, the enhanced immune response and heat shock response that fever produces could explain the benefit seen with in vitro and animal studies. But can these animal models be translated to human patients?

While animal studies suggest a beneficial effect with fever, no controlled human studies evaluating the benefit of fever exist. Most of the published studies in human patients have been case-control series.[23] Early retrospective studies indicate a beneficial effect of fever in patients with gram-negative sepsis and spontaneous bacterial peritonitis.[25,26] Patients who were afebrile, however, were also more likely to receive inappropriate antibiotic therapy, thereby making the determination of a causal relationship impossible. Nevertheless, it is difficult to argue against the notion that the evolutionary preservation of fever and HSPs indicate that some beneficial effect may indeed be present.

While fever may have beneficial effects, there are clearly situations in which fever is detrimental to patients. Body temperatures over 41°C lead to cellular dysfunction and death, and therefore urgent treatment is clearly indicated. Oxygen consumption increases by approximately 10% per degree Celsius.[27] Thus, patients in shock may be adversely affected by fever. In patients with any form of acute brain injury, elevated core temperature may significantly worsen the injury.[28–31] Therefore, clinical judgment becomes the most important role in determining whether or not treatment of fever itself is beneficial to the patient.

● Etiology of Fever in Critically Ill Patients

The presence of fever in critically ill patients often leads to an assumption of infection as the underlying cause (Table 22.1). However, there are numerous non-infectious causes of fever. Conversely, almost half of septic patients present with normothermia or hypothermia.[32] Therefore, a thorough approach to the assessment of febrile patients is as essential as is a constant vigilance for non-febrile infections.

Table 22.1 – Causes of Fever

1. Infection
2. Central Nervous System (intracranial bleeds, seizures)
3. Cardiovascular (myocardial infarction, Dressler's syndrome)
4. Pulmonary (chemical pneumonitis, pulmonary embolus, ARDS)
5. Gastrointestinal (pancreatitis, ischemic bowel, inflammatory disease)
6. Hepatobiliary (acalculous cholecystitis, non-infectious hepatitis)
7. Rheumatologic (vasculitis, gout, collagen vascular disease)
8. Integumentary (hematoma, burns)
9. Endocrine/Metabolic (adrenal insufficiency, thyroid, alcohol withdrawal)
10. Other (transfusion reaction, iatrogenic heating, cholesterol emboli, neoplasm)

The timing and severity of fever are important clues in determining the etiology of fever in critically ill patients. For unknown reasons, with few exceptions (see Table 22.2), non-infectious causes of fever rarely produce temperatures greater than 38.9°C.[33] A high fever should alert the physician to rule out infectious causes first before making the presumption of a non-infectious source. Except for drug fevers, the non-infectious causes of high fever are often clinically recognizable. Therefore, if no infectious cause is apparent, a thorough review of the patient's drug profile is in order.

As fever is part of the immune response of the body, any procedure that causes a significant inflammatory response has the potential to cause fever. Postoperative patients often develop a low-grade fever on the first or second day. These patients often account for the majority of febrile patients in general ICUs, with studies suggesting they are responsible for approximately 70% of these episodes. Classically, the fever was attributed to atelectasis. This belief is incorrect, as studies clearly demonstrate there is no relationship between fever and atelectasis in the absence of pulmonary infection.[34,35] Present belief suggests postoperative fever occurs as a non-specific inflammatory response to tissue injury. Likewise, with manipulation of any tissue, such as with catheterization or instrumentation, the presence of fever should not be alarming in the absence of other signs suggestive of sepsis. Interestingly, almost all fevers that did not persist after the first 72 hours postoperatively were not infectious in origin.[3]

Clinical clues as to the source of fever may be obtained from the timing of the onset of fever. Fever beginning more than 48 hours after intubation makes ventilator-associated pneumonia (VAP) a prime suspect. Likewise, persistent fever arising more than five days post-laparotomy should alert the physician

Table 22.2 – Causes of High Fever (> 38.9°C)

1. Infection (most likely)
2. Drug Fever
3. Transfusion Reaction
4. Extensive Tissue Necrosis
5. Neuroleptic Malignant Syndrome
6. Central Fever

to the possibility of an intra-abdominal abscess. Fever arising after more than seven days of broad-spectrum antibiotic use should always raise the possibility of fungal superinfection or pseudomembranous colititis.

Evaluation of fever in the critically ill patient must include an awareness of the issue of colonization. Many of the devices present in critically ill patients (e.g., endotracheal tubes, catheters, intravenous catheters, etc.) breach the normal host defences. Given enough time, all critically ill patients become colonized with the same bacteria and fungi responsible for causing infection in the ICU.[36] Routine cultures in patients with no signs of active infection have little value. The presence of abundant WBCs in a gram stain would however suggest concomitant inflammation and a greater likelihood that the organism is pathogenic rather than simply a colonizing agent. However, this generalization only applies to patients who can mount an inflammatory response (i.e., immunocompetent patients). Although the correlation of WBCs to likelihood of infection is suggestive, it is not pathognomonic. One must consider the overall clinical picture of critically ill patients when evaluating culture results to determine the likelihood of colonization versus infection.

● Infectious Causes of Fever in Critically Ill Patients

The most common causes of infection in critically ill patients arise from the lungs, indwelling catheters, urosepsis, and intra-abdominal sources. Although community acquired pneumonia (CAP) is the most common pneumonia, nosocomial and ventilator-associated pneumonia are important and distinct causes of fever. In addition to pneumonia, pleural effusions are often seen in critically ill patients and can be a hidden source of infection. Prosthetics, including indwelling catheters, represent a prime portal of entry for bacteria to invade the body. Organisms that are not normally pathogenic due to their inability to penetrate and invade the skin (e.g., Staphylococcus epidermidis), can produce bacteremia and sepsis by infecting an indwelling catheter. While infection often occurs at the entry site in the first two weeks after catheter insertion, intraluminal infection of access ports is often the source of infection in long-term catheters.[37] Although bacteriuria is a common

phenomenon, the lower genitourinary (GU) tract is rarely implicated as the source of urosepsis.[38] Bacteriuria however leads to bacteremia in less than 3% of patients.[39] Sepsis, often termed urosepsis if there is a GU source, is more likely due to the presence of ascending tract infection, obstruction or abscess (e.g., pyelonephritis, nephrolithiasis). Intra-abdominal sources of infection occur in patients who have undergone recent abdominal surgery or who are at risk for intra-abdominal infections (e.g., pancreatitis, portal hypertension, etc.). Some conditions, such as localized abscesses or spontaneous bacterial peritonitis, will not manifest with signs of peritoneal inflammation but will produce fever. Finally, patients who receive antibiotics and develop diarrhea may have fever due to Clostridium difficile colitis (pseudomembranous). Therefore, a high index of suspicion is essential in diagnosing intra-abdominal sources of infection in febrile patients with risk factors for such complications.

Although there are numerous other infectious causes of fever, these sites are considerably less common. Sinusitis has been reported to be present after a week of intubation in 85% of nasally intubated patients[40] and can occur if there is an indwelling nasogastric tube present.[41-43] Meningitis and encephalitis are possible sources of fever in patients presenting to hospital. These entities should be ruled out in patients with central nervous system (CNS) findings on exam. Except in patients with indwelling ventricular shunts or CNS trauma, nosocomial meningitis is uncommon. Persistent blood cultures, with or without fever, should raise the spectre of possible endocarditis. Intravenous drug abusers and patients with vascular grafts or prosthetics (e.g., valves) are at higher risk of developing infective endocarditis. In the absence of risk factors, endocarditis is an uncommon event. Soft tissue and skin infections are more commonly seen on presentation to the hospital but any invasion of the skin or soft tissue can lead to infection. With the increasing incidence of invasive soft tissue infections (e.g., necrotizing fasciitis), and the associated high morbidity and mortality, consider this source in the appropriate clinical setting. Febrile patients with severe soft tissue infections generally fall into two groups. The first, cases of invasive group A streptococcus (Streptococcus pyogenes), has been well publicized. The second important type of soft tissue infection is patients with polymicrobial necrotizing infections of the deep tissues. Cellulitis from Staphylococcus aureus can cause septic shock and fever without tissue necrosis. Surgical exploration and debridement of tissue remains paramount if a necrotizing infection is suspected.

There are two special groups of patients in which fever due to infection can occur: patients treated with antibiotics and patients with compromised immune systems. Any patient on broad-spectrum antibiotics for over a week who develops fever and signs of sepsis may have fungal superinfection. Estimates of fungal infections comprise anywhere from 7 to 17% of nosocomial ICU infections.[44,45] Since fungal colonization is common, it again is often difficult to distinguish colonization versus infection. Due to the high mortality of untreated fungal infection, consider empiric therapy in septic patients who develop fungemia or two or more positive culture sites for fungus. The presence of candidal endopthalmitis and hepatosplenic candidiasis would confirm the occurrence of disseminated candidiasis. Patients with compromised immune systems can develop numerous types of unusual infections. Febrile neutropenia patients deserve special mention. Unlike immunocompetent patients, febrile neutropenic patients can develop sepsis from even transient bacteremia. The gastrointestinal tract has been recognized as a source of fever and infection in febrile neutropenia because bacterial translocation is well documented in neutropenic patients. However, bacterial translocation is a diagnosis of exclusion, and all other potential sources of infection must be ruled out prior to making this diagnosis. While investigation of a febrile neutropenic patient is important, given the extent of immunosuppression, empiric therapy is recommended for all cases.

Non-infectious Causes of Fever in Critically Ill Patients

Non-infectious causes of fever will typically produce low-grade fevers.[1] Drugs are a common but often unrecognized cause of fever in critically ill patients. Antibiotics are most commonly implicated, but many other drugs can cause fever (e.g., neuroleptics). The fever can be high grade and often occurs at specific time intervals that coincide with the regular drug administration schedule. Other incidental findings include a drug rash (often papulomacular and diffuse) and eosinophilia on blood differentials.

Since these are non-specific findings, the only reliable diagnosis occurs with discontinuation of the drug and subsequent resolution of the fever. Drug withdrawal can also cause fever. Signs of delirium, agitation and sympathetic nervous system activation (e.g., tachycardia, hypertension, etc.) are helpful in supporting the diagnosis of withdrawal. Given the non-specific nature of these symptoms, an appropriate index of suspicion in patients dependent on alcohol, stimulants, sedatives or narcotic medications is indicated.

Febrile episodes can occur as the result of blood product transfusions. The fever typically occurs approximately 30 minutes after starting the transfusion and can last up to 24 hours. Leukocytosis may also be seen during this time but it should resolve within 12 to 24 hours. Deep venous thrombosis has been suggested as a potential cause of fever in the ICU. In the immobilized patient, DVT should be excluded for persistent fever with no other apparent cause. Acalculous cholecystitis is a source of infection in critically ill patients that can develop during hospitalization. The triggering mechanism appears to be a combination of local ischemia, bile stasis and depressed immune function. Infection is not the primary process but rather occurs as a secondary event. This problem is more common in patients on total parenteral nutrition. The remainder of the clinical conditions associated with fever in Table 22.1 should be clinically evident. It is important to remember that fever may persist as a result of a prolonged inflammatory response both during the acute illness and during the recovery phase. In these cases clinical features are essential in determining whether further investigation is warranted.

Assessment and Investigation of Fever in Critically Ill Patients

The Society of Critical Care Medicine (SCCM) and the Infectious Diseases Society of America (IDSA) developed guidelines on the evaluation of fever in critically ill patients.[5,46] These recommendations are based almost entirely on expert opinion in combination with non-randomized studies. These guidelines, along with subsequent expert reviews on evaluation of fever,[32,33] all rely on clinical expertise. This expertise has been underlined as the most important element in guiding investigation of fever in the critically ill patient, and should not be set aside in favour of an all-encompassing "shotgun" diagnostic approach.

As with all critically ill patients, prior to investigating the source of fever, resuscitation is the first priority. Attention to the ABC's, adequate volume replacement and hemodynamic stabilization are the mainstays of initial treatment in patients with fever. Patients should never be sent for investigations without prior stabilization. In many instances, it may be appropriate to place patients on hemodynamic and ventilator support to ensure stability while undergoing subsequent investigations.

After initiation of measures to stabilize patients, perform a directed history and physical exam with particular emphasis on the most likely sites of infection. As with the infectious causes of fever, the clinical situation is often extremely helpful in identifying the various non-infectious causes of fever (Table 22.1). A review of patient medications should be performed in the presence of unexplained fever. Due to mechanical ventilation, examination of the lungs often fails to reveal specific findings. While clinical features of peritonitis on the abdominal exam are extremely helpful, these signs are often absent in critically ill patients due to sedatives, analgesics, immunosuppressed states or altered levels of consciousness. Further examination and investigation should be directed based on the clinical presentation. A patient who is deteriorating rapidly requires a more aggressive approach than one who is simply febrile.

Initial investigations in febrile critically ill patients (Table 22.3) include a complete blood count, electrolytes, creatinine, coagulation profile, chest x-ray and electrocardiogram. In cases of severe shock, consider ordering liver enzymes and lipase to assess hepatic and pancreatic status. Elevation of liver enzymes may raise clinical suspicion for cholecystitis, cholangitis or hepatitis. Elevated lipase levels are suggestive of pancreatitis. Patients should have blood cultures drawn, preferably from two different sites. Additional culture sites should be performed according the clinical presentation. A sputum culture with gram stain is appropriate for patients presenting with respiratory symptoms or those ventilated for more than 48 hours. Particular attention should be paid to the gram stain of the sputum, as the presence of WBCs would suggest a higher likelihood of active infection. The role of bronchoscopy is controversial but should be considered if an unusual pathogen is

suspected (e.g., Pneumocystis carinii, mycobacteria, etc.).[47,48] In febrile patients with pleural effusions and no other identifiable source, thoracentesis or thoracostomy drainage are indicated to rule out empyema. Patients with diarrhea should have stool sent for C. difficile toxin assay.

Any investigation of fever should include a review of catheters and their insertion sites. Patients with suspected catheter-related infections should have the catheter removed. In all instances, catheter tips should be sent for culture. The presence of greater than 15 colony-forming units (CFUs) suggests an infected site whereas negative cultures or those with less than 15 CFUs are considered to be clean. In some select cases where intravenous access is difficult, catheter exchange over a guide wire may be considered. Consideration of sources of infection should include a review of all prosthetic material in patients (e.g., heart valves, joints, etc.).

Radiographic investigations are important tests to find sources of infection. A chest x-ray is indicated in virtually all febrile patients. Radiographic views of the abdomen can demonstrate the presence of free air indicative of viscous organ perforation. Ultrasonography may detect intra-abdominal or pelvic abscesses or biliary tract disease, but CT scans are generally the superior method to detect intra-abdominal pathology. Aspiration of known fluid collections under radiographic guidance may assist in diagnosis and the treatment of intra-abdominal abscesses. Although positive findings are helpful, all of these investigations have relatively low sensitivity. Ultimately, the definitive test is a diagnostic laparotomy, and early consultation with the General Surgery service for assistance is appropriate. If urosepsis is suspected as a cause for fever, imaging of the entire system is necessary to confirm the diagnosis and to rule out pathology in ascending tract involvement.

In the postoperative patient, fever alone within the first 48 to 72 hours does not typically warrant investigation. In cases of persistent fever or worsening clinical status, careful exploration of the surgical wound site is an important but often overlooked step in evaluating the septic patient. Exploration and drainage of infected tissue is essential for both diagnosis and treatment of wound infection.

The diagnosis of acalculous cholecystitis is a difficult one since there are no specific features. It should always be considered in critically ill

Table 22.3 – Investigations of Fever in Critically Ill Patients

Source	Investigations	Comments
Initial Screen	History & physical examination CBC, electrolytes, urea, creatinine, coagulation screen, liver enzymes, blood cultures, chest x-ray, electrocardiogram	Important in assessment of severity of sepsis; look for clinical sites of infection
Pneumonia	Sputum sample (tracheal aspirate) +/- bronchoscopy (2nd line)	Consider bronchoscopy if unusual organism suspected
Pleural Effusion	Thoracentesis and/or Thoracostomy tube drainage	Drainage essential if suspected source of infection
Line Sepsis	Removal of intravenous catheter	Change of site ideal therapy
Intra-Abdominal Sepsis	CT abdomen +/- pelvis U/S abdomen (fluid collections) Contrast studies (anastomotic leak) Surgical exploration	CT & other radiographic tests insensitive; if index of suspicion high, must consider surgical exploration
Urosepsis	U/S abdomen (hydronephrosis) IVP +/- cystogram/cystoscopy	Rule out obstruction, nephrolithiasis and/or abscess
Sinusitis	Sinus x-rays (plain vs. CT) Sinus aspiration if present	Consider if purulent drainage and source of nasal obstruction present
Fungal Infection	Cultures in blood or 2+ tissue sites	Consider if broad-spectrum antibiotic or immunosuppression
CNS	Lumbar puncture +/- CT head EEG +/- MRI (encephalitis)	Do not delay treatment! CT if increased ICP suspected
Skin/Soft Tissue	Surgical exploration Consider CT/MRI	First priority is assessment for surgical exploration
Endocarditis	Repeated blood cultures	Diagnosis difficult; based on clinical and microbiological data

CBC = complete blood count; IVP = intravenous pyelogram; EEG = electroencephalogram; MRI = magnetic resonance imaging; ICP = intracranial pressure; U/S = ultrasound; CT = computed tomography

patients, especially those patients on parenteral nutrition. The clinical examination, however, is often unimpressive. Ultrasound may demonstrate an increase in gallbladder wall thickness or distension, although this is a non-specific finding. A normal scan virtually rules out the possibility of acalculous cholecystitis. The diagnosis must therefore be made on both clinical and radiographic findings. The treatment for suspected acalculous cholecystitis in the majority of patients is percutaneous cholecystostomy. Although there is no clear consensus on empiric antibiotic therapy, in cases with high risk of bacterial translocation due to necrosis or perforation, broad-spectrum antibiotic therapy appears reasonable.

Patients with suspected meningitis need immediate evaluation and investigations. Controversy exists on the role of routine CT scans to ensure that a lumbar puncture can be safely performed. Clearly, a CT scan is indicated if there is a clinical suspicion of increased intracranial pressure or an intracerebral lesion. If there is to be any delay in diagnosis, treatment should be instituted prior to these investigations, given the risk of neurologic morbidity and mortality with any delay in therapy.

Echocardiography (trans-thoracic or esophageal) can be helpful to detect valvular vegetations. Clinical examination and CT scans may demonstrate areas with embolic complications but such investigations have low sensitivity. Most importantly, the diagnosis of endocarditis requires clinical, microbiological and/or echocardiographic criteria to be present.

Unfortunately, diagnosis of sinusitis in critically ill patients is especially difficult, given that radiological evidence of sinusitis correlates very poorly with the presence of infectious sinusitis.[41-43] Sinus films, including a Waters view, often demonstrate the presence of fluid levels, as do CT scans. The presence of sinus fluid is non-specific, and aspiration of the fluid should be considered if it is the only possible source of fever present and the diagnosis remains in doubt.

● Management of Fever in the Critically Ill Patient

Management of critically ill patients should focus on three key elements: resuscitation, the decision to use empiric therapy if infection is suspected and the value of actual treatment of the fever itself. A concurrent management strategy in critically ill patients mandates that resuscitation always remain the first priority. As always, ABC assessment and stabilization remain the highest priorities. In keeping with a concurrent management approach, assessment and management of fever in critically ill patients takes place in conjunction with the resuscitation process.

The decision to begin empiric antibiotic therapy ultimately rests on the clinical suspicion of the physician. Remember, in many types of infection, early treatment affects both mortality and morbidity. Given the risks involved in withholding therapy, this often results in the use of empiric antibiotic therapy. It is crucial, however, that the physician employ clinical judgment to guide empiric antibiotic therapy. Given the wide variety of antibiotics and their differing spectrums of antimicrobial coverage, identifying the most likely sources of infection and tailoring empiric therapy towards these sources is essential.

Physicians should be aware of several caveats regarding empiric therapy for critically ill patients. Empiric antibiotics simply encompass the recommendations, a summary of several consensus statements and expert opinions. Presently there are no globally accepted guidelines for empiric antibiotic selection. Regional variations in microbiological spectrum of infecting organisms, new antibiotics and increasing antibiotic resistance have made a uniform set of guidelines impossible to implement. Furthermore, as these patterns of infection change, recommendations can become obsolete in a matter of years. The second caveat is that therapy is guided on probability. The physician therefore must be ready to alter empiric therapy based on culture results, *in the appropriate clinical setting*. In the face of changing clinical and culture information, the diagnosis should be revisited and re-evaluated. Empiric therapy should never simply continue "because the patient got better on that therapy"; rather, continuation reflects an inability to further narrow treatment because of negative culture results or the discovery of an organism only treated by that empiric choice. Patients who are clinically worsening on appropriate empiric antibiotic therapy should have their diagnosis and the choice of antibiotics revisited (Table 22.4). Clinical judgment should serve as the foundation to guide empiric therapy and modify therapy when new information indicates a change is in order.

The role for treatment of fever in adult patients remains unclear. Although in vitro and animal studies suggest there are beneficial effects from elevated body temperature, the lack of human studies demonstrating clear benefit makes a general recommendation for or against active treatment of fever difficult. There are circumstances in which fever can have detrimental effects if not treated. Patients with fevers greater than

---

Table 22.4 – Causes of Antibiotic Failure

1. Incorrect Diagnosis (non-infectious problem, drug fever)
2. Inappropriate Dosing
3. Inadequate Drug Penetration (e.g., abscess, blood brain barrier, foreign body)
4. Inadequate Empiric Coverage
5. Incorrect Spectrum (in vivo differs from in vitro results)
6. Superinfection (especially fungal)
7. Drug Interactions (antibiotic inactivation, antagonism)
8. Untreatable Infectious Disease
9. Unusual Pathogen (e.g., Rickettsia, Chlamydia, parasites)

41°C should be treated, since there is a risk of cellular dysfunction and death. Similarly, febrile patients in refractory shock would benefit from the reduction in oxygen consumption achieved by the reduction of core body temperature. In addition, given the current evidence suggesting potential benefit with hypothermia, reduction of fever in patients with acute brain injury should also be undertaken.

Present therapies for cooling patients include antipyretic agents and physical cooling. Since they exert their cooling effects by different mechanisms (central action versus increased heat loss), critically ill patients are usually treated with both therapies. More invasive measures used to warm patients in severe hypothermia (e.g., intravenous solutions, irrigation of visceral organs, cardiopulmonary bypass) are not routinely used with febrile patients, given the morbidity associated with each measure and the unclear benefits of temperature reduction.

Finally, temperature reduction and empiric antibiotic therapy are not the only aspects of treatment for patients with a suspected source of infection. The discovery and definitive treatment of the source of infection as well as aggressive supportive therapy are just as important as antibiotics in the treatment of febrile patients. Likewise, the discovery of a non-infectious cause of fever mandates the prompt institution of definitive therapy for these non-infectious entities whenever possible.

● Summary

The evaluation and management of fever in critically ill patients can be challenging. Although non-infectious causes of fever are possible, the possibility of infection should always be considered, especially when the temperature is greater than 38.9°C. Patients should always be appropriately resuscitated prior to a clinically directed investigation for the source of fever. Empiric antibiotic therapy is often used but should be refined once additional information is obtained. Antibiotic therapy is however only one component for the management of infection, since many infections require drainage or removal of infected material. Furthermore, patients should always be re-evaluated and the diagnosis challenged if they deteriorate despite therapy. Treatment of fever itself is controversial but is clearly indicated in some settings. Ultimately, decisions on evaluation and management of fever in critically ill patients rely not on the use of diagnostic algorithms or batteries of laboratory tests, but on a rational use of these resources guided by sound clinical judgment.

Key Points

- Fever (over 38.3°C) is an extremely common problem in critically ill patients.
- The gold standard for measurement is from the pulmonary artery but rectal and ear thermometry are also acceptable.
- Animal studies suggest fever is beneficial, but no controlled human studies evaluating its benefit exist.
- Fever treatment is controversial but is indicated if the patient's temperature is over 41°C, the patient is in shock or there is acute brain injury.
- Non-infectious causes of fever rarely produce temperatures over 38.9°C.

- Common infectious sources are the lungs, indwelling catheters, urosepsis and abdominal sources.
- Patients must be resuscitated prior to clinically investigating sources of fever.
- Antibiotics are only part of management, since infections require drainage or removal of infected material.
- Empiric antibiotics are based on consensus statements, and recommendations change frequently.
- Be ready to alter empiric therapy once additional information is obtained.

References

1. Cunha BA, Shea KW: Fever in the intensive care unit. *Inf Dis Clin North Amer* 1996;10:185–209.

2. Arons MM, Wheeler AP, Bernard GR, et al: Effects of ibuprofen on the physiology and survival of hypothermic sepsis. Ibuprofen in Sepsis Study Group. *Crit Care Med* 1999;27:699–707.

3. Circiamaru B, Baldock G, Cohen J: A prospective study of fever in the intensive care unit. *Intens Care Med* 1999;25:668–73.

4. Mackowiak PA, Wasserman SS, Levine MM: A critical appraisal of 98.6 degrees F, the upper limit of the normal body temperature, and other legacies of Carl Reinhold August Wunderlich. *JAMA* 1992;268:1578–80.

5. O'Grady NP, Barie PS, Bartlett J, et al: Practice parameters for evaluating new fever in critically ill adult patients. Task Force of the American College of Critical Care Medicine of the Society of Critical Care Medicine in collaboration with the Infectious Diseases Society of America. *Crit Care Med* 1998;26:392–408.

6. Schmitz T, Bair N, Falk M, Levine C: A comparison of five methods of temperature measurement in febrile intensive care patients. *Amer J Crit Care* 1995;4:282–92.

7. Milewski A, Ferguson KL, Terndrup TE: Comparison of pulmonary artery, rectal and tympanic membrane temperatures in adult intensive care unit patients. *Clin Pediatr* 1991;30(4 suppl):13–16.

8. Nierman DM: Core temperature measurement in the intensive care unit. *Crit Care Med* 1991;19:818–23.

9. Erickson RS, Kirklin SK: Comparison of ear-based, bladder, oral and axillary methods for core temperature measurement. *Crit Care Med* 1993;21:1528–34.

10. Hayward JS, Eckerson JD, Kemna D: Thermal and cardiovascular changes during three months of resuscitation from mild hypothermia. *Resuscitation* 1984;11:21–33.

11. Shiraki K, Konda N, Sagawa S: Esophageal and tympanic temperature responses to core blood temperature changes during hyperthermia. *J Appl Physiol* 1986;61:98–102.

12. Shiraki K, Sagawa S, Tajima F, et al: Independence of brain and tympanic temperatures in an unanesthetized human. *J Appl Physiol* 1988;65:482–6.

13. Leon LR: Invited review: Cytokine regulation of fever: Studies using gene knockout mice. *J Appl Physiol* 2002;92:2648–55.

14. Boulant JA: Role of the preoptic-anterior hypothalamus in thermoregulation and fever. *Clin Infect Dis* 2000;31(suppl 5):S157–61.

15. Bernheim HA, Kluger MJ: Fever and antipyresis in the lizard Dipsosaurus dorsalis. *Am J Physiol* 1976;231:198–203.

16. Jampel HD, Duff GW, Gershon RK, et al: Fever and immunoregulation: III. Hyperthermia augments the primary in vitro humoral immune response. *J Exp Med* 1983;157:1229–38.

17. van Oss CJ, Absolom DR, Moore LL, et al: Effect of temperature on the chemotaxis, phagocytic engulfment, digestion and O_2 consumption of human polymorphonuclear leukocytes. *J Reitculoendothel Soc* 1980;27:561–5.

18. Biggar WD, Gohn DJ, Kent G, et al: Neutrophil migration in vitro and in vivo during hypothermia. *Infect Immunity* 1984;46:857–9.

19. Azocar J, Ynis EJ, Essex M. Sensitivity of human natural killer cells to hyperthermia. *Lancet* 1982;1(8262):16–7.

20. Muschenheim C, Duerschrer DR, Hardy JD: Hypothermia in experimental infections: III. The effect of hypothermia on resistance to experimental pneumococcus infection. *J Infect Dis* 1943;72:187–96.

21. Strouse S: Experimental studies in pneumococcal infections. *J Exp Med* 1909; 11:743–61.

22. Kluger MJ, Kozak W, Conn CA, et al: The adaptive value of fever. *Infect Dis Clin North Am* 1996;10:1–20.

23. Ryan M, Levy MM: Clinical review: Fever in intensive care unit patients. *Crit Care* 2003;7:221–5.

24. Kiang JG, Tsokos GC: Heat shock protein 70 kDA: Molecular biology, biochemistry, and physiology. *Pharmacol Ther* 1998;80:183–201.

25. Bryant RE, Hood AF, Hood CE, Koenig MG: Factors affecting mortality of gram-negative rod bacteremia. *Arch Int Med* 1971;127:120–8.

26. Weinstein MP, Iannini PB, Stratton CW, Eickhoff TC: Spontaneous bacterial peritonitis: A review of 28 cases with emphasis on improved survival and factors influencing prognosis. *Am J Med* 1978;64:592–8.

27. Manthous CA, Hall JB, Olson D, et al: Effect of cooling on oxygen consumption in febrile critically ill patients. *Am J Respir Crit Care Med* 1995;151:10–4.

28. Bernard SA, Buist M: Induced hypothermia in critical care medicine: A review. *Crit Care Med* 2003;31:2041–51.

29. Cairns CJ, Andrews PJ: Management of hyperthermia in traumatic brain injury. *Curr Opin Crit Care* 2002;8:106–10.

30. Natale JE, Joseph JG, Helfaer MA, Shaffner DH: Early hyperthermia after traumatic brain injury in children: Risk factors, influence on length of stay, and effect on short-term neurologic status. *Crit Care Med* 2000;28:2608–15.

31. Hickey RW, Kochanek PM, Ferimer H, et al: Hypothermia and hyperthermia in children after resuscitation from cardiac arrest. *Pediatrics* 2000;106:118–22.

32. Marik, PE: Fever in the ICU. *Chest* 2000;117:855–69.

33. Cunha, BA: Fever in the critical care unit. *Crit Care Clin* 1998;14:1–14.

34. Engoren, M: Lack of association between atelectasis and fever. *Chest* 1995;107:81–84.

35. Lansing AM, Jamieson WG: Mechanism of fever in pulmonary atelectasis. *Arch Surg* 1963;87:168–174.

36. Bergen GA, Toney JF: Infection versus colonization in the critical care unit. *Crit Care Clin* 1998;14:71–90.

37. O'Grady NP, Alexander M, Dellinger EP, et al: Guidelines for the prevention of intravascular catheter-related infections. *Am J Infect Control* 2002;30:476–89.

38. Stark RP, Maki DG: Bacteriuria in the catheterized patient: What quantitative level of bacteriuria is relevant? *N Engl J Med* 1984;311:560–4.

39. Krieger JN, Kaiser DL, Wenzel RP: Urinary tract etiology of bloodstream infections in hospitalized patients. *J Infect Dis* 1983;148:57–62.

40. Hansen M, Poulsen MR, Bendixen DK, Hartmann-Andersen F: Incidence of sinusitis in patients with nasotracheal intubation. *Br J Anaesth* 1988;61:231–2.

41. Grindlinger GA, Niehoff J, Hughes SL, et al: Acute paranasal sinusitis related to nasotracheal intubation of head-injured patients. *Crit Care Med* 1987;15:214–7.

42. Deutschaman CS, Wilton P, Sinow J, et al: Paranasal sinusitis associated with nasotracheal intubation: A frequently unrecognized and treatable source of sepsis. *Crit Care Med* 1986;14:111–4.

43. Rouby JJ, Laurent P, Gosnach M, et al: Risk factors and clinical relevance of nosocomial maxillary sinusitis in the critically ill. *Am J Respir Crit Care Med* 1994;150:776–83.

44. Vincent JL, Bihari DJ, Suter PM, et al: The prevalence of nosocomial infection in intensive care units in Europe: Results of the European Prevalence of Infection in Intensive Care (EPIC) Study. EPIC International Advisory Committee. *JAMA* 1995;274:639–44.

45. Beck-Sague C, Jarvis WR: Secular trends in the epidemiology of nosocomial fungal infections in the United States, 1980–1990. National Nosocomial Infections Surveillance System. *J Infect Dis* 1993;167:1247–51.

46. O'Grady NP, Barie PS, Bartlett J, et al: Practice guidelines for evaluation new fever in critically ill adult patients. Task Force of the Society of Critical Care Medicine and the Infectious Diseases Society of America. *Clin Inf Dis* 1998;26:1042–59.

47. Luna CM, Vujacich P, Niederman MS, et al: Impact of BAL data on the therapy and outcome of ventilator-associated pneumonia. *Chest* 1997;111:676–85.

48. Rello J, Gallego M, Mariscal D, et al: The value of routine microbial investigation in ventilator-associated pneumonia. *Am J Respir Crit Care Med* 1997;156:196–200.

ANTIMICROBIAL THERAPY

R. Bruce Light

You are asked to see a 63-year-old man who was brought to the hospital because of confusion. He has a blood pressure of 80/40 mm Hg, heart rate of 120/ min, tachypnea at 35/min, and has a temperature of 39.5˚C. You begin to resuscitate him using the ABC's and practice concurrent management along with frequent reassessments. It is becoming clear that he likely has sepsis but it is unclear where the focus is. Should you start him on antibiotics? If so, when and which drugs?

Antimicrobial therapy that is both appropriate and timely is a crucial element in the chain of survival for patients with severe sepsis or septic shock, a chain that also includes prompt recognition of the presence of severe sepsis, rapid resuscitation where required, a careful diagnostic approach to the cause of sepsis, timely control of the source of sepsis by surgery or other means and thoughtful application of endocrinologic or metabolic supportive measures. The two key elements of delivery of adequate antimicrobial therapy—appropriateness and timeliness—have somewhat different determinants, which need to be separately addressed to avoid the two most common errors: rapidly delivering the wrong therapy, or delivering optimal therapy too late to do any good.

Antimicrobial therapy for severe sepsis or septic shock should be selected to ensure a near 100% probability of covering the responsible pathogen. It has been repeatedly shown that, in patients with severe sepsis or bacteremia, administration of an antimicrobial ineffective against the pathogen, doubles the risk of septic shock and, in patients who are already in shock, doubles the risk of death.[1-5] In order to minimize the risk of making this error, the physician must synthesize the available information bearing on the likelihood of involvement by different groups of pathogens in the individual patient and knowledge about the likely antimicrobial susceptibility patterns for those pathogens, and adopt a conservative antimicrobial selection approach, erring on the side of wider rather than narrower coverage in the initial instance. Information that bears on which pathogens are likely and their probable susceptibility pattern include: the likely site of the infection; the types of pathogens usually causing infection at that site; the usual antimicrobial susceptibility of those pathogens; the local or regionally specific antimicrobial susceptibility/resistance patterns for those pathogens; and the risk that the patient has become colonized with resistant pathogens (e.g., hospitalization, prior antimicrobial exposure).

Effective antimicrobial therapy for severe sepsis or septic shock should be administered as quickly as possible after the presumptive diagnosis is made. Even the most intelligent choice of therapy may be ineffective if given too late. There is now increasing evidence that every hour of delay in delivering an effective antimicrobial is associated with a measurable increase in the risk of death,[6–9] and increasingly it is being recognized that many hospital systems are failing to meet the test of timeliness for getting drugs from the pharmacy shelf to the patient. Delay can occur for many reasons: physicians spend time trying to better define the diagnosis before writing an antimicrobial prescription; order processing by staff takes time to do or is down the list of competing priorities; pharmacies take time to fill prescriptions or fail to prioritize urgent requests; transport delays occur; or slow preparation and administration of drug occur due to competing nursing task priorities at the bedside of these complex cases. While addressing these problems should be a system priority, in individual cases it falls to the attending physician to pay some specific attention to ensuring that prescribed treatment happens immediately in this highly vulnerable patient group.

In this chapter, we will review which pathogens are most important at which sites, which antimicrobials are generally effective against the different pathogen groups, and the factors that place patients at increased risk of infection with resistant pathogens. A brief review of selected antimicrobials is presented. Finally, an approach to the antibiotic selection for certain septic presentations is discussed.

● Overview of Antimicrobial Agents

In this section we will briefly review the commonly used antimicrobials, emphasizing their specific spectra of antimicrobial activity, common areas of use, relevant aspects of pharmacology and pharmacokinetics, and common misconceptions or pitfalls in the use of these agents. There will be no attempt to be comprehensive in covering all the agents in the different classes; rather, the most commonly used and widely available agents in each class will be discussed.

A. Beta-Lactam Antibiotics

As their name suggests, these antibiotics share the common feature of having the beta-lactam ring in their structure. The beta-lactams act by interfering with bacterial cell wall synthesis and are thus considered to be bactericidal. The beta-lactams are typically divided into three categories: penicillins, cephalosporins and carbapenems.

1. Penicillins[10]

Although there are a large number of penicillins and derivatives available, for practical purposes only three are regularly used in the treatment of severe sepsis: ampicillin, cloxacillin (and similar agents such as methicillin or nafcillin), and piperacillin (usually together with the beta-lactamase inhibitor tazobactam).

a. ampicillin – This is an aminopenicillin administered parenterally with activity against most Streptococcal spp. with the exception of some enterococci and penicillin-resistant pneumococci, meningococci, Listeria, and most anaerobes (except the Bacteroides fragilis group). Ampicillin has activity against the majority of community-acquired Hemophilus spp. and enteric gram-negatives, but cannot be relied upon for these, because resistance rates can be 20–30%. It is not active against bacteria that produce beta-lactamases, including most staphylococci.

Despite its long usage, ampicillin still has a number of legitimate uses in the treatment of severe sepsis, usually as part of a multi-drug treatment regimen. Even in the era of relative penicillin resistance among pneumococci, ampicillin often is included in regimens for the initial treatment of acute bacterial meningitis, along with a third generation cephalosporin and/or vancomycin. The recommendation for its use reflects the fact that it has good activity against meningococcus and most pneumococcus and is also an effective agent for Listeria.

Ampicillin has activity against most enterococci and thus is often used along with other agents in biliary sepsis, intra-abdominal sepsis and urinary tract infections. For the biliary tract and intra-abdominal infections additional drugs are added to better cover enteric gram-negatives (i.e., cephalosporin, quinolone, aminoglycoside) as well as beta-lactamase producing anaerobes such as Bacteroides fragilis (e.g., metronidazole). In urinary tract infections, ampicillin with an aminoglycoside is still a very good choice providing good coverage for both the enterococci and nearly all enteric gram-negatives commonly causing these infections.

Since ampicillin is excreted in the urine, its usual dosing must be reduced in the presence of significant renal insufficiency (Table 23.1). Failure to make this adjustment can lead to drug accumulation with attendant neurotoxicity, signaled by muscular irritability, myoclonic jerks and eventually seizures. The only other significant adverse reaction problems are those related to hypersensitivity, including both anaphylaxis and fixed drug eruption (relatively common but does not preclude use of the drug when the indication is solid). Importantly, ampicillin is frequently (up to 8%) implicated in causing morbilliform fixed drug eruptions occurring a few days after starting the drug, a reaction that is not immunologically mediated. While ampicillin may have to be stopped when this occurs, a history of past occurrence of this rash is not a contraindication to ampicillin or to later therapy with other pencillins or cephalosporins.

b. cloxacillin – This penicillinase-resistant penicillin, along with similar drugs such as nafcillin, has excellent activity against Staphylococcus aureus. Aside from the methicillin resistant Staphylococcus aureus (MRSA) strains, cloxacillin can be considered the drug of choice when this is the leading diagnostic consideration. In the doses used for severe sepsis (Table 23.1), it is generally sufficient to treat Streptococcus pyogenes, which is usually in the differential diagnosis of sepsis due to soft-tissue infections. Cloxacillin shares the usual modest risk of hypersensitivity reactions associated with penicillins, and has also occasionally been implicated in a delayed hypersensitivity reaction causing interstitial nephritis. Unlike most other beta-lactam antibiotics, cloxacillin does not require dosage adjustment for renal insufficiency.

c. piperacillin – This drug alone or in combination with tazobactam has come to be the most commonly used antimicrobial among the group of anti-pseudomonal or extended-spectrum penicillin, which also includes ticarcillin, carbenicillin, azlocillin and mezlocillin.[11] The anti-bacterial spectrum of piperacillin includes all of the microbes covered by ampicillin, but extends coverage to many ampicillin-resistant gram-negatives including many Pseudomonas spp. and most anaerobes. The addition of the beta-lactamase inhibitor tazobactam to piperacillin further extends the spectrum to many other beta-lactamase producing enteric gram-negatives, anaerobes and methicillin-susceptible Staphylococcus aureus. However, the beta-lactamases of Pseudomonas spp., Enterobacter spp. and some other related gram-negatives with inducible beta-lactamases are *not* susceptible to tazobactam, making it is unwise to solely rely on piperacillin for these infections; treatment should also include an aminoglycoside or fluoroquinolone.

Due to the wide spectrum of anti-bacterial activity, piperacillin/tazobactam has become a common choice for empiric "broad-spectrum" coverage for sepsis of unclear origin or for intra-

Table 23.1 – Dosages of Selected Penicillins Used to Treat Severe Sepsis

	Usual Dose for Severe Sepsis	Dose Adjustment for Renal Insufficiency
Ampicillin	2 g iv q6h	CrCl < 10 ml/min - 2–3 g iv q12h
Cloxacillin	2 g iv q4h	no change
Piperacillin/ Tazobactam	3.375 g iv q4–6h*	CrCl < 50 ml/min - 3.375 g iv q12h

*For suspected Pseudomonas spp. sepsis use higher dosing frequency and combine with an aminoglycoside or quinolone.

abdominal sepsis. It is well suited to these uses but requires supplementation with additional agents if the patient is at risk for MRSA, ampicillin-resistant enterococcus, Pseudomonas spp., Enterobacter spp. or other related organisms.

Since piperacillin is renally excreted, dose regimens require adjustments in the presence of renal insufficiency (Table 23.1). Adverse drug reactions for piperacillin are similar to other penicillins and, like ampicillin, fixed drug eruptions are somewhat more common with piperacillin. Drug accumulation can cause neurotoxicity and, less commonly, inhibition of platelet function.

2. Cephalosporins[12]

As a group, the cephalosporins are the most widely used class of antibiotics in the initial treatment of severe sepsis. They are generally classified into four "generations," based on their historical order of appearance and their antimicrobial spectrum. As a general rule, first (cefazolin) and second generation (cefuroxime, cefoxitin) cephalosporins have good activity against gram-positives such as staphylococci and non-enterococcal streptococci but limited activity against enteric gram-negatives. The third generation agents (cefotaxime, ceftriaxone) have better gram-negative activity with relatively preserved gram-positive coverage. Some of the third generation drugs (ceftazidime) have excellent gram-negative and pseudomonal activity, but reduced coverage of gram-positives. So-called fourth generation agents such as cefipime combine the anti-pseudomonal effect with gram-positive activity similar to first generation cephalosporins.

As a group, the cephalosporins are generally non-toxic with the main problem being allergic reactions. The majority of these agents require dosage adjustment for renal insufficiency (Table 23.2) and all share a similar propensity to produce hypersensitivity reactions. There is a pervasive and persistent myth that cephalosporins need to be avoided in all patients with a history of reactions to penicillins. In fact, evidence of predictable cross-reactivity is extremely sparse (though, of course, any patient can coincidentally be allergic to two different drugs), and there is no good reason to withhold these agents from penicillin-allergic patients with severe sepsis for whom these would normally be the preferred choice.[13,14]

Although there are a great many other cephalosporins available other than those listed below, and many have definite merits, it is suggested that clinicians and hospitals be very familiar and comfortable with a few selected agents, in order

Table 23.2 – Cephalosporin and Carbapenem Doses for Severe Sepsis

	Usual Dose for Severe Sepsis	Dosage Adjustment for Renal Insufficiency*
Cefazolin	2 g iv q8h	CrCl < 50 ml/min - 2 g iv q12h CrCl < 25 ml/min - 1 g iv q24h CrCl < 10 ml/min - 0.5 g iv q24h
Cefuroxime	1.5 g iv q8h	CrCl < 25 ml/min - 0.75 g iv q12h CrCl < 10 ml/min - 0.75 g iv q24h
Cefotaxime	2 g iv q6-8h	CrCl < 25 ml/min - 2 g iv q8h CrCl < 10 ml/min - 2 g iv q12h
Ceftriaxone	2–4 g iv q24h	no change
Ceftazidime	2 g iv q8h	CrCl < 50ml/min - 1.5 g iv q12h CrCl < 25 ml/min - 1.5 g iv q24h CrCl < 10 ml/min - 1 g iv q24h
Cefepime	2 g iv q12h	
Meropenem	1 g iv q8h	

*Initial dose should be the full usual dose in all cases, followed by doses reduced appropriately for renal function.

to avoid errors due to confusing one agent and its properties with another similar or similarly spelled agent. For example, consider the similar spelling but differing properties of cefotaxime, cefoxitin and ceftizoxime: ceftizoxime has useful anti-pseudomonal activity, while the others do not; cefoxitin is a useful anti-anaerobic agent while the others are not; cefotaxime penetrates the cerebral spinal fluid and is a good agent for meningitis, while cefoxitin is not.

In general, the antibacterial spectrum of the cephalosporin generations together with the risks associated with under-treating a severe infection dictate the choice of cephalosporin. First and second generation agents, because they do not provide good coverage for relatively resistant common enteric gram-negatives, are mainly used in less severely ill patients with skin and soft tissue infections likely due to staphylococci or streptococci (cefazolin) or less severe respiratory infections likely due to the common upper respiratory bacterial flora (cefuroxime). Although cefuroxime has some cerebral spinal fluid penetration, it, along with other first and second generation cephalosporins, cannot be relied upon for treatment of central nervous system (CNS) infections. The third generation agents, cefotaxime or ceftriaxone, are best used for more severe infections where possibilities include, in addition to the above, enteric gram-negatives that may be resistant to generations one and two. Anti-pseudomonal coverage is generally required only in patients at particular risk for this infection, based on the presence of patient risk factors such as long-standing structural lung disease, or epidemiologic factors such as a long hospital stay in an intensive care unit (ICU) with prior exposure to broad-spectrum antibiotics.

a. cefazolin – This is the prototype first generation parenteral cephalosporin. It has excellent activity against methicillin susceptible Staphylococcus aureus and non-enterococcal streptococci. It also covers a limited range of enteric gram-negatives such as community-acquired E. coli and Klebsiella spp., but does not have useful activity against Hemophilus spp., Moraxella spp., more resistant gram-negatives, or anaerobes. Thus, cefazolin is used primarily for skin and soft-tissue infections likely to be due to staphylococci or streptococci, or as part of a multi-drug regimen for less severe intra-abdominal infections in patients unlikely to be infected with more resistant pathogens.

b. cefuroxime – This second generation agent has activity against the same organisms as cefazolin with the addition of beta-lactamase producing strains of Hemophilus spp and Moraxella spp., making this a useful agent for less-sick patients with respiratory tract infections likely to be due to one of the usual relatively susceptible community-acquired respiratory pathogens.

c. cefoxitin – This is another second generation cephalosporin that has activity similar to cefazolin. The additional effect of cefoxitin is its activity against most anaerobes, making it a useful drug for mixed aerobic/anaerobic infections (e.g., intra-abdominal infections, diabetic foot infections) in which the risk of relatively resistant enteric gram-negatives is low.

d. cefotaxime and **ceftriaxone** – These drugs are both third generation cephalosporins that combine reasonably good gram-positive activity with coverage of the most common respiratory and enteric gram-negative bacteria (but without anti-pseudomonal activity). They are among the most commonly prescribed agents for "basic" empiric treatment of severe sepsis arising from the respiratory tract, skin and soft-tissue, and from intra-abdominal sources (combined with an additional agent for anaerobic coverage).
Cefotaxime's pharmacokinetics are similar to most other cephalosporins thus resulting in a recommendation for three to four daily doses and dose adjustment for renal insufficiency (Table 23.2). Ceftriaxone, however, is more highly protein bound, giving it a longer serum half-life, and is excreted largely by non-renal clearance. Ceftriaxone can therefore be given as a single daily dose without adjustment for renal function, making it easy to dose and convenient to use. Ceftriaxone is especially useful in situations where a long interval between doses may occur, such as transport of a septic patient from a remote location. Both drugs have minimal toxicities associated with their use aside from the usual risk of hypersensitivity associated with all beta-lactams.

e. ceftazidime – This drug is another third generation cephalosporin with an activity spectrum similar to others of this class with two important differences: good anti-pseudomonal coverage but poor activity against Staphylococcus aureus. The enhanced activity against Pseudomonas spp. makes ceftazidime one of the drugs of choice for this group of organisms. The reduced activity against Staphylococcus aureus is significant to the extent that if this organism is a serious consideration, a second agent should be added to the treatment regimen to cover it.

f. cefepime – This so-called fourth generation cephalosporin combines the anti-gram-negative and anti-pseudomonal activity of ceftazidime with the aerobic gram-positive activity similar to first generation cephalosporins, making it quite useful when both of these are in the differential diagnosis. However, when treating suspected Pseudomonas spp. infection, as with other beta-lactam agents it is best to include a second agent of a different class to increase efficacy (i.e., an aminoglycoside or quinolone).

3. Carbapenems[12]

The carbapenem group of antibiotics (i.e., imipenem/cilastatin, meropenem, ertapenem) are highly resistant to nearly all bacterial beta-lactamases and very diffusible across gram-negative cell wall structures, making them widely active against nearly all classes of bacteria, gram-positive and -negative, aerobic and anaerobic. The spectrum, however, does not extend to MRSA or ampicillin-resistant enterococci, and increasingly there are strains of resistant pseudomonas appearing. Carbapenems have useful anti-pseudomonal activity making them one of the drugs of choice for these resistant gram-negative infections, although, as with other beta-lactam agents, it is generally wise to add a second active agent (a quinolone or an aminoglycoside) in the initial therapeutic regimen.

The carbapenems have a toxicity profile similar to other beta-lactams, and require dosage adjustment in renal insufficiency to avoid CNS toxicity in the form of seizures, particularly in those with underlying pre-existing CNS disease (Table 23.2). Notably, for carbapenems there *is* significant cross-reactivity with penicillins for serious allergic reactions to the extent that these agents should usually be avoided when there is a good history of accelerated reactions to penicillins.[15]

a. meropenem – This drug is currently the most widely used carbapenem with particular utility in situations in which multiple organisms of varying susceptibility are likely to be involved, such as mixed-flora soft tissue infections and intra-abdominal infections.[16]

B. Aminoglycosides

The aminoglycosides, one of the oldest classes of antimicrobials still available, remain extremely useful agents in severe sepsis. They act by inhibiting bacterial protein synthesis under aerobic conditions, resulting in both concentration-dependent killing and in a protracted post-antibiotic effect (sustained inhibition after the drug is no longer present), particularly in gram-negative bacilli. In many hospitals these agents remain among the most reliable for aerobic gram-negative bacilli, including most pseudomonas. However, because of this relatively narrow spectrum of activity they must almost always be used in combination with other agents directed at aerobic gram-positives or anaerobes as appropriate.

The major problem with aminoglycosides has been their low therapeutic:toxic ratio. Excreted via the kidney, they accumulate in the presence of renal insufficiency and compound the problem by being nephrotoxic. They also accumulate in the endolymph of the inner ear causing both ototoxicity and vestibulotoxicity, with both problems being less predictable from drug levels than is nephrotoxicity. Dosage adjustment for renal insufficiency is imperative along with monitoring of both drug levels and renal function (Table 23.3).

Although many clinicians have come close to abandoning the aminoglycosides because of toxicity concerns, I would suggest two strategies to mitigate toxicity while continuing to exploit their still-useful antibacterial activity. First, in severe sepsis, maximize efficacy and minimize toxicity by using once-daily dosing, always beginning with a full loading dose regardless of renal function, adjusting the dose on the second day as appropriate.[17-20] Second, since nearly all aminoglycoside toxicity is due to drug accumulation and is highly duration dependent, use the aminoglycoside only for the first few days of the treatment regimen, stepping down to less toxic agents for the remainder of the treatment course whenever possible. Among the available aminoglycosides, gentamicin is the most widely used. In areas in which aminoglycoside-inactivating enteric gram-negatives are prevalent, amikacin may have preserved activity and remain useful.

Table 23.3 – Aminoglycosides and Quinolones for Severe Sepsis

	Usual Dose for Severe Sepsis	Dose Adjustment for Renal Insufficiency
Gentamicin	5 mg/kg iv q24h	CrCl < 75 ml/min - 4 mg/kg iv q24h* CrCl < 50 ml/min - 3 mg/kg iv q24h* CrCl < 25 ml/min - 4 mg/kg iv q48h*
Amikacin	15 mg/kg iv q24h	CrCl < 75 ml/min - 12 mg/kg iv q24h* CrCl < 50 ml/min - 8 mg/kg iv q24h* CrCl < 25 ml/min - 8 mg/kg iv q48h*
Ciprofloxacin	400 mg iv q12h	CrCl < 25 ml/min - 400 mg iv q24h
Levofloxacin	750 mg iv q24h	
Gatifloxacin	400 mg iv q24h	

* Monitor serum drug levels and adjust dose to achieve pre-dose "trough" levels of < 3 mg/L for gentamicin and < 10 mg/L for amikacin.

C. Quinolones[21]

All quinolones work by binding in varying ways to bacterial DNA complexes with type II DNA topoisomerase enzymes thereby inhibiting DNA synthesis leading to rapid cell death. Variations in the ring structure and side chains have led to the development of a bewildering array of quinolones with, in most cases, fairly slight but sometimes important differences in antibacterial spectrum. Unfortunately, because of widespread overuse of these agents in less serious infections, the last few years have seen rapid emergence of resistance in many pathogen groups to the extent that, today, in the setting of serious sepsis they must almost always be used in combination with other agents. Since quinolones have a propensity to induce chromosomal mutations that can lead to the development of resistance during treatment, it is usually unwise to rely on these drugs as single agents, particularly in hard-to-treat infections with high bacterial loads and limited tissue penetration of the antimicrobial (e.g., abscess, poor vascular supply).

Most quinolones require some dose adjustment in the presence of significant renal insufficiency (Table 23.3). In patients with severe infections, there are few concerns about significant adverse effects of these agents; hypersensitivity reactions, CNS side effects and gastrointestinal (GI) symptoms can all occur but are seldom severe.

a. ciprofloxacin – Although it is one of the older agents, ciprofloxacin is still one of the most useful quinolones. It remains the most active against gram-negative bacilli, including Pseudomonas aeruginosa, has activity against many Staphylococcus aureus, and is active against most of the causes of atypical pneumonia, Legionella spp. in particular. However, it does not have dependable activity against many streptococcal spp. including pneumococcus, and is not a reliable anti-anaerobic agent.

b. levofloxacin and gatifloxacin – These newer quinolones are often termed the "respiratory quinolones" because their spectrum includes pneumococcus and other streptococci, atypical pneumonia agents and anaerobes, while retaining significant gram-negative activity. In recent years, these have been widely used as single agents for community-acquired pneumonia, however, the appearance of quinolone resistance among pneumococci in many jurisdictions has led to treatment failures, mandating combination therapy with a beta-lactam in patients with severe pneumonia or with associated sepsis.[22]

D. Macrolides[23]

There are three macrolide antibiotics currently available: erythromycin, clarithromycin and azithromycin. All macrolides act by inhibiting bacterial protein synthesis by binding to the 50S ribosomal subunit. The differences between them in the antimicrobial spectrum are relatively minor in that all have activity against most of the major community-acquired pneumonia pathogens, including most Streptococcus pneumoniae, Hemophilus influenzae, Moraxella spp. and the main atypical pneumonia pathogens including Legionella spp. Of the three, azithromycin has the most activity against Legionella spp., and it is also better against some other gram-negative bacteria. This, along with its lesser propensity to cause GI upset, has made erythromycin virtually obsolete. In most areas of North America, 10–30% of Streptococcus pneumoniae strains are macrolide resistant, and a strain resistant to one of these agents is resistant to all.[24,25] Thus, the only indication for azithromycin in critical illness is in patients with severe community-acquired pneumonia, and then only in combination with a beta-lactam antibiotic.

The usual dose of azithromycin for severe pneumonia (where Legionella is a consideration) is 500 mg iv od for 5–10 days; because the drug is taken up into tissues and slowly excreted, therapeutic levels of drug will continue to be present for twice the period of administration. Dosage adjustment for renal dysfunction is not necessary. Adverse effects are mainly GI upset, occasional CNS disturbances and, rarely, severe allergic reactions.

E. Clindamycin[26]

Like the macrolides, clindamycin binds to 50S ribosomal binding sites in susceptible bacteria, inhibiting microbial protein synthesis. It has clinically important antibacterial activity for nearly all aerobic gram-positive cocci other than enterococci and for most anaerobic bacteria. It has two main roles in the treatment of serious sepsis: 1) as the anti-anaerobe/anti-gram-positive component of a treatment regimen for mixed infections of the respiratory tract or intra-abdominal infections (always in combination with another agent for enteric gram-negatives); and 2) as a second agent along with a beta-lactam in the treatment of soft tissue infections due to Streptococcus pyogenes (i.e., necrotizing fasciitis) or the streptococcal toxic shock syndrome, aiming to reduce toxin formation by inhibiting bacterial protein synthesis.[27]

The increasing use of clindamycin for streptococcal toxic shock syndrome brings with it an important caveat: Staphylococcal infection is usually in the differential diagnosis in this situation, and about 10–20% of Staphylococcus aureus strains are either resistant to clindamycin or have a propensity to develop it due to prior erythromycin resistance.[28]

For seriously ill patients the usual dose of clindamycin is 600–900 mg iv q8h depending on patient size; no dose adjustments are required for renal dysfunction but the dose is reduced if there is concomitant hepatic insufficiency, in which case the dose should be roughly halved. Tissue penetration of the drug is excellent with most tissues, even into abscesses, with the exception that CNS penetration is poor, precluding its use when this is a consideration.

Adverse effects include occasional severe hypersensitivity reactions, usually mild hepatic dysfunction (e.g., elevated enzymes) and antibiotic-associated diarrhea. The most significant adverse effect is the development of Clostridium difficile colitis, which can occur in up to 10–15% of cases and can be associated with serious morbidity and even mortality. In hospitals with a high incidence of this problem, systematic limitation of clindamycin use has sometimes been necessary.

F. Vancomycin[29]

Vancomycin is a glycopeptide antibiotic that works by inhibiting formation of peptidoglycan in bacterial cell walls. It is active against nearly all gram-positive bacteria, but *only* gram-positive bacteria. Vancomycin has therefore become a mainstay of therapy for otherwise difficult-to-treat infections due to methicillin-resistant Staphylococcus aureus, coagulase-negative staphylococci, and ampicillin-resistant streptococci such as Enterococcus faecium.

In patients with severe sepsis, empiric use of this agent should be limited to those with suspected MRSA or ampicillin-resistant enterococcal infections. This suspicion generally arises on the basis of known prior colonization with one of these organisms or sepsis in a hospital or unit with known ongoing nosocomial spread of these organisms. For cases of sepsis of less severe degree, in which infection with resistant but less aggressive gram-positive pathogens is suspected (such as coagulase-negative staphylococci causing line sepsis), it is generally not necessary to use vancomycin empirically. It is reasonable to wait for the culture and sensitivity result, prescribing vancomycin only when the necessity for its use has been demonstrated. This practice is advised to try to limit vancomycin use to only those infections in which its use is really necessary, since heavy use of the drug has been associated with the emergence of vancomycin-resistant strains of enterococci and MRSA.

An important point to remember is that although vancomycin is a drug to which most resistant gram-positives remain susceptible, it is not the most effective drug for organisms that are actually susceptible to beta-lactam or other agents. Because of this, when vancomycin is used empirically, it is good practice to include in the regimen a beta-lactam drug directed at susceptible staphylococci as well, so as not to deny optimal therapy to these patients.

Oral vancomycin is also used in the treatment of Clostridium difficile colitis when metronidazole has failed (dose usually 125 mg po q6h). When using it in this way, it is good to remember that it is not absorbed from the GI tract, acts only as a local treatment for the GI mucosa and depends on GI motility to deliver it to the colon. In patients with serious sepsis due to pseudomembranous colitis, parenteral systemic antibiotics to treat systemic sepsis must also be given with it, and if GI motility problems cause doubt about delivery of the drug to the site of infection, administration of concomitant intravenous metronidazole is prudent.

Although it is currently customary to dose-adjust vancomycin in the presence of renal dysfunction and to monitor levels to maintain peaks of less than 30 mg/L and troughs of less than 10 mg/L, I find that it is not necessary to be as rigid about drug level limits with vancomycin as with aminoglycosides. Most recent studies of this drug have been unable to demonstrate convincing evidence that it is a significant nephrotoxin, and ototoxicity has generally not been a major problem. In patients with serious MRSA infections, the risk of under-treatment with vancomycin by too rigorous limitation of dose for renal insufficiency is probably greater than the risk of toxicity. For serious sepsis with reasonably preserved renal function it is best to start with 1g iv q12h, reducing to 1g q24h for more significant renal insufficiency and even down to 1g iv as a single dose for anephric patients, re-dosing based on levels. Subsequently, check peak and trough serum levels for dose adjustment; troughs in the 10–30 mg/L and peaks in the 30–50 mg/L range have not been shown to have significant toxicity and may be associated with improved efficacy.[30]

The most common adverse reaction to vancomycin is the "red-man" syndrome, characterized by immediate onset of facial and torso flushing accompanied by a prickly sensation of the skin and scalp and sometimes hypotension. It reverses after minutes to an hour or two after ceasing infusion. It is an acute histamine release phenomenon usually caused by excessively rapid infusion of the drug not an allergic reaction. It can generally be prevented by pre-treatment with an antihistamine and by infusing the drug slowly (over an hour or more). However, actual allergic reactions in the form of fixed drug eruptions also occur in 10% of vancomycin-treated patients, and when this diagnosis is made an alternative regimen should be sought.

G. Metronidazole[26,31]

A 5-nitroimidazole compound known to inhibit bacterial DNA synthesis, metronidazole is active against virtually all obligate anaerobic bacteria and *only* obligate anaerobic bacteria. Since anaerobes are almost never the sole players in serious infections, this drug is generally combined with other agents aimed at covering the aerobic gram-positives and gram-negatives involved. Used in this way, it is a mainstay of many regimens for acute intra-abdominal infections, necrotizing soft tissue infections due to mixed aerobes and anaerobes and mixed-flora necrotizing pneumonias. It is also, of course, the drug of choice for Clostridium difficile colitis.

Used acutely for serious infections metronidazole has really no substantial toxicity problems, and a requirement for dosage adjustments with hepatic or renal dysfunction has not been demonstrated. The usual dose is 500–750 mg iv q8h. Other advantages of the drug include low cost and, because it is very well absorbed from the GI tract, the ability to use it enterally as well as parenterally if the GI tract is functional. In Clostridium difficile colitis, enteral metronidazole is the preferred route but unlike vancomycin, it has some effect if given parenterally.

● Major Pathogen Groups in Severe Sepsis

The major pathogens responsible for severe sepsis can usefully be grouped into a few categories based on their expected antimicrobial susceptibilities and on their epidemiology. Grouping these pathogens in this way helps the clinician to quickly get to a "short list" of pathogens that have to be included in an empiric antimicrobial regimen based on the suspected site and nature of the infection along with the patient's epidemiologic features, which may importantly affect the microflora involved.

A. Community-Acquired Respiratory and Skin Pathogens

The first group of organisms are all, at least some of the time, normal flora of the upper respiratory tract of humans (Table 23.4). All can cause acute community-acquired pneumonia with associated sepsis but a few of them are responsible for nearly all primary community-acquired bacteremias (bacteremia without an anatomic focus) and meningitis. Some organisms move from the respiratory tract to the skin and are responsible for the majority of skin and other soft tissue infections. They include Streptococcus pneumoniae, Hemophilus influenzae, Neisseria meningitides, Streptococcus pyogenes (group A beta-hemolytic streptococcus) and methicillin-susceptible Staphylococcus aureus. This group is still mostly susceptible to second and third generation cephalosporins, which is why these agents remain the backbone of most empiric antimicrobial regimens.

B. Community-Acquired Enteric Gram-Negative Pathogens

The second group include Escherichia coli, Klebsiella spp., Proteus spp. and a number of other somewhat less commonly isolated organisms (Table 23.5). Normal flora of the large intestine and colonizing the perineum, they are always involved in infections arising from the lower bowel and are the most common causes of urinary tract infections and infections of bowel appendages (gall bladder, pancreas, etc.) in otherwise healthy people. Normally confined to the GI tract and adjacent structures, they are *opportunistic pathogens* elsewhere: that is, they will colonize sites such as the upper respiratory tract of debilitated patients or those receiving antimicrobials and chronic wounds such as diabetic foot and leg ulcers. This makes them important causes of nosocomial infections and pneumonia in the debilitated elderly and bone and soft tissue infections in chronic wounds. This group is still mostly susceptible to second and third generation cephalosporins, but it must be borne in mind that resistance is increasing substantially in some geographic areas. They are usually susceptible to aminoglycosides and to quinolones, so when cephalosporin resistance is a concern, and particularly in cases in which under-treatment might prove

Table 23.4 – Community-Acquired Respiratory and Soft Tissue Pathogens

	Sepsis/ Meningitis	Primary Bacteremia	Pneumonia	Soft Tissue Infections
Streptococcus pneumoniae	++++	+++	++++	+
Neisseria meningitides	++++	+++	+	+
Hemophilus influenzae		+	++	+
Streptococcus pyogenes		++	+	++++
Staphylococcus aureus		++++	++	++++

Table 23.5 – Community-Acquired Enteric Gram-Negative Pathogens

Organisms	Associated Infection Syndromes
Escherichia coli	Urinary tract infections: acute pyelonephritis, abscess, prostatitis
Klebsiella spp.	Intra-abdominal infections: appendicitis, diverticulitis, peritonitis post-perforation
Proteus spp.	Female genital tract infections: endometritis/myometritis
Others	Nosocomial and nursing-home-acquired pneumonia
	Polymicrobial necrotizing soft tissue infections

catastrophic (e.g., shock), it is often reasonable to treat these infections initially with more than one class of agent.

C. Anaerobic Pathogens

Anaerobes are implicated in virtually all polymicrobial infections arising from the lower GI tract and necrotizing polymicrobial soft tissue infections (Table 23.6), generally along with enteric gram-negatives or streptococci. Anaerobes are also always present in the upper airway and are implicated in aspiration-associated anaerobic pleuro-pulmonary infections and abscesses. However, they are almost never important contributors to acute community-acquired or nosocomial pneumonia with severe sepsis, even if aspiration has been involved in its genesis. The exception is pneumonia occurring acutely after aspiration of feculent gastric contents in the setting of bowel obstruction. Although most anaerobes are actually susceptible to a wide range of antimicrobials, including penicillin, the choice of agent is generally driven by penicillin-resistant Bacteroides fragilis group organisms, which are involved in most anaerobic infections. The prototype anaerobic agent is metronidazole which is effective against nearly all anaerobes but only anaerobes. Some potential alternatives are some specific cephalosporins effective against most anaerobes (e.g., cefoxitin, cefotetan), beta-lactam/beta-lactamase combinations, carbapenems and clindamycin.

D. Antimicrobial-Resistant Conventional Bacteria

The fourth group is unlike the other groups (Table 23.7). The first three groups include organisms that are normal flora in humans, and become implicated in infections by ending up in the wrong place at the wrong time or when a structural problem leads to an infection. The fourth group is somewhat diverse, but has in common the fact that the patient generally has a reason to have acquired the pathogen. The most common reasons include being debilitated or cared for in a health-care institution, antimicrobial exposure, and having undergone treatments that have not gone smoothly, thereby providing opportunities for acquisition of these pathogens.

The first, and perhaps most important of this group, is methicillin-resistant Staphylococcus aureus (MRSA). It can cause any infection that MSSA (methicillin-sensitive Staphylococcus aureus) can, and therefore must be covered empirically when a patient has a serious infection in which it may be implicated due to known colonization with MRSA or exposure to MRSA endemic environments. The mainstays of therapy are vancomycin and, more recently, linezolid. Trimethoprim/sulfamethoxazole (TMP/SMX or Septra®) and clindamycin are also sometimes effective, when the susceptibility is known.

Resistant gram-negative bacteria, such as Pseudomonas spp. and extended-spectrum beta-lactamase producing enteric gram-negatives (ESBLs) should also be considered with this group. These will be resistant to the usual first-choice cephalosporins and mandate inclusion of a carbapenem, often with another class of agent such as an aminoglycoside or quinolone, in the empiric regimen. Enterococcus spp., although it is also a component of normal bowel flora, is also considered along with this group, because the range of treatment options is extremely limited (vancomycin, linezolid, or ampicillin/aminoglycoside) and because, other than in the setting of acute urinary tract infection, it is seldom an important cause of sepsis other than in the setting of a complicated nosocomial intra-abdominal or soft-tissue infection.

Table 23.6 – Anaerobic Pathogens

Organisms	Associated Infection Syndromes
Bacteroides fragilis group Clostridium spp. Peptostreptococcus spp., Fusobacterium spp., etc.	Intra-abdominal infections Female genital tract infections Polymicrobial necrotizing soft tissue infections

Table 23.7 – Antimicrobial-Resistant Bacterial Pathogens

Organism	Associated Infections and Clinical Context
Methicillin resistant Staphylococcus aureus (MRSA)	Infection spectrum similar to MSSA Known colonization with MRSA Infection acquired in MRSA-endemic area
Pseudomonas spp. Other resistant gram-negatives	Pneumonia: Underlying structural lung disease, prior antimicrobial therapy, long-term ICU stay UTI: Recurrent UTI, prior antimicrobials, chronic instrumentation Soft tissue infection: chronic wound, prior antimicrobials Intra-abdominal sepsis: tertiary peritonitis (see text)
Enterococcus spp.	UTI: occurs in healthy population, more common with recurrent UTI or structural abnormality Intra-abdominal sepsis: tertiary peritonitis (see text), biliary tract Soft tissue infection: polymicrobial chronic wound infections, necrotizing soft tissue infections

MSSA = methicillin sensitive Staphylococcus aureus; MRSA = methicillin resistant Staphylococcus aureus; ICU = intensive care unit; UTI = urinary tract infection

E. Non-conventional Sepsis Pathogens

The final group of pathogens to be considered in designing an empiric antimicrobial infection for severe sepsis is what I will term the non-conventional sepsis pathogens (Table 23.8). These are non-conventional bacteria or non-bacterial pathogens for which the usually selected antimicrobials for sepsis are ineffective. Most often, there is an epidemiologic clue which, if noted, will cue the physician to include in the regimen an agent that may have activity or to perform specific diagnostic investigations.

Among pneumonia pathogens, the most important in this group is, of course, Legionella spp. which is not detectable by routine bacteriologic methods and for which beta-lactam drugs are ineffective. Severe pneumonia with sepsis in which there is not an evident conventional bacterial diagnosis must, therefore, always be treated with an agent for Legionnaire's disease (i.e., quinolone or macrolide). For severe Q-fever pneumonia, the clue is usually an animal exposure, particularly in a part of the country where cases are occurring. The addition to the empiric antimicrobial regimen in these circumstances would be to include doxycycline. Viruses to consider in this context include Hantavirus, severe influenza, and severe adenoviral infection. These viruses usually produce diffuse bilateral infiltrates, and there are often other clues in the clinical course, exposures and hematologic results that will trigger the appropriate additional investigation. For apparent severe sepsis without an evident focus, the travel history will most often provide a clue to suspecting malaria (leading to blood smear examination followed by anti-malarial drug therapy), ehrlichiosis (doxycycline) and rickettsioses such as Rocky Mountain Spotted Fever (doxycycline), and lead to appropriate additional investigation and empiric antimicrobial treatment.

● Empiric Antimicrobial Selection for Severe Sepsis

For most patients with acute onset of sepsis associated with organ dysfunction or shock, antimicrobials must be prescribed promptly and, nearly always, empirically. The information we have at hand to determine what to include in the therapeutic regimen consists only of our clinical assessment of the likely focus of the infection (based on the history, physical examination and laboratory assessment) and our knowledge of the microbial pathogens likely to be involved. After a definitive clinical and microbiologic diagnosis has been made, usually two to three days later, treatment can be modified appropriately;

Table 23.8 – Non-conventional and Non-bacterial Pathogens Causing Severe Sepsis

Organism	Associated Clinical/Epidemiologic Features
Legionella spp.	Severe pneumonia, otherwise undiagnosed; relative immunocompromise
Q-Fever (Coxiella burnettii)	Atypical pneumonia syndrome; headache; animal exposure in endemic area
Malaria	Travel history leading to blood smear examination
Ehrlichiosis	Travel history in south-central USA, tickbite, relative immunocompromise, otherwise non-localizing sepsis syndrome; leukopenia
Rickettsiosis (e.g., Rocky Mountain Spotted Fever, typhus)	Travel history in south-central USA, tickbite (RMSF), otherwise non-localizing sepsis with fever, headache, with or without rash

however, in this section we will deal only with suggested empiric initial regimens.

A. Primary Sepsis (Sepsis without an Obvious Focus)

a. community acquired – A patient who comes from the community with severe sepsis without a definable focus or the potential for an atypical pathogen exposure most often has a bacteremia caused by one of the several pathogens that intermittently colonize the upper respiratory tract. Staphylococcus aureus bacteremia is the most common; about 50% of such bacteremias have no definable source at presentation, though in many cases one becomes obvious later (e.g., endocarditis). Similarly, Neisseria meningitides and Streptococcus pneumoniae can produce primary bacteremia, though meningitis is also often present. Hemophilus influenzae is less frequent, often associated with prior splenectomy. A third generation cephalosporin is generally the most appropriate choice; first and second generation cephalosporins are discouraged because of the possibility of associated incipient meningitis. Suspicion that there may be an undiagnosed intra-abdominal process not yet evident (e.g., early bowel ischemia) should prompt addition of an anti-anaerobic agent such as metronidazole or clindamycin.

b. Nosocomial – The patient with nosocomial primary sepsis is less common and more often this is eventually traced to a specific focus, particularly intravascular catheters, urinary catheters that were infected and subsequently manipulated or occult post-surgical sources such as abscesses or perforations not yet clinically evident. When the episode of sepsis occurs early in the hospital course, it is reasonable to treat with a third generation cephalosporin, since the likely pathogens will be Staphylococcus aureus or relatively susceptible enteric gram-negatives. However, in longer-stay patients who have previously been exposed to antibiotics, ICU or surgery, it is necessary to consider whether the patient is at risk for one of the microbes on the resistant pathogen list, particularly pseudomonas and MRSA. In this setting, a carbapenem or piperacillin/tazobactam, possibly with an aminoglycoside or quinolone initially, is a safer choice, and the addition of vancomycin must be at least considered.

B. Meningitis[32]

Streptococcus pneumoniae and Neisseria meningitides account for most cases of acute meningitis associated with severe sepsis. While both are most often susceptible to the full range of available beta-lactam antimicrobials, including penicillin, in most parts of North America about 15% of pneumococci have developed "intermediate" resistance to beta-lactams, and up to 1–2% have high-level resistance. While intermediate resistance has not affected beta-lactam response rates or outcome outside the CNS, it has led to treatment failure in meningitis. Accordingly, both vancomycin and a third generation cephalosporin should be included in the empiric treatment regimen until the organism and its susceptibility are known. Ampicillin may also be included in cases where listeriosis is a consideration (less severe meningitis/

sepsis, negative gram-stain or small-gram-positive cocci or bacilli seen, immunocompromised).

C. Pneumonia

a. Community Acquired – The management of community-acquired pneumonia has been the subject of several sets of widely used guidelines.[33–35] For severely ill patients, the target pathogens are essentially the upper airway colonizers plus Legionella spp., and most guidelines suggest a second or third generation cephalosporin together with a quinolone (or azithromycin). Although some have suggested a respiratory quinolone alone (e.g., levofloxacin, moxifloxacin, gatifloxacin) may be acceptable, this is now inadvisable because of increasing resistance to these agents among pneumococci world-wide; this is also true of azithromycin. In addition, there is some recent evidence that in severe pneumococcal pneumonia, therapy with more than one active agent may favourably influence outcome.[36,37]

b. nosocomial – The management of nosocomial pneumonia has also been the subject of guideline writing.[38,39] The principal pathogens are community upper airway colonizers in addition to what the patient is likely to have acquired in hospital. Thus, for early onset pneumonia of lesser severity a third generation cephalosporin is probably acceptable, since the likely acquired pathogens would be mainly susceptible enteric gram-negatives. However, for severely ill patients or those with risks for acquiring more resistant pathogens such as pseudomonads, an anti-pseudomonad beta-lactam (e.g., ceftazidime, a carbapenem or piperacillin/tazobactam) usually with an aminoglycoside or quinolone is best. If there is a possibility of acquisition of MRSA, the use of vancomycin should be considered. For most patients, Legionella spp. coverage is not necessary, but in particular hospitals (with high local incidence) or particular patients (steroids, suggestive features, non-prophylaxed transplant recipients), the addition of a quinolone is advised.

D. Intra-abdominal Sepsis (Including Female Genital-Tract Infections)[40,41]

The concept of primary, secondary and tertiary peritonitis is a useful notion in thinking about antimicrobial selection for the diverse infections occurring in the abdomen. Primary refers to peritonitis occurring without surgical intra-abdominal pathology, secondary is an infection acutely associated with such pathology and tertiary refers to late infections related to failure of surgical therapy.

a. primary peritonitis – This problem, also called *spontaneous bacterial peritonitis*, occurs in the setting of underlying ascites that then becomes infected by translocation of organisms from the GI tract or by transient bacteremia. The usual organisms are upper airway colonizers reaching the GI tract by swallowing and enteric gram-negatives; hence the usual treatment is with a third generation cephalosporin such as cefotaxime.

b. secondary peritonitis – In acute secondary peritonitis, such as a perforated appendix, the pathogens are mixed enteric gram-negatives, generally not particularly resistant to antimicrobials in patients coming from the community, enteric gram-positives and anaerobes. A number of regimens are reasonable and acceptable: ampicillin/metronidazole/gentamicin; clindamycin/cefotaxime; piperacillin/tazobactam with or without ciprofloxacin or an aminoglycoside, among others. Regimens such as this are also used for postpartum endometritis or parametritis, diverticulitis, colonic perforation and other infections likely to have similar microflora.

c. tertiary peritonitis – When initial surgical treatment of one of these infections fails, as may occur with anastamosis failure, for example, the initial antimicrobial therapy will have eliminated most of the important pathogens initially present, leaving behind a mainly antimicrobial-resistant minority, which will then become the dominant microflora causing tertiary peritonitis. The microbiology of these infections is very hard to predict, but often involves resistant gram-negatives such as Pseudomonas spp., enterococci and yeast. A carbapenem such as meropenem is usually the best basic regimen, and addition of vancomycin and an antifungal agent (e.g., fluconazole) should be considered. Earliest possible acquisition of specimens for culture to define the problem more clearly is strongly advised.

E. Urinary Tract Infection[42]

Severe sepsis due to acute pyelonephritis presenting from the community without a prior history of repeated UTI and antimicrobial therapy is most often due to enteric gram-negatives, and less commonly to enterococus or Staphylococcus saprophyticus. For this reason, ampicillin with an aminoglycoside remains a very good choice for initial treatment for most patients. About 30% of community-acquired Escherichia coli are ampicillin resistant, but gentamicin will usually cover this eventuality, and the combination provides reasonable initial coverage for the gram-positives. It should be borne in mind that severe sepsis secondary to UTI is often associated with obstruction so, in addition to prompt antimicrobials, renal imaging should be done to determine whether a drainage procedure is also needed.

For patients with more complicated urosepsis histories that involve recurrent infectious episodes with antimicrobial therapy or chronic instrumentation of the urinary tract, relatively resistant gram-negatives are much more likely. In this setting, initial treatment with piperacillin/tazobactam or meropenem with an aminoglycoside or with a quinolone is more appropriate.

F. Soft Tissue Infections

Most soft tissue infections beginning acutely in otherwise healthy tissue as an acute cellulitis or skin infection are due to Staphylococcus aureus or Streptococcus pyogenes.[43] These are seldom associated with a severe sepsis syndrome unless there is an associated bacteremia, although antigen-mediated toxic-shock syndrome can occur with either, even with a relatively trivial-appearing infection. Any of the several different beta-lactam antimicrobial regimens is acceptable for community-acquired cellulitis caused by these organisms: cloxacillin, cefazolin, a second or third generation cephalosporin or a beta-lactam/beta-lactamase inhibitor.

Streptococcus pyogenes infections, often starting from relatively minor skin injuries, can produce the streptococcal toxic shock syndrome or result in the rapidly-advancing soft-tissue infection called *necrotizing fasciitis*. Although this organism is highly susceptible to penicillin and most other beta-lactams, addition of clindamycin to the antimicrobial regimen has been advocated. The addition of clindamycin is based on the notion that an antibiotic that inhibits bacterial protein synthesis might reduce toxin production and limit the systemic effects of the infection.[27] If a penicillin with clindamycin is used in this way for streptococcal toxic-shock syndrome or necrotizing fasciitis (often along with an infusion of human immunoglobulin,[44] also aimed at mitigating toxin effects), it must be borne in mind that if Staphylococcus aureus infection is also a possibility it may not be adequately covered. Up to 20% of staphylococci may be resistant to clindamycin, so relying on this agent for coverage in a patient with severe sepsis is unwise; another beta-lactam with anti-staphylococcal activity should be included in the regimen.

Another major category of soft tissue infections is polymicrobial infection due to anaerobes combined with aerobic streptococci and enteric gram-negatives.[45] These can cause necrotizing fasciitis arising from a contaminated traumatic injury or from a chronically infected wound such as a decubitus ulcer or diabetic foot ulcer. They also occur arising from perineal lesions or abdominal wounds leading to the necrotizing infections termed Fournier's gangrene and Meleney's synergistic gangrene. More limited infections of this type can result in localized myonecrosis. All of these infections should be treated with antimicrobial regimens similar to those used for mixed aerobic/anaerobic intra-abdominal infections.

● Summary

Timely effective antimicrobial therapy is a crucial element in the treatment of severe sepsis and septic shock and must be thought of as part of the early resuscitation effort. In selecting therapy, while it is important to carefully consider what the likely pathogens involved might be, based on the clinical syndrome being treated and on specific patient risk factors, it is also important to recognize that getting "a drug on the bug" at the beginning is a major key to survival. Initially broad or aggressive therapy can later be tailored or reduced based on a more specific diagnosis and on microbiological results as they become available.

Key Points

- Parenteral antimicrobial therapy should be initiated as soon as possible after the diagnosis of severe sepsis or septic shock is seriously considered.
- Antimicrobial therapy should target microbial pathogens likely to be involved in the infection, based on the clinical syndrome being treated and the pathogens usually involved in those infections.

- Always adjust antimicrobial therapy in consideration of specific risk factors for less usual or antimicrobial resistant pathogens.
- Antimicrobial therapy should be selected so as to ensure adequate coverage of all potential pathogens of more than trivial likelihood.
- Antimicrobial doses should initially be at the high end of the recommended dose range and later be adjusted for renal or other organ system function or according to microbiologic results.

References

1. Young LS, Martin WJ, Meyer RD, et al: Gram-negative rod bacteremia: Microbiologic, immunologic, and therapeutic considerations. *Ann Intern Med* 1977;86:456–71.

2. Kreger BE, Craven DE, McCabe WR: Gram-negative bacteremia: IV. Re-evaluation of clinical features and treatment in 612 patients. *Am J Med* 1980;68:344–55.

3. Romero-Vivas J, Rubio M, Fernandez C, Picazo JJ: Mortality associated with nosocomial bacteremia due to methicillin-resistant Staphylococcus aureus. *Clin Infect Dis* 1995;21:1417–23.

4. Kollef MH, Sherman G, Ward S, Fraser VJ: Inadequate antimicrobial treatment of infections: A risk factor for hospital mortality among critically ill patients. *Chest* 1999;115:462–74.

5. Ibrahim EH, Sherman G, Ward S, et al: The influence of inadequate antimicrobial treatment of bloodstream infections on patient outcomes in the ICU setting. *Chest* 2000;118:146–55.

6. Meehan TP, Fine MJ, Krumholz HM, et al: Quality of care, process, and outcomes in elderly patients with pneumonia. *JAMA* 1997;278:2080–4.

7. Aronin SI, Peduzzi P, Quagliarello VJ: Community-acquired bacterial meningitis: Risk stratification for adverse clinical outcome and effect of antibiotic timing. *Ann Intern Med* 1998;129:862–9.

8. Miner JR, Heegaard W, Mapes A, Biros M: Presentation, time to antibiotics, and mortality of patients with bacterial meningitis at an urban county medical center. *J Emerg Med* 2001;21:387–92.

9. Lodise TP, McKinnon PS, Swiderski L, Rybak MJ: Outcomes analysis of delayed antibiotic treatment for hospital-acquired Staphylococcus aureus bacteremia. *Clin Infect Dis* 2003;36:1418–23.

10. Wright AJ, Witkowska CJ: The penicillins. *Mayo Clin Proc* 1999;74:1050–1.

11. Sanders WE Jr, Sanders CC: Piperacillin/tazobactam: A critical review of the evolving clinical literature. *Clin Infect Dis* 1996; 22:107–23.

12. Asbel LE, Levison ME: Cephalosporins, carbapenems, and monobactams. *Infect Dis Clin North Am* 2000;14:435–47.

13. Anne S, Reisman RE: Risk of administering cephalosporin antibiotics to patients with histories of penicillin allergy. *Ann Allergy Asthma Immunol* 1995;74:167–70.

14. Kelkar PS, Li JT: Cephalosporin allergy. *N Eng J Med* 2001;345:804–9.

15. Prescott WA Jr, DePestel DD, Ellis JJ, Regal RE: Incidence of carbapenem-associated allergic-type reactions among patients with versus patients without a reported penicillin allergy. *Clin Infect Dis* 2004;38:1102–7.

16. Hurst M, Lamb HM: Meropenem: A review of its use in patients in intensive care. *Drugs* 2000; 59:653–80.

17. Moore RD, Smith CR, Lietman PS: The association of aminoglycoside plasma levels with mortality in patients with gram-negative bacteremia. *J Infect Dis* 1984;149:443–8.

18. Moore RD, Smith CR, Lietman PS: Association of aminoglycoside plasma levels with therapeutic outcome in gram-negative pneumonia. *Am J Med* 1984;77:657–62.

19. Chelluri L, Jastremski MS: Inadequacy of standard aminoglycoside loading doses in acutely ill patients. *Crit Care Med* 1987;15:1143–5.
20. Craig WA: Once-daily versus multiple-daily dosing of aminoglycosides. *J Chemother* 1995;7(suppl 2):47–52.
21. O'Donnell JA, Gelone SP: Fluoroquinolones. *Inf Dis Clin North Am* 2000;14;489–513.
22. Conton R, Morosini M, Enright MC, Morrissey I: Worldwide incidence, molecular epidemiology and mutations implicated in fluoroquinolone-resistant Streptococcus pneumoniae: data from the global PROTEKT surveillance programme. *J. Antimicrob Chemother* 2003;52:944–52.
23. Zhanel GG, Dueck M, Hoban JDH, et al: Review of macrolides and ketolides: focus on respiratory tract infections. *Drugs* 2001;61:443–98.
24. Zhanel GG, Palatnick L, Nichol KA, et al: Antomicrobial resistance in respiratory tract Streptococcus pneumoniae isolates: results of the Canadian Respiratory Organism Susceptibility Study, 1197 to 2202. *Antimicrob Agents Chemother* 2003;47:1867–74.
25. Jacobs MR: Streptococcus pneumoniae: epidemiology and patterns of resistance. *Am J Med* 2004;117(suppl 3A):3S–15S.
26. Falagas ME, Borbach SL: Clindamycin and metronidazole. *Med Clin North Am* 1995;79:854–67.
27. Stevens DL: Streptococcal toxic shock syndrome associated with necrotizing fasciitis. *Ann Rev Med* 2000;51:271–88.
28. Schreckenberger PC, Hendo E, Ristor KL: Incidence of constitutive and inducible clindamycin resistance in Staphyococcus aureas and coagulase-negative staphylococci in a community and tertiary care hospital. *J. Clin Microbiol* 2004;42:2777–9.
29. cunha BA: Vanconycin. *Med Clin North Am* 1995;79:817–31.
30. Zimmerman AE, Katona BG, Plaisance KI: Assocation of vancomycin serum concentrations with outcomes in patients with gram-positive bacteria. *Pharmacotherapy* 1995;15:85–91.
31. Freeman CD, Klutman NE, Lamp KC: Metronidazole. A therapeutic review and update. *Drugs* 1997;54:679–708.
32. Quagliarello VJ, Scheld WM: Treatment of bacterial meningitis. *N Engl J Med* 1997;337:793–4.

33. Bartlett JG, Dowell SF, Mandella LE, et al: Practice Guidelines for the management of community-acquired pneumonia in adults. *Clin Infect Dis* 2000;31:347–82.
34. Mandell LA, Marrie TJ, Grossman RF et al: Canadian guidelines for the initial management of community-acquired pneumonia: an evidence-based update by the Canadian Infectious Disease Society and the Canadian Thoracic Society. *Clin Infect Dis* 2000;31:383–421.
35. Neiderman MA, Mandell LA: Guidelines for the management of adults with community-acquired pneumonia. *Am J Respir Crit Care Med* 2001;163:1730–54.
36. Waterer GW, Somes GW, Wunderink RG: Monotherapy may be suboptimal for severe bacteremic pneumococcal pneumonia. *Arch Intern Med* 2001;161:1837–42.
37. Baddour LM, Yu V, Klugman KP, et al: Combination antibiotic therapy lowers mortality among severly ill patients with pneumococcal bacteremia. *Am J Respir Crit Care Med* 2004;170:440–4.
38. Mandell LA, Marrie TJ, Niederman MS, et al: Initial antimicrobial treatment of hospital-acquired pneumonia. *Can J Infect Dis* 1993;4:317–21.
39. The American Thoracic Society: Hospital-acquired pneumonia in adults: Diagnosis, assessment of severity, initial antimicrobial therapy, and preventive strategies. A consensus statement. *Am J. Respir Crit Care Med* 1996;153:1711–25.
40. McClean KL, Sheehan GJ, Harding GKM: Intraabdominal infection: a review. *Clin Infec Dis* 1994;19:100–16.
41. Mazuski JE, Sawyer RG, Nathens AB, et al: The surgical infection society guidelines on antimicrobial therapy for intra-abdominal infections. *Surg Infect* 2002;3:161–73.
42. Stamm WE, Hooton TM: Management of urinary tract infections in adults. *N Engl J Med* 1993;329:1328–34.
43. Swartz MN: Cellulitis. *N Engl J Med* 2004;350:904–12.
44. Kaul R, McGeer A, Norrby-Teglund A, et al: Intravenous immunoglobulin therapy for streptococcal toxic shock syndrome — a comparative observational study. *Cin Infect Dis* 1999;28:800–7.
45. Chapnick EK, Abter EI: Necrotizing soft tissue infections. *Infect Dis Clin North Am* 1996;10:835–55.

Apneic - 6, 116
Apoptotic cell death - 213
Aprotinin - 173
APRV - *see Airway pressure release ventilation*
Arachidonic acid - 212
ARDS - *see Acute Respiratory Distress Syndrome*
ARDSNetwork - 134, 136-137, 140
Arrhythmias - 140, 150, 181, 185, 195, 219
Arterial blood gas (ABG) - 96-97, 118, 133, 196, 217
Arterial line - 8, 139, 151, 161-163, 188, 194, 196, 216-218
Arterial oxygen content - 88-89, 95, 97, 147, 162
Arterial oxyhemoglobin saturation - 88
Arterial thrombosis - 188
Aspergillosis - 229
Aspiration - 5, 38, 43, 45-47, 52, 56-57, 65-68, 71, 79, 81-82, 101-102, 117-118, 136, 139, 150, 230, 240-242, 257
Aspirin - 93, 172
Assist/control (AC) mode - 108, 110, 112, 137, 139
Assisted ventilation - 80, 101
ATC ™ - *see Automatic tube compensation*
Atelectactic trauma - 134
Atelectasis - 103, 126, 139, 229, 233, 237
Atenolol - 93
Auscultation - 6-7, 21, 43, 47, 78, 99, 114, 149, 187-188
Autoflow ™ - 109
Autologous transfused blood - 168, 175
Automatic tube compensation - 109
Auto-PEEP - 113-115, 122, 124-127, 136, 138-139
Azithromycin - 207, 216, 233, 253-254, 260
Babesia - 228
Bacillary angiomatosis - 228
Bacillus cereus - 231
Bacterial peritonitis - 236, 238, 260
Bacterial translocation - 134, 239, 241
Bactericidal - 228, 230, 233, 248
Bacteriuria - 238
Bacteroides fragilis - 248-249, 257
Bag & mask ventilation - 5-7, 9, 37, 40-42, 45, 51, 68-73, 78-79, 81, 101, 103, 150
- Anesthesia mask - 41-42
- Clear mask - 41
BAL - *see Bronchoalveolar lavage*
Bandemia - 160
Barotrauma - 49, 108, 134, 138
- Interstitial emphysema - 134
- Pneumomediastinum - 134
- Pneumothorax - 5-8, 12-13, 21, 99, 102-103, 126, 134, 136, 138-139, 146, 149, 179, 190
Bartonella - 228
Benziodiazepines - 58, 60-61
- Diazepam - 58, 60
- Lorazepam - 60, 77, 102
- Midazolam - 58-61, 70
Beta agonist - 147, 181-182
Beta blocker - 53, 59, 70, 182, 209-210
- Atenolol - 93
- Esmolol - 59, 69, 70
Beta-lactam antibiotics - 229-230, 233, 248-249, 251-255, 257-261

- Carbapenems - 233, 248, 250, 252, 257, 259-260
- Cephalosporins - 232-233, 248-252, 256-257, 259-261
- Penicillins - 216, 223, 232-234, 248-250, 252, 257, 259, 261

BiLevel ® - 109
Biliary sepsis - 249
Bilirubin - 174, 211
Biotrauma - 134
BiPAP ® - 38, 109, 116-117
Blastomycosis - 228-229
Blood bank - 167, 169-171, 174
Blood brain barrier - 232-233, 242
Blood glucose - 222
Blood groups – 169-170
- Duffy - 169
- Kell - 169
- Kidd - 169
- Rh - 169
Blood pressure - 3, 6-9, 11, 20-21, 40, 55, 60, 69-71, 73, 95, 112-113, 115, 139-140, 145-152, 155-156, 159, 162, 179-180, 182, 187-188, 198-199, 207, 211, 216-219, 221, 223, 247
- Arterial catheter - 188, 217
- Auscultation - 6-7, 21, 43, 47, 78, 99, 114, 149, 187-188
- Oscillometric method - 118
Blood products - 151, 159-160, 167-169, 171-173, 175-176, 185
- Packed red blood cells (PRBC) - 158, 161, 168-169, 171-172, 174-175, 219
- Plasma - 157-159, 168, 171, 174, 211, 215, 219, 221, 228
- Platelets - 167-171, 173, 175, 207, 214, 216, 222
Blood viscosity - 148
Blood warmer - 173
Body surface area (BSA) - 147, 195
Bradycardia - 61-62
Breath stacking - 108
Broad-spectrum antibiotics - 213, 235, 238-239, 241, 251
Bronchoalveolar lavage (BAL) - 230
Bronchoscope - 46-47, 50-51, 80-81
Bronchospasm - 56, 59, 101-103, 115, 118, 122, 138-139
BSA - *see Body surface area*
Budesonide - 93
BURP - 43, 67-68
Calibration - 188
Candidal endopthalmitis - 239
Candidosis - 229
CAP - *see Community acquired pneumonia*
Capnocytophaga - 228
Carbapenem - 233, 248, 250, 252, 257, 259-260
- Ertapenem - 252
- Imipenem - 232-233, 252
- Meropenem - 232-233, 250, 252, 260-261
Cardiac compliance - 156, 163
Cardiac glycosides - 182
- Digoxin - 182
Cardiac index (CI) - 163, 185, 195-196, 198-200, 211

Difficult mask ventilation (DMV) - 78-80
Digoxin - 182
Dinamap® - 188
Diplococci - 216
Disproportionate hypofibrinogenemia - 171
Disseminated intravascular coagulopathy (DIC) - 170-171, 173-174, 215, 229
Diverticulitis - 260
DMV - see Difficult mask ventilation
DNA viruses - 228
- Cytomegalovirus - 175, 228
- Epstein Barr - 228
- Herpes simplex - 228
- Varicella-Zoster - 228
Dobutamine - 8, 151-152, 161, 181-182, 184-185, 216, 218
Dopamine - 8, 151-152, 179, 182-185, 219
- Cardiac dose – 183
- Renal dose - 183
- Vasopressor dose - 183
Doxycycline - 258
Drug fever - 229, 237, 242
Dynamic compliance - 124
Dynamic pressure volume loops - 129
Dyspnea - 98, 117-118, 230
Dysrythmias - 97, 173
Dysynchrony - 114, 133, 138-139
Echocardiography - 138, 241
- Esophageal - 241
- Trans-thoracic - 241
ECS ™ - see Emergency Care Simulator ™
Ecthyma gangrenosum - 228-229
Ehrlichiosis - 258-259
Elastance - 123, 127-128
Elastic recoil - 123, 126-127
Elastic work - 126
Emergency Care Simulator ™ (ECS ™) - 21-22
EMLA ® - 51
Empiric oxygen - 99
Encephalitis - 238, 241
Encephalopathy - 217
End organ dysfunction - 96, 168
End organ function - 149, 151-152, 181, 185
End tidal CO_2 - 73, 97
Endocarditis - 231, 238, 241-242, 259
Endotoxemia - 229
Endotoxin - 211-214, 236
Endotracheal tube placement - 7, 37, 43, 68
Endotracheal tube (ETT) - 5, 7, 37-40, 42-43, 45-51, 53, 55-56, 65-66, 68-71, 73, 77, 80, 82, 91, 97, 102-103, 115, 127, 139, 238
Engineering fidelity - 18
Enterobacter - 230, 249-250
Enterococcus - 257-258
Eosinophil - 229, 239
EPAP - see Expiratory positive airway pressure
Ephedrine - 6, 8, 14, 52, 60, 71, 183-184, 191
Epinephrine - 151-152, 183-185
Epistaxis - 42
Epstein Barr - 228

Equation of motion - 123, 127-128
Ertapenem - 252
Erythromycin - 189, 233, 253-254
Erythropoietin (Epo) - 17
Escherichia coli - 256, 261
Eschmann bougie - 81
Esmolol - 59, 69, 70
Ethylated starches - 157
- Hetastarch (Hespan®) - 157-158, 219
- Pentastarch (Pentaspan®) - 157-158
Etomidate - 70
ETT - see Endotracheal tube
Euvolemia - 8, 57
Euvolemic - 151
Exotoxin - 211, 229, 231
Expiratory phase - 108, 110-112, 114-115, 122
Expiratory positive airway pressure (EPAP) - 116-118
Expiratory time (TE) - 114, 122, 138-139
External PEEP - 114-115
Extracellular fluid - 156
- Intravascular fluid – 156
- Interstitial fluid – 156
Extracorporeal membrane oxygenation - 137
Extubation - 82, 102, 117
Exudative phase - 136
Fasciitis - 223, 232, 238, 254, 261
- Group A strep fasciitis - 232
- Necrotizing fasciitis - 223, 232, 238, 254, 261
Febrile - 149, 175, 207, 210, 235-240, 243
Fentanyl - 58-59, 61, 69-70, 102
Fever - 91, 137, 148, 158, 170, 174, 207-208, 210-212, 228-231, 233, 235-243, 258-259
FFP - see Fresh frozen plasma
Fiberoptic bronchoscope - 47, 81
Fiberoptic intubation - 50-52
Fibrinogen - 214
Fibroproliferative phase - 136
Fick's equation - 162
Fidelity - 15, 18-23
- Engineering fidelity - 18
- Functional fidelity - 18
- High-fidelity - 15, 18-23
- Intermediate-fidelity - 21
- Low-fidelity - 18
- Physical fidelity - 18
- Psychological fidelity - 18
Fixation error - 4-5, 13, 15, 159
Flora - 223, 251, 255, 260
Flow triggering - 108
Fludrocortisone - 221
Fluid bolus - 55, 60, 151- 152, 179, 200
Fluid resuscitation - 155, 159-160, 162-189, 218-219
Fluid therapy - 150-151, 156, 162, 185, 189, 219
Fluoroquinolones - 233
Foley catheter - 161-162
Ford manoeuvre - 43, 48
Fournier's gangrene - 261
FP24 - Frozen plasma 24 hours
Fresh frozen plasma (FFP) - 157-159, 168, 171, 174, 211, 215, 219, 221, 228
Frozen plasma 24 hours (FP24) - 171

Functional fidelity - 18
Fungal infection - 229, 239, 241
- Aspergillosis - 229
- Blastomycosis - 228-229
- Candidosis - 229
- Coccidioidomycosis - 229
- Cryptococcosis - 229
- Histoplasmosis - 228-229
- Paracoccidioidomycosis - 229
- Pneumocystosis - 229

Fungal superinfection - 238-239
Fusobacterium - 257
Gangrene - 261
- Fournier's gangrene - 261
- Meleney's synergistic gangrene - 261

Gastric aspiration - 45- 46, 101
Gastric distension - 66, 117-118
Gatifloxacin - 253
Gentamicin - 230, 233, 252-253
Glasgow Coma Score - 38
Glycemic control - 222
Glycopyrrolate - 51
Gram stain - 216, 232, 238, 240, 260
Group A strep fasciitis - 232
Group A streptococcal (GAS) toxic shock syndrome - 223
Gum elastic bougie - 48
Haemate ® P - 172
Haemophilus influenzae - 228, 231, 233, 254, 256, 259
Haldane effect - 101
Hantavirus - 258
Haptoglobin - 174
Hawthorne effect - 23
Hct - *see Hematocrit*
Heat shock proteins (HSP) - 236
Heat shock response - 236
Hematinic levels - 172
Hematinics - 172
- Ferrous sulphate - 172
- Folic acid - 172
- Vitamin B_{12} - 172

Hematocrit (HCT) - 161, 168, 171, 218
Hematoma - 30, 38-39, 188, 190, 237
Hemodilution - 172, 219
Hemodynamic complications - 41
Hemodynamic compromise - 13, 68
Hemodynamic effect(s) - 52, 70, 107, 112-113, 126, 181, 183
Hemodynamic monitoring - 163, 187
- Blood pressure - 3, 6-9, 11, 20-21, 40, 55, 60, 69-71, 73, 95, 112-113, 115, 139-140, 145-152, 155-156, 159, 162, 179-180, 182, 187-188, 198-199, 207, 211, 216-219, 221, 223, 247
- Central venous pressure - 7-8, 20, 113, 151, 156, 184, 188-191, 193, 196-197, 218-219
- Pulmonary artery catheter - 8, 156, 160, 162-163, 169, 188-192, 194-201, 217, 236

Hemodynamic parameters - 6, 163, 211
Hemodynamics - 6-7, 68, 103, 159, 194
Hemoglobin - 87-90, 93, 101, 137, 147-148, 162, 167-169, 172, 174, 216

Hemoglobin transfusion - 168
Hemolysis - 172-174
Hemophilia - 173
Hemophilus influenzae - *see haemophilus influenzae*
Hemorrhage - 117, 139, 145, 170-174, 188, 215
Hemorrhagic shock - 152, 159
Hemostasis - 170, 173
Heparin - 170, 223
Heparin induced thrombocytopenia & thrombosis (HITT) - 170
Hepatic dysfunction - 254
Hepatitis - 174, 237, 240
Hepatoslpenic candidiasis - 239
Herpes simplex - 228
Hetastarch (Hespan®) - 157-158, 219
High-fidelity - 15, 18-23
Histoplasmosis - 228-229
HITT - *see Heparin induced thrombocytopenia & thrombosis*
Hoover's sign - 94, 99
HPS ® - *see Human Patient Simulator ™*
HSP - *see Heat shock proteins*
Human Patient Simulator ™ (HPS ®) - 21
Humoral immunity - 227-228
Hydrocephalus - 232
Hydrocortisone - 221-222
Hydrostatic pressure - 156-157
Hypercapnia - 87, 90-91, 94-96, 100, 102, 117, 135-136, 138
Hypercarbia - 78, 94, 101, 118
Hyperglycemia - 211, 221-222
Hyperkalemia - 57, 59, 62
Hypermetabolism - 218
Hypernatremia - 159
Hyperosmolarity - 159
Hypertonic saline - 158-159, 219
- Bleeding - 159
- Central pontine myelinolysis - 159
- Hypernatremia - 159
- Hyperosmolarity - 159

Hyperventilation - 62, 72, 89, 95, 110
Hypobarism - 95
Hypocapnia - 38, 91, 96
Hyponatremia - 172
Hypotension - 4, 6-7, 9, 52-53, 57-61, 70-71, 94, 97, 112-113, 138, 140, 145-146, 149-150, 152, 161-162, 175, 181-182, 187, 198, 208-211, 215, 218-219, 223, 255
Hypotensive - 6, 8, 17, 52, 70, 94, 103, 113, 140, 145, 152, 179, 187, 217-218
Hypothermia - 173, 208, 210-211, 237, 243
Hypoventilation - 89, 95
Hypoventilatory failure - 95-96, 98, 101
- Central hypoventilary failure - 96, 98
- Peripheral hypoventilary failure - 96

Hypovolemia - 6-8, 57, 60, 146, 160-162, 184, 219
Hypoxemia - 12, 52, 70, 72, 77-78, 80, 87-91, 94-97, 101-102, 104, 107, 113, 117-118, 136-139, 145, 151, 175, 194, 211
Hypoxemic failure - 95-96
Hypoxia - 4-5, 87-89, 94, 100, 160, 162, 174, 195, 216, 218
Hysteresis - 128

Ibuprofen - 207, 212
ICU - *see Intensive care unit*
IFR - *see Inspiratory flow rate*
IL - *see Interleukins*
ILMA - *see Intubating laryngeal mask airway*
Imipenem - 232-233, 252
Immunoglobulins - 174, 212, 222, 232, 261
Immunohematology - 169
Immunomodulation - 159
Immunosuppression - 159, 168, 174-175, 212, 239, 241
Indrawing - 5, 94, 98
Infrared ear thermometry - 236
Inodilators - 181
Inotropes - 8, 147, 150, 161, 163, 179, 181-185, 187, 191, 199-200, 218
- Amrinone - 181-182
- Beta agonists - 147, 181-182
- Dobutamine - 8, 151-152, 161, 181-182, 184-185, 216, 218
- Milrinone - 8, 151-152, 181-182, 184-185
- Phosphodiesterase inhibitors - 147, 181-182
Inspiratory flow rate (IFR) - 110, 122
Inspiratory phase - 109-112, 114-115
Inspiratory positive airway pressure (IPAP) - 116-118
Inspiratory time (TI) - 103, 109, 111-112, 115, 121-122, 125, 127, 129, 131
Insulin - 221-222
Intensive care unit (ICU) - 9, 93, 159, 210, 216, 218, 223, 235, 238-239, 251, 258-259
Interferon-γ - 211-212
Interferons - 211-212, 236
Interleukins (IL) - 211-212, 236
Intermediate-fidelity - 21
Interstitial emphysema - 134
Interstitial fluid - 156
Intracardiac shunt - 90, 101, 113, 138, 195
Intracellular fluid - 156, 166
Intracellular organisms - 228
- Bartonella - 228
- Legionella - 228-231, 233, 253-254, 258-260
- Listeria - 228-229, 232-234, 248-249
- Mycobacteria - 228-229, 233-234, 240
- Nocardia - 228-229, 232, 234
- Rhodococcus - 228-229, 232, 234
- Rochalimaea – 228
- Salmonella - 228, 233
Intrapulmonary shunt - 89-90, 101, 136
Intravascular fluid - 156
Intrinsic PEEP - 107, 114
Introducer sheath - 8, 50
Intubate - 4-7, 9, 14, 38-42, 45, 48, 51-53, 55-56, 59-61, 68, 70-72, 77-78, 81-82, 89, 93, 97, 102-103, 107, 133, 145, 149, 174, 187, 216, 238
Intubating Laryngeal Mask Airway (ILMA) - 46-47
Intubation - 5-7, 9, 12, 19-22, 37-43, 45-53, 55-62, 65-72, 77-82, 101-103, 112, 115, 117-118, 126, 138-139, 148-150, 161, 179, 210, 216-217, 237-238
- Endotracheal intubation - 65
- Fiberoptic intubation - 50-52

- Nasotracheal intubation - 66
- Rapid sequence intubation (RSI) - 52, 65, 69
- Retrograde intubation - 50
Inverse ratio ventilation (IRV) -122
IPAP - *see Inspiratory positive airway pressure*
Ipratropium - 93
Iron lung - 116
IRV - *see Inverse ratio ventilation*
Ischemic colitis - 228
Isotonic - 6, 150, 159, 179
Jet ventilation - 48, 50, 53, 81-82
Jugular venous pressure (JVP) - 151, 161, 164, 184-185
Ketamine - 58-59, 61, 70, 73
Ketoacidosis - 159
Klebsiella - 228, 231, 233, 251, 256
Kortokoff sounds - 187
Kyphoscoliosis - 96, 126
Lactate acidosis - 222
Laerdal SimMan ™ - 21
Laerdal Trachlight ® - 49
Laparotomy - 170, 173, 237, 240
Laryngeal axis - 40-41
Laryngeal Mask Airway (LMA) - 45-46, 72, 79, 81, 83
- LMA Classic ™ - 45-47, 81
- LMA Fastrach ™ - 46, 80-81
- LMA ProSeal ™ - 47, 81
Laryngoscope - 39-43, 46, 48, 53, 56, 68-69, 71, 79-81
- Macintosh blade - 40, 81
- Miller blade - 40, 81
Laryngoscopy - 38, 40, 43, 48-50, 52, 56, 59, 66-73, 79-82
Left ventricular end diastolic filling pressure (LVEDP) - 192-193, 197
Left ventricular end diastolic volume (LVEDV) - 192-193, 195
Left ventricular stroke work (LVSW) - 196-198
Legionella - 228-231, 233, 253-254, 258-260
Leukocytosis - 160, 208, 210-211, 231, 239
Leukodepletion - 175
Leukopenia - 160, 208, 211, 259
Levofloxacin - 253, 260
Lidocaine - 51-53, 58-59, 62, 69-70
Lighted stylet - 47-49, 81
Linezolid - 233
Listeria - 228-229, 232-234, 248-249
Listeriosis - 259
LMA Classic ™ - 45-47, 81
LMA Fastrach ™ - 46, 80-81
LMA ProSeal ™ - 47, 81
LMA ™ - *see Laryngeal mask airway*
Lorazepam - 60, 77, 102
Low-fidelity - 18
LRM – *see Lung recruitment manoeuvre*
Lumbar puncture (LP) - 170, 232, 234, 241
Lung protective ventilation - 134-136
Lung recruitment manoeuvre (LRM) - 137, 140
LVEDP - *see Left ventricular end diastolic filling pressure*
LVEDV - *see Left ventricular end diastolic volume*
LVSW - *see Left ventricular stroke work*
Lymphatic flow - 156

Lymphocyte - 159, 211-213, 228-229, 232

Lymphotoxin - 216

Macintosh blade - 40, 81

Macrolides - 230, 233, 253-254, 258
- Azithromycin - 207, 216, 233, 253-254, 260
- Clarithromycin - 233, 253
- Erythromycin - 189, 233, 253-254

Macrophage - 159, 211-212, 214, 222, 236

Malaria - 175, 258-259

Mannequins - 18-24

MAP - *see Mean arterial blood pressure*

Mean airway pressure - 125-126

Mean arterial blood pressure (MAP) - 156, 160-161, 163, 184-185, 188, 196-199, 201, 216, 218, 222

Mechanical ventilation - 7, 38, 101-103, 107, 109, 115-116, 119, 124-125, 127, 129, 133-139, 148, 150, 159, 162, 218, 240

Medical Educational Technologies Incorporated (METI) - 21

Medical error(s) - 27-32

MedSim-Eagle Patient Simulator ® - 20

Meleney's synergistic gangrene - 261

Meningitis - 230, 232-234, 238, 241, 248, 251, 256, 259

Meningococcal sepsis - 210

Meningococcus - 228, 233, 248
- M. tuberculosis - 229-230, 232

Meperidine - 61

Meropenem - 232-233, 250, 252, 260-261

Methicillin resistant Staphylococcus aureus (MRSA) - 249-250, 252, 254-255, 257-260

Methicillin susceptible Staphylococcus aureus (MSSA) - 251, 256

Methylprednisolone - 221

METI Simulators - *see Medical Educational Technologies Incorporated*

MIC - *see Minimum inhibitory concentration*

Microvasculature - 208, 210, 213-216

Midazolam - 58-61, 70

Miller blade - 40, 81

Milrinone - 8, 151-152, 181-182, 184-185

Minimum inhibitory concentration (MIC) - 233

Minute ventilation (MV) - 87, 91, 101, 114, 121-122, 126, 135, 208, 213
- Alveolar ventilation - 88-91, 135
- Dead space ventilation - 91, 101, 112, 135, 197

Mitochondrial dysfunction - 216

Mitral stenosis - 193

Mitral valve - 193

Mixed venous oxygen saturation - 90, 137, 162, 211, 218-219

Morphine - 61

MRSA - *see Methicillin resistant Staphylococcus aureus*

Mucormycosis - 229

Muscle relaxant - 52, 59-62, 70-71
- Rocuronium - 62, 69-70
- Succinylcholine - 57, 59-62, 69-70, 73

MV - *see minute ventilation*

Mycobacteria - 228-229, 233-234, 240

Myocardial ischemia - 5, 139, 147, 180-181, 183, 185, 199

Myocardial oxygen consumption - 147, 150, 152, 180-181, 199

Myocardial wall tension - 148, 200

Myonecrosis - 261

Myopathy - 96, 138

Naloxone - 56, 101

Narcotic(s) - 53, 58, 61, 70, 96, 98, 101, 112, 239
- Fentanyl - 58-59, 61, 69-70, 102
- Meperidine - 61
- Morphine - 61

Nasal airway - 42, 49, 70

Nasal cannulae - 80, 94, 100

Nasotracheal intubation - 66

Necrosis - 118, 183, 213, 237, 239, 241

Necrotizing fasciitis - 223, 232, 238, 254, 261

Negative pressure ventilation - 60, 134

Negative pressure ventilator - 116

Negligence - 28, 30

Neisseria - 228, 256, 259
- N. meningitides - 256, 259

Neoplasia - 168

Nephrotoxic - 252

Neuroleptics - 239

Neuromuscular relaxant - 137-138

Neutropenia - 227-228, 230, 233, 239

Neutropenic enterocolitis - 228

Neutrophil chemotaxin - 212

Neutrophil function - 227

Neutrophils - 207, 212, 214-215, 227

NiaStase® - 169, 173

Nitric oxide - 103, 137, 215-216, 223

Nitroglycerine - 52, 59-60

Nocardia - 228-229, 232, 234

Non-conventional sepsis pathogens - 258
- Coxiella burnettii - 259
- Ehrlichiosis - 258-259
- Legionella sp. - 228-231, 233, 253-254, 258-260
- Malaria - 175, 258-259
- Rickettsiosis - 259

Non-invasive positive pressure ventilation (NPPV) - 101-103, 115-118

Non-invasive ventilation - 37, 101-102, 116
- Bag & mask ventilation - 5-7, 9, 37, 40-42, 45, 51, 68-73, 78-79, 81, 101, 103, 150
- Non-invasive positive pressure ventilation (NPPV) - 101-103, 115-118

Non-rebreathing mask - 8, 100

Non-steroidal anti-inflammatory drugs (NSAID) - 232, 236

Norepinephrine - 8, 151-152, 179, 181, 184-185, 216, 219

Normal saline - 6, 9, 73, 150, 155, 157, 159, 216

Nosocomial pneumonia - 257, 260

NPPV - *see Non-invasive positive pressure ventilation*

NSAID - *see Non-steroidal anti-inflammatory drugs*

Oncotic pressure - 156-158

Opportunistic pathogens - 256

Opsonization - 228

Oral airway - 5, 12, 40, 42, 46, 79

Organ dysfunction - 96, 146, 159, 168-169, 209-211, 217, 220, 223, 258

Organ hypofusion - 218

Situational awareness - 12-13, 15
Sniff position - 39-41, 43, 67, 69, 71, 73, 79
Soft tissue infections - 231, 234, 255-258, 261
- Cellulitis - 228, 232, 238, 261
- Necrotizing fasciitis - 223, 232, 238, 254, 261
- Polymicrobial infection - 229, 257, 261
- Streptococcal toxic shock syndrome - 254, 261
Specific compliance - 124
Spirometer - 78
Spontaneous/time (S/T) mode - 116-117
Staphylococcus - 228, 232, 238-239, 249, 251-254, 256-259, 261
- Methicillin-resistant Staphylococcus aureus (MRSA) - 249-250, 252, 254-255, 257-260
- Methicillin-susceptible Staphylococcus aureus (MSSA) - 251, 256
- Staph. aureus - 228-233
- Staph. epidermis - 231
Starling equation - 156-157
Starling's law of the heart - 180, 199-200
Static compliance - 124-125
Static pressure volume loops - 128-129
- Inspiratory occlusion technique - 128
- Quasi-static method - 128
- Super syringe method - 128
Streptococcal toxic shock syndrome - 254, 261
Streptococcus – 228, 238, 249, 254, 256-257, 259, 261
- Group A strep (GAS) - 223, 228-229, 231-233, 238
- Strept. pneumoniae - 228, 254, 256, 259
- Strept. pyogenes - 238, 249, 254, 256, 261
- Strep. viridans - 228
Stridor - 5, 78, 99
Stroke volume - 147-148, 150, 162, 180, 195-200
Strong ion theory - 159
Stylets - 43, 48, 81
- Gum elastic bougie - 48
- Laerdal Trachlight ® - 49, 81
- Lighted stylet - 47-49, 81
Subdural hematoma - 30
Succinylcholine - 57, 59-62, 69-70, 73
Sulfa drugs - 230
Superantigens - 229, 231
Supranormal minute ventilation - 208
Surgical hemostatis - 173
SVR - see Systemic vascular resistance
Swan-Ganz catheter – see pulmonary artery catheter
Synchronized intermittent mandatory ventilation (SIMV) - 103, 108-110, 112
Systemic inflammatory response syndrome (SIRS) - 159-161, 163, 208-210, 213, 217, 223
Systemic vascular resistance (SVR) - 146-148, 180, 195-198, 200
Systole - 147, 180, 189, 195, 200
Systolic blood pressure (SBP) - 156, 161-162, 188, 211,
Tachycardia - 4, 6, 56, 59, 97, 150, 155, 160, 181, 195, 208, 210, 212, 219, 239
Tachypnea - 95, 97-98, 118, 138-139, 160, 208, 210-212, 247
Tamponade - 6-7, 113, 146, 179, 190, 201
Tazobactam - 248-250, 259-261

TBW - see Total body water
TE - see Expiratory time
Tension pneumothorax - 6-7, 99, 126, 146, 149, 179
Tetracycline - 230, 233
Thermodilution technique - 195
Thiopental - 59-60, 70
Thoracentesis - 99, 240-241
Thoracostomy - 140, 240-241
Thrombin - 173, 214-215
Thrombocytopenia - 170, 172, 195, 211
Thrombomodulin - 214
Thrombotic thrombocytopenic purpura (TTP) - 170-1
Thromboxane A_2 - 212
Thyromental distance - 39, 73
TI - see Inspiratory time
Tidal volume - 71, 88, 91, 103, 108-112, 115, 118, 121-122, 124-125, 128-130, 133-138, 140
Time constant - 124, 129-131
Tissue dysoxia - 159, 168
TNF-α - see Tumor necrosis factor
TNF-β - see Tumor necrosis factor
Tobramycin - 230, 233
Toll-like receptors - 213
Total body water (TBW) - 156-157
Total parenteral nutrition (TPN) – 8, 189
Toxic shock syndrome - 223, 254, 261
- Streptococcal toxic shock syndrome - 254, 261
Toxoplasmosis - 228, 234
TPN – see Total parenteral nutrition
Tracheal stenosis - 39
Tracheotomy - 39, 50
TRALI - see Transfusion related acute lung injury
Tranexamic acid - 169, 172-173
Transducer - 188-189
Transfusion - 148, 158-159, 162, 167-175, 218, 237, 239
- Platelet transfusion – 170
- Red blood cells transfusion - 168
Transfusion related acute lung injury (TRALI) - 175
Trans-tracheal procedures - 49
Trendelenberg position - 138, 192
Trimethoprim/sulfamethoxazole (TMP/SMX) - 257
TTP - see Thrombotic thrombocytopenic purpura
Tumor necrosis factor - 212, 236
- TNF-α - 211-212, 216, 236
- TNF-β - 216
TUMS - 39, 80
Typhlitis - 228
U/O - see Urine output
Uremia - 171-172
Urinary catheter - 162-163, 259
Urinary tract infection (UTI) - 249, 256-258, 260
Urine output (U/O) - 145, 149, 151, 156, 160-163, 181, 185, 198, 211, 216, 218-219
Urosepsis - 155, 238, 240-241, 261
UTI - see Urinary tract infection
V/Q mismatch - 89-91, 101
VAP - see Ventilator-associated pneumonia
Varicella - 228-229